Prognosis of epilepsies

ISBN : 2-7420-0435-1

Éditions John Libbey Eurotext
127, avenue de la République
92120 Montrouge, France.
Tél : 01 46 73 06 60
e-mail : contact-@john-libbey-eurotext.fr
http//www.john-libbey-eurotext.fr

John Libbey Eurotext Ltd
42-46 High Street
Esher, Surrey
KT 10 9QY United Kingdom

© John Libbey Eurotext, Paris, 2003

Il est interdit de reproduire intégralement ou partiellement le présent ouvrage sans autorisation
de l'éditeur ou du Centre français d'exploitation du droit de copie (CFC), 20, rue des Grands-Augustins, 75006 Paris.

PROGNOSIS OF EPILEPSIES

Editor
Pierre Jallon

Associate editors
Anne Berg, Olivier Dulac, Allen Hauser

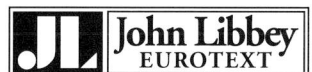

The last book of prognosis of epilepsies was written by Rodin in 1968. For the next 35 years, many original papers or chapters in textbooks have been published on this complex topic. Most of these endeavours, reflecting the clinician's highly detailed point of view are based on selected cases with little concern for the epidemiological context or upon the epidemiologist's population-based approach which tends to ignore important clinical details. Until quite recently, fundamental epidemiological aspects of epilepsy, as it is understood by clinicians, have not been explored, and clinicians viewed population-based epidemiology as relatively irrelevant to their daily practice.

It is for this reason that I organized this workshop which took place in Chamonix (France) during the last days of June 2002. During this workshop, epidemiologists and clinicians met and tried to synthesize their respective approaches and understanding of epilepsy.

This book is divided into two major parts. Presentations in the first part address methodological issues regarding prognostic studies (including remission and mortality) as well as results from long-term cohort studies. The second part contains presentations on the clinical aspects and prognosis of several individual epilepsy syndromes as well as presentations about the prognosis of status epilepticus and the outcome of frontal and temporal lobe surgery. This book is the result of delightful, animated discussions and close collaborations between epidemiologists and clinicians. It is intended to provide an up-to-date overview of the field from the combined perspectives of epidemiology and clinical epileptology.

Pierre Jallon

Participants to the workshop (Chamonix, France, 26-29 juin 2002)

Willem F.M. Arts
Department of Paediatric Neurology,
Erasmus MC/Sophia Children's Hospital,
PO Box 2060,
3000 CB Rotterdam, The Netherlands

Alexis Arzimanoglou
Head of the Epilepsy Program,
Child Neurology and Metabolic Diseases Department,
University Hospital Robert-Debré,
48, boulevard Serurier,
75019 Paris, France

Giuliano Avanzini
Department of Experimental Neurophysiology,
C. Besta Neurological Institute,
Via Celoria 11,
20133 Milano, Italy

Ettore Beghi
Istituto "Mario Negri",
Via Eritrea, 62,
20157 Milano, Italy

Anne T. Berg
BIOS – NIU,
Dekalb,
Illinois 60115, USA

Catherine Billard
Department of Neuropaediatrics,
Bicêtre Hospital,
94275 Le Kremlin-Bicêtre, France

Christine Bulteau
Fondation Ophtalmologique A.-de-Rothschild,
Service de neurochirurgie pédiatrique et chirurgie de l'épilepsie,
25-29, rue Manin,
75940 Paris Cedex, France

Peter and Carol Camfield
Department of Pediatrics, Division of Neurology,
IWK Health Centre,
PO Box 3070, Halifax,
Nova Scotia, Canada, B3J 3G9

Arturo Carpio
School of Medicine and Research Institute,
PO Box 0101 719,
University of Cuenca,
Ecuador

Catherine Chiron
Neuropediatric dpmt,
Hôpital Saint-Vincent-de-Paul,
82, avenue Denfert-Rochereau,
75674 Paris Cedex, France

Amadou Gallo Diop
Clinique Neurologique,
Centre Hospitalier Universitaire de Fann,
BP 5035, Dakar, Senegal

Olivier Dulac
Neuropediatric dpmt,
Hôpital Saint-Vincent-de-Paul,
82, avenue Denfert-Rochereau,
75674 Paris Cedex, France

Charlotte Dravet
Centre Saint-Paul,
300, boulevard Sainte-Marguerite,
13009 Marseille, France

Lars Forsgren
Department of Pharmacology and Clinical Neuroscience,
Section of Neurology,
Umeå University Hospital,
SE-901 85 Umeå, Sweden

Simone Garrel
174, chemin de la Faurie,
F 38410 Vaulnaveys-le-Haut, France

Pierre Genton
Centre Saint-Paul,
300, boulevard Sainte-Marguerite,
13009 Marseille, France

Marja-Liisa Granström
Epilepsy Unit, Department of Child Neurology,
Hospital for Children and Adolescents,
BOX 280, FIN 00029HUS, Finland

Allen Hauser
Columbia University,
Gertrude H. Sergievsky Center,
630 West 168th Street, P&S Unit 16,
New York, NY 10032, USA

Dale Hesdorffer
Columbia University,
Gertrude H. Sergievsky Center,
630 West 168th Street, P&S Unit 16,
New York, NY 10032, USA

Édouard Hirsch
Clinique Neurologique,
1, place de l'Hôpital,
67091 Strasbourg, France

Pierre Jallon
Epilepsy and EEG Unit,
Hôpital Cantonal Universitaire,
CH 1211 Genève 14, Suisse

Peter W. Kaplan
Department of Neurology,
The Johns Hopkins Bayview Medical Center,
4940 Eastern Avenue,
Baltimore, MD 21224, USA

Pierre Loiseau
4, allée du Carabin,
33460 Arsac, France

Jérôme Loiseau
University Hospital Pellegrin,
33076 Bordeaux Cedex, France

Jacques Motte
Unité de neurologie pédiatrique,
American Memorial Hospital,
49, rue Cognac-Jay,
51092 Reims Cedex, France

Elias Olafsson
Department of Neurology,
National University Hospital (Landspitali),
108 Reykjavik, Iceland

Hervé Outin
Réanimation médicale,
Hôpital de Poissy,
CHI Poissy/Saint-Germain-en-Laye,
78303 Poissy, France

Marie-Christine Picot
University Hospital Arnaud-de-Villeneuve,
371, av. du doyen-G.-Giraud,
34295 Montpellier Cedex 5, France

Perrine Plouin
Neurophysiologie Clinique,
Hôpital Saint-Vincent-de-Paul,
82, avenue Denfert-Rochereau,
75014 Paris, France

Pierre-Marie Preux
Institut d'Épidémiologie neurologique et de Neurologie tropicale,
2, rue du Dr-Marcland,
87025 Limoges Cedex, France

Josemir Was Sander
Department of Clinical and Experimental Epilepsy,
Institute of Neurology,
University College London,
Queen Square,
London WC1N 3BG, UK

Franck Semah
Service Hospitalier Frédéric-Joliot,
CEA,
4, place du Général-Leclerc,
91401 Orsay Cedex, France

Matti Sillanpää
Departments of Child Neurology and Public Health,
20014 Turku University, Finland

Pierre Thomas
Unité Fonctionnelle EEG/Épileptologie,
Service de neurologie, Hôpital Pasteur,
30, voie Romaine, BP 69,
06002 Nice, France

Torbjörn Tomson
Department of Clinical Neuroscience,
Division of Neurology,
Karolinska Institute,
Stockholm, Sweden

Suzanne Trottier
INSERM U573,
Centre Paul-Broca,
2 ter, rue d'Alésia,
75014 Paris, France

Laurent Vercueil
Service de Neurophysiologie,
Hôpital Michallon,
BP 217 X,
38700 Grenoble Cedex, France

Hervé Vespignani
Faculté de Médecine de Nancy,
Avenue de la Forêt,
BP 184, 54505 Vandœuvres Cedex, France

Jean-Guy Villemure
Service de Neurochirurgie,
CHUV,
CH 1011, Lausanne, Suisse

H. Gregor Wieser
Department of Neurology,
Universitätsspital,
CH 8091, Zurich, Suisse

Contents

Part 1. Methodology and cohort studies

Methods in prognosis studies
    Dale C. Hesdorffer, Giancarlo Logroscino 3

Mortality studies in epilepsy
    Torbjörn Tomson, Lars Forsgren 12

Prognosis of first seizure
    Ettore Beghi 21

Prognosis of epileptic syndromes: EPIGIR study
    Jerôme Loiseau, Marie-Christine Picot and Pierre Loiseau 29

Determining prognosis of epilepsy from a prevalence cohort
    Elias Olafsson, Örn Olafsson and Allen Hauser 39

Long term prognosis of first epileptic seizures: EPIGEN study
    Pierre Jallon, Jean Sébastien Landry 44

Prognosis of epilepsy: The Rochester Studies
    Allen Hauser 55

The prognosis of epilepsy in the national general practice study of epilepsy
    Samden D. Lhatoo, Josemir W. Sander 64

Prognosis of epilepsy based on epidemiological studies from Västerbotten, northern Sweden
    Lars Forsgren 73

The ecuadorian study of prognosis of epilepsy
    Arturo Carpio 85

The dutch study of epilepsy in childhood
    Willem FM Arts 101

Nova Scotia pediatric epilepsy study
    Peter and Carol Camfield 113

Long-term prognosis in Finnish childhood-onset epilepsy
   Matti Sillanpää 127

Prognosis of epilepsy in Africa
   Amadou Gallo Diop, Fatou Sene-Diouf, Léopold Boissy, Pierre-Marie Preux,
   Ibrahima Pierre Ndiaye 135

Prognosis of temporal lobe epilepsy after surgery
   H. Gregor Wieser 147

Prognosis of frontal lobe epilepsy after surgery
   Suzanne Trottier, Jean-Marie Scarabin 167

Identification of epilepsy syndromes at diagnosis and modification with time
   Anne T. Berg 185

Part 2. Prognosis of epilepsy syndromes

Prognosis of neonatal seizures
   Perrine Plouin, Emmanuel Raffo, Talvany de Oliveira 199

Prognosis of infantile spasms
   Marja-Liisa Granström 210

Prognosis of febrile seizures
   Anne T. Berg 221

Prognosis of myoclonic-astatic epilepsy
   Olivier Dulac and Anna Kaminska 231

Prognosis of severe myoclonic epilepsy in infancy (Dravet syndrome)
   Catherine Chiron 239

Prognosis of idiopathic absence epilepsies
   Jérôme Guiwer, Maria Paula Valenti, Ahmed Bourazza, Édouard Hirsch,
   Pierre Loiseau 249

Prognosis of idiopathic myoclonic epilepsies
   Pierre Genton, Philippe Gelisse, Pierre Thomas, Charlotte Dravet 258

Prognosis of idiopathic localisation-related epilepsies
   Christine Brasselet, Jacques Motte 265

Prognosis of Lennox-Gastaut syndrome
    Alexis Arzimanoglou 277

Prognosis of Landau Kleffner syndrome and other forms of cognitive epilepsy
    Catherine Billard... 289

Prognosis of epileptic encephalopathy with electric status epilepticus during sleep
    Christine Bulteau 295

Prognosis of convulsive status epilepticus
    Hervé Outin, Pierre Thomas.. 300

Prognosis in non-convulsive status epilepticus
    Peter W. Kaplan... 311

Concluding remarks
    Anne Berg, Olivier Dulac, Allen Hauser 326

Part 1

Methodology and cohort studies

Methods in prognosis studies

Dale C. Hesdorffer, Giancarlo Logroscino

Why look at prognosis of a disease?

The study of disease prognosis is important for several reasons. It is important for clinicians who wish to understand the natural history of a disease, for characterization of factors affecting prognosis, and for understanding changes in the natural history of disease due to the introduction of treatment. Clearly, comprehending the natural history of a disease is important if for evaluation of treatment effects. For some disorders, treatment may be so common that the natural history is unobservable. In the case of seizures, we are better able to observe the natural history for a first unprovoked seizure than for epilepsy, because first unprovoked seizures are largely untreated in some regions. Prognosis is articulated in quantitative terms [1]. Prognosis can also help to address the public health impact of a disease, particularly when the disease has a serious prognosis (e.g., cardiovascular and cerebrovascular disease), or affects specific groups (e.g., children for cerebral palsy or homosexuals and bisexual males or drug users for AIDS), or leads to an increased need for services.

Natural history

Knowing the natural history of epilepsy is important when studying the prognosis of epilepsy. This natural history begins at the time of the disease's biologic onset, which may or may not be recognized *(figure 1)*. After this, pathologic evidence of the disease emerges, and subsequently signs and symptoms may develop. Medical care may be sought, a diagnosis made, and treatment begun. There are several different possible prognostic outcomes to be assessed at this point, including remission of disease, social impact of the disease, and death.

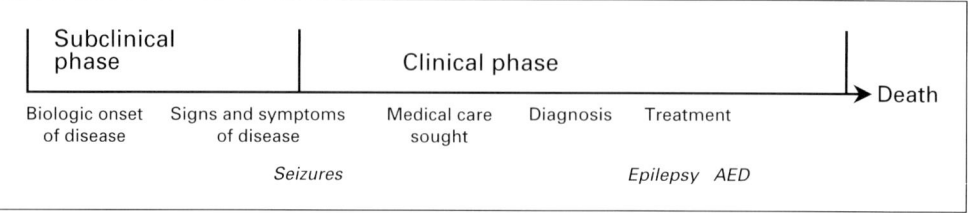

Figure 1. Natural history of disease.

Outcomes

Possible outcomes for prognosis studies of epilepsy have included death, remission, intractability, educational achievement, marriage, and employment. *Death* is measured by mortality. The expectation of life is adversely affected in epilepsy, predominantly among those with symptomatic etiology (remote symptomatic and progressive symptomatic cases). However, it is unclear if epilepsy by itself adds an additional risk of death over and above that due to the underlying disease (e.g., stroke, brain tumor). Additionally, some individuals who have seizures at least once a month may be at risk for sudden unexplained death in epilepsy. Studies of mortality are difficult in the elderly who have a high baseline risk of death. *Remission* is a disease-free period, which has been variously defined in epilepsy as 2-years or 5-years seizure-free. *Intractability*, a clear manifestation of epilepsy severity and a major contributor to the burden of epilepsy, is measured in terms of seizure frequency over a specified time period after a certain number of adequate trials of antiepileptic drugs at correct dosages have failed to stop seizures. There is little agreement on the number of seizures, the time period, or the number of drugs that must be tried before a patient is considered intractable. *Educational outcomes* are defined as the number of grades completed and attendance at special schools. Educational achievement may be poorer for individuals with epilepsy than for unaffected individuals, even if the disorder does not have a clear etiology and epilepsy has remitted [2]. *Employment* is defined as working in a part-time or full-time job for pay. *Marriage* is defined as a legal union. Although outcomes such as employment and marriage are easy to measure, they may be affected as much by the person's epilepsy as by societal stigma.

Definitions of outcome must be applied uniformly to all members of a study population. This can be difficult when the endpoint is intractability because some seizure types are quite difficult to count accurately (e.g., simple partial seizures without motor manifestations). Undercounting of seizures may cause underascertainment of intractability. The resultant misclassification of outcome will lead to estimates of effect biased toward the null when predictors of intractability are evaluated, unless the underascertainment is related to the predictor. In such cases, the direction of the bias may vary.

The evolution of syndromes is an unexplored *outcome* in studies to date. Due to the difficulty of precisely classifying syndromes at onset of epilepsy, it may be interesting to study syndromes as an outcome.

Public health impact of epilepsy

Epilepsy impacts upon public health. Epilepsy is a common disorder with a prevalence of active epilepsy of 6 per 1 000 population [3], and it affects specific groups. Incidence in males is greater than incidence in females. Epilepsy occurs early in life (incidence = 90/100 000 under 1 year) and over the last decades, the incidence is increasing in the elderly [4]. In specific age groups like infants or elderly, studies of prognosis can establish groups that need specific attention for public health intervention.

Selection of cases for studies of prognosis

Generally in studies of disease prognosis, what we would like to observe is the natural history of the disease from the moment the disease makes itself manifest. As the moment a disease begins may be unclear in reality, what we observe is the medical history of a disease from the moment of diagnosis *(figure 1)*.

There are two types of cohorts that can be followed to determine prognosis in epilepsy. The first is an *incident cohort* of new cases. The second type of cohort is a *prevalent cohort* of existing cases. The existing cases are new and old (mostly old cases). Therefore prevalent cases are survivors with epilepsy, and these individuals may have a substantially different prognosis from incident cases.

After the onset of the clinical phase of the disease with sign and symptoms, the patient seeks medical attention and the diagnosis is made. This moment represents the inception of incident cases. For epilepsy, defined as two or more unprovoked seizures, the inception of incident cases differs by seizure type because different seizure types have their own characteristic lag time from manifestation of the first seizure to the moment of diagnosis. The diagnosis of epilepsy relies upon the patient's ability to recognize their seizures, seek medical care, and be diagnosed. While the formal definition of epilepsy is two or more unprovoked seizures, in reality the recognition of subtle seizure types may occur after many seizures. As a result, the inception of incident cases of epilepsy is heterogeneous, depending upon seizure type, and upon the interval between the first and the second seizure. Identification of pure incident cases may be possible for convulsive seizure types only. In contrast, nonconvulsive seizure types are identified after many seizures have occurred, and these cases may be more similar to prevalent cases of convulsive seizures. Such misclassification of the onset of epilepsy (start of the follow-up period) and heterogeneity of the case mix is therefore a problem in prognosis studies of epilepsy.

To circumvent this difficulty when examining prognosis of epilepsy, investigators have defined incident epilepsy as the first diagnosis of epilepsy and others have studied only seizures that are identified at their first occurrence [5]. It is important to recognize, however, that such subtle distinctions in incident case definition may yield spurious differences in prognosis by seizure type and true incident cohorts may only be possible for motor seizures. Hypothetically, there may be some forms of absence or complex partial seizures that occur so infrequently that they are never diagnosed. This may lead to incomplete ascertainment for nonconvulsive seizure types but not for convulsive seizure types, and to possible overestimation of the severity of nonconvulsive forms of epilepsy. Thus, it is important to stratify by seizure type in studies of epilepsy prognosis.

The cases that are incepted some time after the diagnosis is made are prevalent case or survivors (new and old). Predictors of recurrent seizures, social and educational outcomes, and mortality will be quite different for prevalent versus incident cohorts. This is because cohorts of prevalent epilepsy exclude individuals whose seizures have remitted and this results in a substantially different distribution of seizure types, age, and gender from that seen in incident cohorts.

As we have already discussed, an incident cohort of epilepsy is completely different from a prevalent cohort of epilepsy. To illustrate this, we compared an incident and a prevalent cohort assembled from the same source population in Rochester, Minnesota, during the same time period. The incident cohort differed from the prevalent on age (more cases among children and in the elderly), gender (more males), etiology (more remote symptomatic, especially vascular) and seizure type (more generalized). Since each of these variables has a prognostic value, a mortality study using incident cases might reach a different conclusion than one using prevalent cases. Prevalent cohorts may underestimate short-term mortality because the more severe cases that die in the early phase of the disease are not included in the calculation of deaths over the period of observation. On the other hand, prevalent cohorts may overestimate or underestimate long-term mortality compared to incident cohorts, depending on the age, gender etiology and seizure type structure of the cohort. For example, prevalent cohorts will overestimate mortality if more benign cases of epilepsy are not included in the cohort, because they did not have a seizure in the last years.

Sources of cases

We can assemble different type of cohorts for prognosis studies, depending upon the source of cases. Cases can be ascertained in single hospitals, in all medical facilities in a defined community (i.e., they are population-based), or based upon general population surveys. As previously mentioned, both incident and prevalent cases are assembled during a specified time period.

Many published studies of mortality in epilepsy are based on clinical series, collected in neurology departments or in tertiary centers specialized in the diagnosis and treatment of epilepsy. There are some reports from institutionalised patients. The problem with these studies results from the increased likelihood that selection of cases is based on a characteristic of the disease (i.e., severity, age) that might affect the results of the study if the characteristic is related to the outcome (e.g., death, in studies of mortality) [6].

More severe cases are likely to be ascertained in clinical settings than in population-based studies. Population-based studies avoid the selection bias that could be present when cases are ascertained in other fashions. This is because population-based studies have the complete spectrum of disease, and include people who are unlikely to present to a tertiary care center because they enter remission immediately after diagnosis.

Ascertainment of predictors

Studies of epilepsy prognosis are usually cohort studies. In a typical cohort study, an exposure and a disease are defined. The study begins when disease-free individuals with and without the exposure are ascertained. These individuals are followed through time to detect disease and the incidence of disease in the exposed is compared to the incidence of disease in the unexposed.

In cohort studies of disease prognosis, the study begins when individuals with the *disease* are ascertained. These individuals are categorized based upon specific baseline characteristics or predictors and then they are followed for defined endpoints. Non-modifiable predictors in studies of epilepsy prognosis may include age at onset, gender, seizure type, etiology, EEG abnormalities, and epilepsy syndrome. Modifiable predictors may include timing of introduction of antiepileptic drugs and timing of epilepsy surgery. Endpoints may include mortality, remission, educational and vocational outcome, and intractability.

Methods used to ascertain predictors must be applied uniformly to all members of the cohort or bias may result. This is not a problem for factors such as age and gender, but may be problematic for epilepsy syndrome [7]. At least in children, syndromes may have little prognostic utility in epidemiological studies, because of the large proportion of children who are partially or completely unclassified (as high as 45% of children in the Bronx) after experiencing two seizures, and because the initial diagnosis may prove incorrect over time (10% of children in the Connecticut study). Another difficulty with using syndromes in studies of epilepsy prognosis relates to how the definitions are applied in the face of descriptions that are sometimes vague, and an individual syndrome may change over time.

Etiology is a predictor that may pose problems when results are compared across studies. It is important to define the group that the ILAE epidemiological classification defines as idiopathic/cryptogenic. This group contains cases of as yet unrecognised cause as well as the cases that may be attributed to genetic etiology. Determination of this group depends, in part, on what definitions are used for the symptomatic group. In the case of remote symptomatic seizures due to stroke for example, some investigators rely upon clinically detected stroke to classify a patient as having epilepsy due to stroke, while others add imaging criteria in the absence of clinically detected stroke. Such differences in definition change the idiopathic/cryptogenic group as well, and compromise our ability to draw conclusions from groups of studies.

Loss to follow-up

Loss to follow-up is a problem that plagues all cohort studies, and retaining cases with epilepsy during the follow-up may be the most daunting task facing the investigator.

Loss to follow-up rates of less than 20% are considered acceptable and are unlikely to cause severe bias, unless the loss is restricted to one prognostic category (e.g., idiopathic/cryptogenic). Rates in excess of 20% are problematic and will likely introduce bias. The problem of loss to follow-up is greatest in places where people tend to relocate far away from the study site.

Measures of prognosis

Descriptive measures of outcome in studies of prognosis: these measures are used predominantly in studies using mortality as the outcome. Different measures are used to describe mortality according to the study design. In a cohort study, the *mortality rate, case fatality, and standardized mortality ratio (SMR)* are used. The *mortality rate* indicates the incidence rate of death in a cohort and is given by the number of deaths divided by person-year at risk. *Case fatality* is the proportion of subjects dying within a cohort and is given by the number of deaths divided by the number of subjects with the disease in the cohort. The mortality rate estimates the individual risk of dying while case fatality is the average risk of dying for a group. A less frequently used measure is the proportionate mortality ratio (PMR). This measure is used when information on deaths is all that is available.

The *SMR* is the ratio of the observed number of deaths in the study group divided by the expected number of deaths [8]. The expected number of deaths are calculated applying the death rate of a general or external population to the gender, age, calendar period distribution of group in the study. SMR is a measure of external comparison because the denominator is the expected deaths that are calculated using the rate of the general population applied to the distribution of the group of interest [8]. The assumptions underlying SMR are that: a) the diagnostic process and the attribution of cause of death is conducted in the same fashion for both the group of interest and the general population; and b) the group of interest and the general population come from the same source population.

Although the SMR is commonly used in studies of mortality in epilepsy, it has some methodological problems. Each SMR is calculated using a different standard that is the age- and gender-distribution of the actual study group. Therefore, the SMR is not really comparable across studies because each SMR use a different standard. Only when the age and gender distribution and the age and gender specific death rates are similar is the SMR comparable across studies.

To illustrate the problem of comparing the SMR across studies, we present data on short-term mortality of acute symptomatic seizure at thirty days in two communities: Washington Heights, a multiethnic urban community in Northern Manhattan, New York and Rochester, a middleclass Caucasian community in North-Eastern Minnesota. The SMR were 149.1 (95% CI: 119.9-184.7) in Rochester and 102.1(95% CI: 79.3-127.8) in Washington Heights. We used the death rates of the South-Eastern Minnesota general population to calculate the SMR for Rochester, and the overall US population to calculate the SMR for Washington Heights. The death rate of the overall US population is three times that of South-Eastern Minnesota. This alone explains the apparently different SMRs.

The SMR is very popular in the epilepsy literature, but we want to emphasize the issue of non-comparability that results from indirect standardization [8]. The method of direct standardization is preferred when comparisons are made within and between studies, especially when the age structure of the populations is significantly different. This is particularly true when the SMR from studies in developing countries are compared with those from studies in the US and Europe.

Proportionate mortality ratio (PMR) is also used in studies of mortality in epilepsy. The PMR is defined as the proportion of deaths due to one cause divided by the proportion of deaths due to other causes. The validity of assigning cause of death is a problem even in the most sophisticated setting of a tertiary care center. Thus, studies using the PMR must be interpreted with caution.

In studies using the PMR, only deaths are considered and there is no follow-up period for study subjects because they are already dead. Consequently, we cannot measure risk. For example, if the PMR from epilepsy in a community is 0.01%, this is the proportion of deaths in that community that are due to epilepsy compared to deaths due to other causes.

Analytic methods: In cohort studies that follow individuals over time for a defined outcome that is either present or absent (intractability, remission, employment), analytic methods must take into account the follow-up time for each individual. Individuals who do not reach the endpoint during the follow-up period are censored at their date of last follow-up or date of death. The analytic methods used in this situation include Kaplan-Meier survival analysis for univariate examinations of the data [9] and Cox Proportional Hazards regression for multivariate analyses [9]. Logistic regression analyses are inappropriate in this setting unless all individuals have been followed for the same duration after epilepsy diagnosis and none are lost to follow-up.

When it is possible to experience the endpoint more than once (e.g., seizure recurrence, remission of seizures), other analytic methods that build upon Cox regression have been developed but have not been used in studies of epilepsy. These analytic methods account for repeated failures (i.e., endpoints that occur more than once such as seizure recurrence) and are described in detail elsewhere [10, 11]. However, they appear to add little useful information beyond what is gained in looking at the second occurrence of the endpoint among people who have experienced the first occurrence.

Cohort effects

A cohort effect is due to the experience that a birth-cohort of one age at a specific point in time has undergone at some earlier time in its journey from its birth year to the year of observation [12]. Thus, disease rates manifested by an age group at a point in time can be due to an age effect (e.g., high rates of epilepsy in the elderly associated with dementia throughout time) a period effect (e.g., HIV infection in the 1980's and 1990's increased the likelihood of central nervous system infection and lymphoma, thereby increasing the risk of epilepsy) or a cohort effect (e.g., In Rochester the birth cohort 1930-34 had a lower incidence of unprovoked seizures than other birth cohorts. These people were born during the height of the depression [13]). A single cross-sectional observation cannot detect a birth cohort effect, yet the age-dependent risk of the disease can vary by birth cohort. Seldom are prognosis studies of epilepsy large enough or long enough to address this problem, but it is important to consider the potential for such effects.

Competing risks

Competing risks are events that "compete" with the outcome of interest to remove persons from the population at risk [14]. An example of competing risks in epilepsy is the relationship between epilepsy and stroke *(figure 2)*. In this example: risk factors are common to epilepsy, stroke and death; stroke increases the risk of epilepsy; epilepsy increases the risk of stroke; and both epilepsy and stroke increase the risk of death. Data support the relationship between stroke and epilepsy. Stroke increases the risk of developing epilepsy [15] and idiopathic/cryptogenic epilepsy in people aged 55 years and older increases the risk for cerebral hemispheric infarct and intracerebral hemorrhage [16].

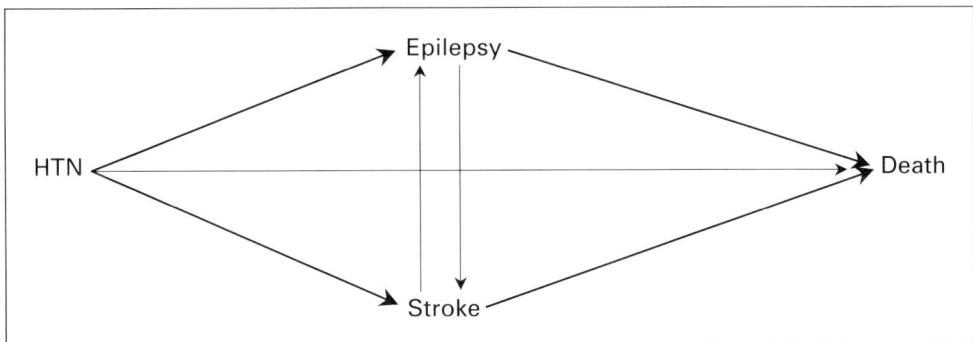

Figure 2. Example of possible competing risks.

Competing risks are particularly important among the elderly who have a high risk of dying. The elderly are also at risk for many diseases that have an increased incidence with advancing age. In this situation, the average time to death for a disease may preclude getting another disease that is itself associated with death.

Risk factors may be shared for many diseases. In the previous example, it is important to point out that severe hypertension in a risk factor for both epilepsy and stroke [17, 18]. Severe hypertension may also increase the risk of death for epilepsy and stroke (i.e., risk factors for the disease are also prognostic factors for people with the disease).

We give another example of competing risks, this time theoretical. If the survival rate for breast cancer increases over time, then as people age they are at risk for brain metastases. These people are not cured but they survive and, as a result, they are at increased risk for epilepsy. Both brain metastases and epilepsy increase the risk for death. Similarly, epilepsy occurs following stroke, because people survive long enough to experience at least two unprovoked seizures. Stroke and epilepsy are each associated with death.

There is a statistical technique for "removing" competing risks [19]. Although this technique is not completely successful, it treats competing risks as censored observations rather than as deaths. Thus, changes in incidence and mortality of a disease over time can result from changes in competing risk. Most of the time, however, we do not know.

Conclusions

Identifying the study question is the first step in studies of the prognosis of epilepsy. The soundest answer to the posited question often comes from a population-based cohort of incident cases. Only this type of cohort permits a complete collection of data and the observation of the clinical phase of the disease from the diagnosis of epilepsy to the outcome of the study. In order to maximize the yield from each study of epilepsy prognosis, investigators should work together to develop uniform definitions of predictors and outcomes. Even after such work has been done, meta-analyses of observational studies are unwise.

Future work: Considerable work has been done on mortality in epilepsy, yet this work not addressed the contribution that epilepsy itself makes to mortality. There are two possible approaches to this question. One is to study mortality in idiopathic/cryptogenic cases, and the other is to compare the mortality of people with incident epilepsy attributable to underlying condition to the mortality of individuals from the same population with the underlying condition alone.

Future work should also explore the utility of syndromes as predictors and as outcomes. As many predictors of prognosis in epilepsy are unmodifiable, focus should turn to further examination of modifiable risk factors such as timing of epilepsy surgery. Additionally, investigators should work together to operationalize the definitions of predictors and outcomes used in prognosis studies of epilepsy. Such work will strengthen the impact of future studies on the accumulation of knowledge about the prognosis of epilepsy.

References

1. Gordis L. *Epidemiology.* Philadelphia: WB Saunders Company, 2000: 77-8.
2. Sillanpaa M, Jalava M, Kaleva O, Shinnar S. Long-term prognosis of seizures with onset in childhood. *N Engl J Med* 1998; 338: 1715-22.
3. Hauser WA, Annegers JF, Kurland LT. Prevalence of epilepsy in Rochester, Minnesota: 1940-1980. *Epilepsia* 1991; 32: 429-45.
4. Hauser WA, Annegers JF, Kurland LT. Incidence of epilepsy and unprovoked seizures in Rochester, Minnesota: 1935-1984. *Epilepsia* 1993: 34: 453-68.
5. Shinnar S, Berg AT, Moshe SL, Petix M, Maytal J, Kang H, Goldensohn ES, Hauser WA. Risk of seizure recurrence following a first unprovoked seizure in childhood: A prospective study. *Pediatrics* 1990; 85: 1076-85.
6. Rothman KJ. *Modern Epidemiology.* Boston: Little Brown, 1986: 83-4.
7. Berg AT. Identification of epilepsy syndromes at diagnosis and modification with time. In: Jallon P, ed. *Prognosis of epilepsies.* Paris: John Libbey Eurotext, 2003: 185-96.
8. Rothman KJ. *Modern Epidemiology.* Boston: Little Brown, 1986: 45-9.

9. Lee ET. *Statistical methods for survival data analysis.* Belmont, CA: Lifetime Learning Publications, 1980.
10. Wei LJ, Lin Dy, Weissfeld L. Regression analysis of multivariate incomplete failure time data by modelling marginal distributions. *J Am Statistical Assoc* 1989; 84: 1065-73.
11. Prentice RL, Willians BJ, Peterson AV. On the regression analysis of multivariate failure time data. *Biometrika* 1981; 68: 373-9.
12. MacMahon B, Trichopoulos D. *Epidemiology: principles and methods.* Boston: Little Brown, 1996: 184-93.
13. Annegers JF, Hauser WA, Lee JRJ, Rocca WA. Secular trends and birth cohort effects in unprovoked seizures: Rochester, Minnesota 1935-1984. *Epilepsia* 1995; 36: 575-9.
14. Rothman KJ. *Modern Epidemiology.* Boston: Little Brown, 1986: 29-31.
15. Hauser WA, Ramirez-Lassepas M, Rosenstein R. Risk for seizures and epilepsy following cerebrovascular insults. *Epilepsia* 1984; 25: 666.
16. So EL, Whisnant JP, Hauser WA, Hesdorffer DC, Annegers JF, O'Brien PC. Late-onset idiopathic seizures are associated with increased risk of subsequent strokes. *Neurology* 1995; 45 (Suppl 4): A423.
17. Hesdorffer DC, Hauser WA, Annegers JF, Kurland LT, Rocca WA. Severe, uncontrolled hypertension and adult-onset seizures: a case-control study in Rochester, Minnesota. *Epilepsia* 1996; 37: 736-41.
18. Bansal BC, Agarwal AK, Rewari BB. Hypertension and cerebrovascular disease. *J Indian Med Assoc* 1999; 97: 226-32.
19. Gooley TA, Leisenring W, Crowley J, Storer BE. Estimation of failure probabilities in the presence of competing risks: new presentations of old estimators. *Statistics in Medicine* 1999; 18: 695-706.

Mortality studies in epilepsy

Torbjörn Tomson, Lars Forsgren

Mortality or survival of the patient is one of the most important aspects of the prognosis of epilepsy. Several studies have addressed this issue through the years. Despite differences in methods and study populations, all demonstrate an increased mortality rate among patients with epilepsy, although to a variable extent. This review will focus on reports of mortality from population-based studies and from some recent large more selected epilepsy cohorts.

Methods and measures

Different studies use different measures of mortality. The appropriateness of the measures depends on the questions to be addressed and the study design. The mortality rate is the number of deaths that occur in a defined population in a specific time divided by the person years at risk in that population. Case fatality is the number of deaths divided by the number of patients with the disease in the study population. The death rate in an epilepsy population can be compared with that of the general population using the standardised mortality ratio (SMR), which is the ratio of observed number of deaths in a population with epilepsy to that expected, based on the age and sex-specific mortality rates in a reference population. All these measures are used in cohort studies. Although SMR is widely used in epilepsy studies, it may be difficult to compare SMRs between studies since the measure depends on the mortality rate in the reference population, which may vary between studies. Proportionate mortality ratio describes the proportions of deaths due to specific causes among cohorts of people with epilepsy. Proportionate mortality compares the relative contribution of different causes to the overall mortality in a specific population, but is not a direct measure of the ratio of rates of death between populations.

Selection of study and reference populations is a critical issue. One type of study design involves analyses of deaths in prevalence cohorts of patients. There are important limitations with this type of studies, the most important being the selection bias. Prevalent cases represent survivors with epilepsy. Patients who enter remission or those who die early after diagnosis will be excluded, and there will be an over-representation of chronic patients with severe epilepsy in such cohorts. Hence, prevalence studies may underestimate short-term mortality and depending on the composition of the cohort probably overestimate long-term mortality. Incident cohorts of new onset cases are therefore preferred in mortality studies.

The source of the study population is also important for the possibility to generalise from the results. Many prevalence cohorts are hospital-based or come from epilepsy centres, thus including selected populations with more severe epilepsy. Potential advantages with this approach might be reliable diagnoses of epilepsy and possibly more accurate classification of the cause of death. However, the ideal approach is a prospective study of a community- or population-based incident cohort with a sufficient number of unselected individuals with epilepsy, where practically all patients in the cohort can be traced allowing a long-term follow-up of the patients.

Definitions of epilepsy and seizure classification may also vary between studies, although the International League Against Epilepsy has published guidelines for epidemiological research [1]. The accuracy of the epilepsy diagnoses and of the classification of cause of death may also differ and is sometimes not assessed. Such differences are likely to affect mortality estimates. The accuracy of the cause of death will depend on whether the classification relies on death certificates only, to what extent these are supported by post mortem examinations, and whether supplementary clinical data are obtained from medical records or by structured interviews of witnesses or relatives, the verbal autopsy.

Overall mortality

As discussed above, population-based studies are likely to provide the death rates and SMRs that are most representative of the epilepsy population in general, although the cohorts and number of observed deaths may be smaller than in some prevalence studies. Seven such studies have been published [2-10]. The first is a prevalence cohort from Warsaw, Poland [2], the others are studies of incident cohorts, the preferred type of epilepsy population, and come from the US [3], the UK [4], Iceland [5], France [6], Sweden [7], and Canada [10]. Hence, all come from the industrialised world and there is no population-based study of mortality in people with epilepsy from the developing world. SMRs in these population-based studies range from 1.6-5.3 *(table I)*. The US study comes from Rochester, Minnesota, and is a retrospective analysis of 618 patients with first diagnosis of epilepsy between 1935-1974 with a variable follow-up time up to more than 30 years [3]. The UK study is a prospective study of 1,091 patients with newly diagnosed or suspected epilepsy identified from 275 general practices throughout the country. Of these, 564 were considered as definite epilepsy, although this included also people with single seizures. The first publication, after a median follow-up of 6.9 years, reported an SMR of 3.0 (2.5-3.7; 95% CI) [4]. In a subsequent report after 11.9 years of follow-up SMR was 2.6 (2.1-3.0) [9]. The study from Iceland is a follow-up of 224 incident cases of unprovoked seizures diagnosed from 1960 through 1964 [5]. By 30 years after diagnosis SMR was 1.6 (1.2-2.2). The French study is a short-term, one-year, follow-up of mortality of 804 patients with a first seizure, provoked or unprovoked, in the region of Gironde [6]. SMR in the 459 patients with unprovoked seizures was 4.1 (2.5-6.2), higher than in other population-based studies. This is largely explained by the short follow-up period. The Swedish study comprised 107 adult residents of the County of Västerbotten, with newly diagnosed unprovoked seizures between 1985 and 1987 followed until death or the end of 1996 [7]. The Canadian study is a follow-up of 686 children from Nova Scotia with onset of epilepsy between 1977 and 1985, while aged from 28 days to 16 years. SMR in this cohort of childhood onset epilepsy was 5.3 (2.3-8.3) 1980-1989, and 8.8 (4.2-13.4) 1990-1999 [10].

Table I. Community based studies of all-cause mortality in epilepsy

Reference	Method	SMR (95% confidence interval)
Poland 1974 [2]	Retrospective analysis of prevalence cohort	1.8 (not available)
US 1980 [3]	Retrospective analysis of incidence cohort	2.3 (1.9-2.6)
US 1984 [8]*	Retrospective analysis of incidence cohort	2.1 (1.9-2.5)
UK 1994 [4]	Prospective analysis of incidence cohort	3.0 (2.5-3.7)
UK. 2001 [9]**	Prospective analysis of incidence cohort	2.6 (2.1-3.0)
Iceland 1998 [5]	Retrospective analysis of incidence cohort	1.6 (1.2-2.2)
France 1999 [6]	Prospective analysis of incidence cohort	4.1 (2.5-6.2)
Sweden 2000 [7]	Prospective analysis of incidence cohort	2.5 (1.6-3.8)
Canada 2002 [10]***	Retrospective analysis of incidence cohort	5.3 (2.3-8.3) first 10 years 8.8 (4.2-13.4) following 10 years

* Extended series and follow-up of [3].
** Extended follow-up of [4].
*** Children with onset of epilepsy from 28 days to 16 years.

The increased SMR was mainly caused by a high mortality among children with neurological comorbidity. Those with disorders sufficient to cause funtional neurological deficit were 22.2 (7.0-69.7) times more likely to die than those without. The SMR for those without severe neurological deficit was not significantly increased, 1.5 (0.2-2.8).

Two additional follow-up studies have recently been published reporting mortality in population-based cohorts of children with epilepsy, although they do not present SMRs. In a prospective study of 17 440 children in the UK, Kurtz *et al.* [11] identified 124 children with a confirmed diagnosis of epilepsy. Nine of the 124 children (7%) with epilepsy had died by age 28. Sillanpää *et al.* [12] studied prospectively the long-term prognosis of 245 (61% incident, 39% prevalent) children with epilepsy in Finland. Sufficient data were available on 220 patients 30 years after diagnosis. Forty-four (20%) of the 220 patients had died, yielding a mortality rate of 6.2 per 1 000 patient-years (95% CI 5.7-6.7), 4.8 (95% CI 4.4-5.3) among incident cases and higher in prevalent cases, 8.4 (95% CI 7.8-9.0).

SMRs for some studies based on selected populations are presented in *table II*. The studies span over five decades and SMRs range from 1.9-3.6. Although this is similar to SMRs in population-based incident cohorts, risk factors and causes of death may be different due to the methodological shortcomings discussed above. In addition to the problems of selection bias towards more chronic, severe epilepsy in hospital-based cohorts, some of the studies also suffer from small numbers of observed deaths. However, there are two recent large-scale hospital-based studies. One comprised all 9 061 patients aged 16 years or more who were admitted and discharged from any hospital in Stockholm, Sweden with a diagnosis of epilepsy during the years 1980-1989. These were followed until the end of 1992, and an SMR of 3.6 (3.5-3.7) was reported [17]. However, review of medical records of a sample of these cases revealed that only 80% fulfilled the criteria for epilepsy. Inclusion of such misclassified cases as well as medical conditions other than epilepsy requiring hospital admission may have contributed to the high mortality in this report. Shackleton *et al.* [18] made a retrospective analysis of mortality in 1 355 patients with epilepsy diagnosed at a Dutch epilepsy centre between 1953 and 1967 and followed until 1994. The mean follow up of these incident cases was 28 years, 38 665 person years were surveyed, and SMR was 3.2 (2.9-3.5).

Difficulties to carry out incidence studies, problems in long-term follow-up, low autopsy rates and less reliable death certificates are contributory causes for the lack of mortality studies in epilepsy from developing countries. However, a hospital-based incident cohort from Ecuador included 412 newly diagnosed epilepsy patients of all ages, of which 33 were lost in follow-up. Seven patients died, yielding a mortality rate of 6.1/1 000 patient-years at risk and an SMR of 6.3 [19].

Table II. All-cause mortality in selected epilepsy populations

Reference	Population	SMR (95% confidence interval)
Alström [13]	Hospital-based case series	2.4 (2.0-2.8)
Henriksen et al. [14]	Hospital-based case series*	2.7 (2.3-3.2)
White et al. [15]	Epilepsy residential centre	3.0 (2.8-3.3)
Klenerman et al. [16]	Epilepsy residential centre	1.9 (1.6-2.3)
Nilsson et al. [17]	Case series based on hospital admissions	3.6 (3.5-3.7)
Shackleton et al. [18]	Incident cases from epilepsy centre	3.2 (2.9-3.5)

* Patients with intractable tumours excluded.

Risk factors for mortality

Although epidemiological studies have demonstrated an increased mortality for people with epilepsy, the risk is not the same for all epilepsy patients. It was noted already by Alström [13] that in contrast to those with epilepsy of known origin, there was no excess mortality among patients with epilepsy of unknown aetiology. Population-based studies of incident cohorts [3-7] also consistently report higher mortality (SMR) in patients with remote symptomatic epilepsy compared with idiopathic cases. In most studies of mortality, the term idiopathic epilepsy is used in the broader sense, indicating epilepsy with unknown cause, and not the more restrictive definition suggested by the International League Against Epilepsy [20]. Although SMR ranges from 1.1-1.8 among patients with idiopathic epilepsy, it was increased significantly only in the Rochester and UK studies, 1.8 (1.4-2.3) and 1.6 (1.0-2.4), respectively [3, 4]. In fact, in the extended follow-up at a median of 11.9 years of the UK cohort, SMR for idiopathic epilepsy was no longer significantly increased, 1.3 (0.9-1.9) in contrast to the first report after 6.9 years follow-up [9]. Highest SMRs are reported in patients with epilepsy and neurodeficit from birth, ranging from 11 to 50 [3, 4, 10]. Taken together these observations demonstrate the importance of the aetiology underlying epilepsy for the increased mortality and suggest that patients without a demonstrated cause for their epilepsy only have a slightly if at all increased mortality. However, there are also observations supporting a substantial role of the epilepsy and the epileptic seizures in some populations. Forsgren et al. [21] studied the influence of epilepsy on mortality in a cohort of patients with mental retardation. SMR for those with mental retardation only was 1.6 (1.3-2.0) compared with 5.0 (3.3-7.5) in patients with mental retardation and epilepsy. The increased mortality was related to seizure type as well as seizure frequency.

While most studies report a trend towards higher mortality among males, overall there are no significant differences in SMRs between males and females in the population-based studies [3-5, 7].

Mortality ratios also depend on the age of the patient. Although most studies [2-4] reveal an increased SMR in all age groups, the excess mortality is more pronounced in children. The high SMR in children is explained by high mortality among patients with epilepsy and congenital neurodeficits [10] and also by the low expected number of deaths in the young population.

The duration of epilepsy is another factor of importance. An increased mortality was found in patients with epilepsy during the first ten years after diagnosis in the Rochester study, and then again after 25 years [3]. A clear time-trend was observed also in the prospective community-based study from the UK, with the highest SMR, 6.6 (4.8-8.7) during the first year after the index seizure. SMR declined during the second, third, fourth, and fourth to ninth year to 2.6, 2.3, 3.1 and 1.5, respectively. There was a trend for an increase again at 9-14 years after onset, SMR being 1.8 (1.1-2.7) [9]. In the Swedish study [7] a significantly increased mortality was found during the first two years, and in accordance with other studies, the increase was most pronounced during the first year (SMR 7.3, 95% CI 4.4-12.1). A late increase after 9-11 years was also found [7]. The study from Iceland [5] demonstrated significantly increased mortality during the first 14 years after diagnosis, but only marginally beyond four years. Hence, the excess mortality is most pronounced the first few years after diagnosis but, with exception of the Icelandic study, long-term follow-up indicates a late increase in SMR 10-25 years after diagnosis.

Cause-specific mortality

Evaluation of cause-specific mortality is more complicated partly since larger cohorts are needed and also because it may be difficult to accurately determine the cause of death in each individual case. Most studies rely on information from death certificates, which to a variable extent are supplemented by autopsy reports. The causes of death among people with epilepsy may be completely independent of their epilepsy, be related to the underlying etiology of epilepsy or to associated handicaps, related to the treatment, or the death could be directly (e.g. status epilepticus and sudden unexpected death in epilepsy, SUDEP) or indirectly caused by seizures (e.g. accidents). From this follows that the cause-specific mortality also depends on the patient population, and differences in the severity and duration of epilepsy will have an impact on the results.

Proportionate mortality has been reported in a number of epilepsy cohorts based on institutions and hospitals as well as community samples *(table III)*. In these, neoplasms have accounted for 12-34% of deaths. Pneumonia has been another dominating cause of death, reported in 5-25% of cases. The highest figures for pneumonia were found in case series from institutions [15, 16]. In contrast, cerebrovascular disorders appear to be a more frequent cause of death in populations based studies (12-17%) [3, 4, 6, 21] compared with some hospital-based cohorts, 5-6% [15, 16]. Heart disease has been reported as a cause of death in 8-19% of people with epilepsy *(table III)*.

Accidents have accounted for 1-20% of deaths *(table III)*. In studies of suicide, the proportionate mortality also varies considerably, ranging from 0 to 9% *(table III)*. Most recent population-based studies report low figures, 1% in the Rochester study and in the UK cohort [3, 9]. The study from Iceland is an exception with 9% of deaths being suicide [22].

Table III. Causes of death in epilepsy (proportionate mortality ratios, %) in population-based studies as well as some selected populations

Cause of death	Study							
	Poland [2]	US [3, 8]	UK [9]	France [6]#	Sweden [17]	UK [15]	UK [16]	Iceland [22]
Cerebrovascular	12	14	16	17	14	6	5	16
Heart disease	16	19	11		16	10	19	16
Neoplasm, all	24	20	34		16	12	26	23
Brain tumors	15	8	11	53	4	0.6	0.8	
Pneumonia	8	8	18		5	12	25	
Suicide	7	1.6	0.7		1.3	3.3	0	9
Accidents	4	6	2.0		3	7	3	20
Seizure related	10	6	0.7			31	12	
SUDEP§	4		0.7				6	
Other	15	25	18	30	41	18	5	25

Unprovoked seizures + progressive symptomatic. § Sudden unexpected death in epilepsy.

As discussed above, proportionate mortality does not demonstrate an increased mortality in comparison to a reference population. This requires ratios such as SMR. Cause-specific SMRs from population-based incident cohorts are summarised in *(table IV)*. Such analyses have demonstrated an increased SMR ranging from 3.5-7.3 for pneumonia [3, 9]. Mortality due to neoplasms is also increased in most studies, SMR ranging from about 2-3.5 [3, 7, 9, 22]. SMR remained significantly increased also when brain tumours were excluded, SMR 1.8-2.4 in the US and UK studies [3, 9]. Mortality is also increased in cerebrovascular diseases, SMR 1.8-4.2, whereas death attributed to heart disease does not seem to be increased. A significantly increased SMR for accidents was reported in the Rochester study, SMR 2.4 [3] and for men in the Iceland cohort, SMR 2.8 [22]. In general, these studies do not distinguish between seizure induced fatal accidents and those that are unrelated to seizures. As for suicide, results are more ambiguous. Only one population-based study of an incident cohort has reported an increased SMR, 5.8 among men, based on four suicides, in the study from Iceland [22].

Table IV. Cause-specific mortality in population-based incident cohorts of epilepsy. SMR (95% confidence interval)

Disease	USA [3, 8]	UK [9]	Sweden [7]	Iceland [22] Men	Iceland [22] Women
Cerebrovascular	2.6 (1.8-3.6)	3.7 (2.3-5.5)	4.2 (2.2-8.0)	3.0 (0.8-7.8)	1.8 (0.4-5.2)
Heart disease	1.1 (0.8-1.5)				
Ischemic		1.1 (0.6-1.7)	1.5 (0.7-3.2)	1.7 (0.7-3.4)	–
Myocardial insufficiency			1.8 (1.2-3.0)		
Other circulatory	7.1 (3.4-13)				
Neoplasms	2.9 (2.1-3.9)	3.5 (2.6-4.6)	3.4 (1.9-5.8)	2.1 (0.9-4.4)	1.2 (0.2-3.4)
Excl brain tumors	1.8 (1.1-2.6)	2.4 (1.7-3.4)			
Pneumonia	3.5 (1.6-6.6)	7.3 (4.8-10.6)			
Accidents	2.4 (1.3-3.7)			2.8 (1.2-5.6)	1.7 (0.02-9.4)

Studies of selected cohorts may provide complementary information although the results cannot be considered representative of the epilepsy population in general. In a large hospital-based study where an estimated 80% of the patients on which calculations were based had true epilepsy, mortality was increased for a wide range of causes [17]. Suicide was significantly more common than expected (SMR 3.5, 95% CI 2.6-4.6). Except for heart disease mortality was also increased for all causes examined in a long-term residential care unit for patients with epilepsy [15]. A later study in the same institution also found an increased mortality for neoplasms (SMR 2.0, 95% CI 1.3-2.9) [16], although only one of the 29 neoplasms was a brain tumor.

Seizure related death

The proportion of deaths that is considered being directly seizure related vary markedly between studies. This is partly due to differences in definitions but mainly depending on the study population although results in population-based incident cohorts also vary. Ficker *et al.* [23] reviewed all deaths in the 1 535 persons whose epilepsy was diagnosed in Rochester between 1935 and 1994. There were nine SUDEPs among 535 deaths (1.7%). In the UK study, one SUDEP was identified among 79 deaths in the 564 patients with definite epilepsy [9]. In addition, there was one death in status epilepticus. Of the 39 deaths among 107 adult patients with epilepsy diagnosed in Västerbotten, Sweden, none was seizure related [7]. It is not clear if there were any SUDEPs or fatalities in status epilepticus in the study from Iceland, although the numbers must be low [22]. Two of in total 21 deaths among 469 patients with unprovoked seizures in the short-term follow-up in Gironde, France occurred during a seizure [6]. Hence, in general the proportion of seizure related deaths is low in population-based incident cohorts.

This is in contrast with observations from cohorts of patients with chronic refractory epilepsy.

Three studies from institutions in Finland and the UK have reported epilepsy as the main cause of death in 19% [24], 31% [15], and 20% [16]. High proportions of epilepsy-related deaths have also been reported in two more recent studies of children with epilepsy. Harvey and co-workers [25] found that death was directly attributable to epilepsy in 22%, and Sillanpää et al. [12] found death to be related to seizures in 45% of the fatalities. In contrast, only two of 26 deaths from the Nova Scotia childhood epilepsy cohort were seizure- or epilepsy related (one status epilepticus and one sudden unexpected death) [10]. Differences in criteria, population at study, age and length of follow-up, may account for the wide range in proportion of deaths attributed to epilepsy.

Sudden unexpected death in epilepsy (SUDEP) is generally considered to be the most frequent epilepsy-related death. Ficker et al. [23] estimated the incidence of SUDEP to 0.35 per 1 000 person years in an unselected cohort of epilepsy patients. SUDEP accounted for 8.6% of deaths in persons 14-44 years of age. SMR for SUDEP was 23.7 (7.7-55.0) compared with SUD in the general population. A direct comparison of incidence rates across studies is hampered by differences with respect to SUDEP criteria. However, it is quite obvious that the incidence varies with the patient population being lowest among incident cases in community-based studies [4, 23]. The highest risk is observed in patients with severe chronic epilepsy [25] and in particular among epilepsy surgery candidates, where the incidence was found to be 9.3 per 1 000 patient years [27]. Follow-up studies confirm that this is a sub-population with a particularly high proportion of epilepsy related deaths also after surgery. In a study of 305 patients who had temporal lobe epilepsy surgery in the UK, 14 of 20 deaths (70%) were considered definitely or possibly epilepsy related, six (30%) were SUDEP [28]. A follow-up of 393 patients who had epilepsy surgery in the US identified 11 deaths of which seven were epilepsy related (six SUDEPs) [29]. Interestingly, none of the 199 patients who became seizure free after surgery died.

The importance of the study population is further illustrated by a recent study based on pooled data from new antiepileptic drug applications submitted to the US Food and Drug Administration [30]. While there were 3.8 SUDEPs per 1 000 person-years in patients with chronic epilepsy participating in add-on trials, there was no SUDEP in 983 person-years among new onset epilepsy patients taking part in monotherapy initiation trials.

Conclusions

Data on mortality in people with epilepsy come almost exclusively from studies carried out in industrialised countries, and we know very little about mortality in epilepsy patients from the developing world. The population-based studies demonstrate an increased mortality, generally 2-3 times that of the general population. This is most evident in patients with remote symptomatic epilepsy, which points to the importance of the underlying cause of epilepsy to explain the excess mortality. Mortality is probably only slightly increased, if at all, in people with idiopathic epilepsy. Highest mortality ratios are seen in young age groups (partly due to the low expected mortality rates) and during the first 5-10 years after seizure onset although long-term follow-up indicates a late increase 10-25 years after diagnosis.

References

1. Commission on Epidemiology and Prognosis, International League Against Epilepsy. Guidelines for epidemiologic studies on epilepsy. *Epilepsia* 1993; 34: 592-6.
2. Zielinski JJ. Epilepsy and mortality rate and cause of death. *Epilepsia* 1974; 15: 191-201.
3. Hauser WA, Annegers J, Elveback L. Mortality in patients with epilepsy. *Epilepsia* 1980; 21: 399-412.
4. Cockerell O, Johnson A, Sander JWAS, Hart Y, Goodridge D, Shorvon S. Mortality from epilepsy: results from a prospective population based study. *Lancet* 1994; 344: 918-21.
5. Olafsson E, Hauser WA, Gudmundsson G. Long-term survival of people with unprovoked seizures: a population-based study. *Epilepsia* 1998; 39: 89-92.
6. Loiseau J, Picot M-C, Loiseau P. Short-term mortality after a first epileptic seizure: a population-based study. *Epilepsia* 1999; 40: 1388-93.
7. Lindsten H, Nyström L, Forsgren L. Mortality in an adult cohort with newly diagnosed unprovoked unprovoked epileptic seizure. A population-based study. *Epilepsia* 2000; 41: 1469-73.
8. Annegers JF, Hauser JF, Shirts SB. Heart disease mortality and morbidity in patients with epilepsy. *Epilepsia* 1984; 25: 699-704.
9. Lhatoo SM, Johnson AL, Goodridge DM, MacDonald BK, Sander JWAS, Shorvon SD. Mortality in epilepsy in the first 11 to 14 years after diagnosis: Multivariate analysis of a long-term, prospective, population-based cohort. *Ann Neurol* 2001; 49: 336-44.
10. Camfield CS, Camfield PR, Veugelers PJ. Death in children with epilepsy: a population-based study. *Lancet* 2002; 359: 1891-95.
11. Kurtz Z, Tookey P, Ross E. Epilepsy in young people: 23 year follow up of the British national child development study. *Br Med J* 1998; 316: 339-42.
12. Sillanpää M, Jalava M, Kaleva O, Shinnar S. Long-term prognosis of seizures with onset in childhood. *N Engl J Med* 1998; 338: 1715-22.
13. Alström CH. A study of epilepsy in its clinical, social and genetic aspects. *Acta Psychiatr Neurol Scand* 1950; Suppl. 63: 1-284.
14. Henriksen B, Juul-Jensen P, Lund M. The mortality of epilepsy. In: Brackenridge RDC, ed. Proceedings of the 10th International Congress of Life Insurance Medicine. London: Pitman, 1970: 139-48.
15. White SJ, McLean AEM, Howland C. Anticonvulsant drugs and cancer. A cohort study in patients with severe epilepsy. *Lancet* 1979; 2: 458-61.
16. Klenerman P, Sander JWAS, Shorvon SD. Mortality in patients with epilepsy: a study of patients in long term residential care. *J Neurol Neurosurg Psychiatry* 1993; 56: 149-52.
17. Nilsson L, Tomson T, Farahmand B, Diwan V, Persson PG. Cause-specific mortality in epilepsy: a cohort study of more than 9,000 patients once hospitalized for epilepsy. *Epilepsia* 1997; 38: 1062-8.
18. Shackleton DP, Westendorp RGJ, Kasteleijn-Nolst Trenité DGA, Vandenbroucke JP. Mortality in patients with epilepsy: 40 years of follow up in a Dutch cohort study. *J Neurol Neurosurg Psychiatry* 1999; 66: 636-40.
19. Carpio A. Mortality of epilepsy in Ecuador. Workshop of Mortality of Epilepsy. International League Against Epilepsy. Commission on the Burden of Epilepsy. Brussels, May 19-20, 2000.
20. Commission on Classification and Terminology, International League Against Epilepsy. Proposal for revised classification of epilepsies and epileptic syndromes. *Epilepsia* 1989; 30: 389-99.
21. Forsgren L, Edvinsson S-O, Nyström L, Blomquist K, Son H. Influence of epilepsy on mortality in mental retardation: an epidemiologic study. *Epilepsia* 1996; 37: 956-63.
22. Rafnsson V, Olafsson E, Hauser WA, Gudmundsson G. Cause-specific mortality in adults with unprovoked seizures. *Neuroepidemiology* 2001; 20: 232-6.
23. Ficker DM, So EL, Shen WK, Annegers JF, O'Brien PC, Cascino GD, Belau PG. Population-based study of the incidence of sudden unexplained death in epilepsy. *Neurology* 1998; 51: 1270-4.
24. Iivanainen M, Lehtinen J. Causes of death in institutionalized epileptics. *Epilepsia* 1979; 20: 485-92.
25. Harvey AS, Nolan T, Carlin JB. Community-based study of mortality in children with epilepsy. *Epilepsia* 1993; 34: 597-603.
26. Nashef L, Fish DR, Garner S, Sander JWAS, Shorvon SD. Sudden death in epilepsy: a study of incidence in a young cohort with epilepsy and learning difficulty. *Epilepsia* 1995; 36: 1187-94.

27. Dasheiff RM. Sudden unexpected death in epilepsy: a series from an epilepsy surgery program and speculation on the relationship to sudden cardiac death. *J Clin Neurophysiol* 1991; 8: 216-22.
28. Hennessy MJ, Langan Y, Elwes RDC, Binnie CD, Polkey CE, Nashef L. A study of mortality after temporal lobe epilepsy surgery. *Neurology* 1999; 53: 1276-83.
29. Sperling MR, Feldman H, Kinman J, Liporace JD, O'Connor MJ. Seizure control and mortality in epilepsy. *Ann Neurol* 1999; 46: 45-50.
30. Racoosin JA, Feeney J, Burkhart G, Boehm G. Mortality in antiepileptic drug development programs. *Neurology* 2001; 56: 514-9.

Prognosis of first seizure

Ettore Beghi

Epilepsy is a chronic clinical condition characterized by the occurrence of repeated unprovoked seizures. More specifically, the disease means two or more unprovoked seizures (including status epilepticus) occurring at least 24 hours apart [1]. This definition reflects the concept that not all epileptic seizures are spontaneous and not all individuals experiencing a first unprovoked seizure will necessarily develop a recurrence during their life. These concepts have practical implications, including the need for specific requirements for the diagnosis of epilepsy in patients with epileptic seizures, the identification of underlying epileptogenic conditions, the assessment of the sociocultural implications of seizure recurrence, and the risk:benefit ratio of pharmacological treatment. Thus, the prognosis of a first epileptic seizure (ie, the risk of recurrence) and the role of all prognostic indicators (including treatment) should be established for all individuals coming to medical attention after a first seizure.

Problems underlying the assessment of the prognosis of a first seizure

The physician asked to define the prognosis of a patient referred with a first seizure faces three major questions: 1. Is the referred episode an epileptic seizure or a nonepileptic event (pseudoseizure, syncope or related condition, etc.)?; 2. Is the attack a first epileptic seizure or a recurrence?; 3. Is it an unprovoked seizure?

The differential diagnosis between epileptic seizures and nonepileptic events is sometimes difficult and subjected to differing interpretation among physicians. Up to 20% of patients referred to epilepsy centers are reported to present pseudoseizures [2] and a high variability can be expected even between neurologists in the clinical interpretaton of a first seizure [3].

Generalized tonic-clonic seizures may be more easily identified as first seizures. By contrast, nonconvulsive events (ie, partial, myoclonic, or absence seizures) tend to be diagnosed only after recurrence. These seizures may also have occurred prior to a first convulsive event.

By definition, unprovoked seizures are the hallmark of epilepsy. An unprovoked seizure is an event occurring in the absence of any acute precipitating factor and is classified as idiopathic, cryptogenic or remote symptomatic depending on the absence, presumed presence, or presence of an underlying *non progressive* epileptogenic condition [1]. Unlike unprovoked seizures, provoked or *acute symptomatic* seizures are seizures occurring in close temporal relationship with an acute systemic, toxic, or metabolic insult which is expected to be the underlying cause [1]. Although acute symptomatic seizures may be a risk factor for the development of epilepsy (see below), their outcome is strictly dependent on the management of the underlying clinical condition.

Risk of relapse of a first unprovoked seizure

Based on published studies, the risk of relapse of a first unprovoked seizure has been reported to range from 23 to 71% [4-15]. Most of the differences among studies can be explained by the different clinical condition, with particular reference to the definition of first seizure (unprovoked and/or provoked), the study design (retrospective or prospective; community-based or clinic-based), the target population (children and/or adults; patients from developed or developing countries), the timing of enrolment (interval between seizure and admission), the type of seizure (generalized tonic and/or clonic, partial and other), the length of follow-up, and the use of antiepileptic drugs. A summary of published reports using actuarial methods for the assessment of the prognosis of the first unprovoked seizure is depicted in *table I*. In these studies, the risk of relapse of a first seizure at one year ranged from 14 to 68%. The corresponding rates at two and five years were 21-69% and 34 ≥ 71%. The study with the highest recurrence rate was that of Elwes and co-workers [6] who assessed retrospectively patients seen at a specialty clinic who were left untreated at the time of the initial seizure. Retrospective enrolment, use of referral patients, and lack of treatment might explain an extraordinarily high risk of seizure recurrence. One of the two studies with the lowest relapse rates [5] dealt with a prolonged interval between first seizure and outpatient visit (range 2-10 weeks; 80% between five and seven weeks), by which time several patients have already presented a seizure relapse. In the other study [10], a high proportion of patients (80%) received drug treatment after the first seizure. Population-based studies [7,11], whether prospective or retrospective, provided more homogeneous relapse rates at one (36-37%) and two years (43-45%) regardless of the different proportion of cases treated after the first seizure (15 and 61%).

In a systematic review of 16 reports [4], the average recurrence risk was 51% (95% Confidence Interval [CI] 49-53%). The risk was 40 and 52% in prospective and retrospective studies. By two years, the recurrence risk was 36 and 47% in prospective and retrospective studies.

Risk factors for seizure relapse

The identification of risk factors for seizure relapse in patients with a first unprovoked seizure is subjected to several methodological drawbacks, including the absence of a systematic search of *all* relevant factors in *all* published reports and the lack of standard methods for the definition and mode of assessment of a given risk factor. A critical view of the methodology of observational studies on the recurrence of a first seizure is given in a separate publication [16].

Based on the systematic review [4] and the results of more recent studies [5-15], the two most consistent predictors of recurrence were a documented etiology of the seizure and an

Table 1. Summary of published studies on the prognosis of the first unprovoked epileptic seizure

Author, yr (ref)	Country	Source	N. pts (age)	Seizure type(s)	Design	Follow-up, (mos)	Relapse (%) (*) 1yr	Relapse (%) (*) 2yr	Relapse (%) (*) 3yr	% treated	Predictors of recurrence (**)
Cleland, 1981 [5]	UK	Regional Neurological Center	70 (adults)	GTC	R, CB	Mean 57	16	35	39	?	Abnormal EEG
Elwes, 1985 [6]	UK	Specialty clinic	133 (adults)	GTC	R, CB	Median 15	62	69	–	–	?
Annegers, 1986 [7]	USA	Local population	424 (all)	All	R, PB	> 24	36	45	56	61	Abnormal EEG^Δ ° Abnormal neuro examination Partial seizures
Hopkins, 1988 [8]	UK	Specialty clinic referrals	408 (adults)	All	P, CB	?	36	45	–	15	Timing of seizures
Boulloche, 1989 [9]	France	Neurology oriented general pediatric unit	119 (children)	GTC	P, CB	> 60	29	30	37	61	Duration of seizures Family history of epilepsy
Hauser, 1990 [11]	USA	Emergency room	244 (all)	All	P, CB	Median 22	14	25	34	80	Known etiology^Δ Abnormal EEG Siblings with seizures
Hart, 1990 [12]	UK	General practitioners	564 (all)	All	P, PB	24-48	37	43	–	15	Known etiology Partial seizures Age < 16 or > 59 Seizure in sleep/awakening Abnormal EEG
van Donselaar, 1991 [13]	Holland	Hospital	165 (adults)	Idiop,	P, CB	24-48	32	40	–	–	Younger age ° Abnormal EEG
Shinnar, 1996 [14]	USA	Hospital, private practice	407 (children)	GTC, partial	P, CB	Mean 75.6	29	37	42	5	Remote symptomatic etiology Prior febrile seizures Todd's paralysis Onset of seizure in sleep
Martinovic, 1997 [15]	Yugoslavia	Hospital	78 (children)	GTC	P, CB	Mean 62.4	68	–	–	42	Epileptiform patterns in first EEG
Ramos Lizana, 2000 [16]	Spain	Hospital	217 (children)	All	P, CB	Mean 45.6	46	57	63	16	° Known etiology Age 3-10
Hui, 2001 [17]	China	EEG laboratory	132 (adults)	GTC	R, CB	Mean 27	30	37	52	–	° Abnormal CT scan

* Actuarial methods; ** Only significant factors; R = Retrospective; PB = Population-based; CB = Clinic-based; P = Prospective; ° Multivariate analysis; GTC = generalized tonic-clonic; ^Δ Only idiopathic seizures.

abnormal (epileptiform and/or slow) EEG pattern. The pooled recurrence risk in patients with idiopathic or cryptogenic first seizures was 32% (95% CI 28-35%) and that of patients with remote symptomatic seizures was 57% (95% CI 51-63%). The recurrence risk ranged from 27% (95% CI 21-33%) in patients with normal EEG tracings to 58% (95% CI 49-66%) in those with epileptiform abnormalities. Where assessed, epileptiform abnormalities tended to be associated with a higher risk of seizure recurrence than nonepileptiform abnormalities. The pooled two-year recurrence risk was lowest in patients with an idiopathic or cryptogenic first seizure *and* a normal EEG (24%; 95% CI 19-29%), intermediate with a remote symptomatic seizure (48%; 95% CI 34-62%) *or* an abnormal EEG (48%; 95% CI 40-55%), and highest with a remote symptomatic seizure *and* an abnormal EEG (65%; 95% CI 55-76%). Seizures while asleep tend to be associated with a higher risk of recurrence both in children and in adults [8,12,16,17]. Partial seizures, which are most frequently associated with a recognized etiology and/or abnormal EEG findings, are also correlated with a higher risk of recurrent seizures. A consistent association between partial seizures and an increased risk of relapse has been confirmed after controlling for etiology and EEG abnormalities [7,17]. A positive correlation between seizure relapse and family history of seizures was confirmed in patients with idiopathic or cryptogenic first seizures in only one study [10]. History of prior provoked seizures has been occasionally found to increase the risk of relapse, while evidence is inconclusive or lacking for sex, age, and status epilepticus [4]. A limited number of observations prevents conclusions about factors like previous provoked seizures, status epilepticus, post-ictal paresis, and abnormal neurological and/or psychiatric symptoms or signs.

Except for etiology and abnormal EEG which, when combined, have been shown to increase significantly the risk of relapse, other variable groupings were not examined to identify patients at high risk of recurrence.

The role of treatment on the risk of recurrence

As several observational studies reported a significant correlation between number of seizures before treatment, multiple recurrences and chance of long-term remission [19-21], suggestions were made for early treatment to be followed by a better long-term prognosis of epilepsy. However, based on the results of comparative studies, no significant difference in the risk of relapse of a first unprovoked seizure was detected between treated and untreated patients [8, 9, 11, 18]. As treatment effects may be confounded by the tendency to treat patients who are more likely to relapse, the issue can be solved only with an experimental design. To the present time, there are three published randomized studies assessing the effects of treatment of the first unprovoked seizure on the risk of relapse [22-25] and the chance of prolonged seizure remission [24, 26]. The results of these studies are consistent in showing that treatment of the first seizure seems to reduce the risk of short-term relapse but is apparently ineffective on the chance of long-term seizure remission. In a small trial of 31 children with a first unprovoked partial or generalized tonic-clonic seizure randomized to treatment (14) or no medication (17), two treated and nine untreated patients had a recurrent afebrile seizure [22]. Ninety-one patients aged 18-50 years with a single generalized tonic-clonic seizure were randomized to receive treatment (45) or to remain untreated (46) and followed until recurrence or 36 months whichever first [23]. There were significantly more seizure-free patients in the treated (10) compared to the untreated group (29) ($p < 0.005$). In a large multicenter trial [24, 25], 397 children and adults, seen within seven days after a first witnessed primarily or secondarily generalized tonic-clonic seizure, were randomized to immediate treatment (204) or to withhold treatment until recurrence (193). Overall, 36 treated and 75 untreated patients had a relapse. The cumulative time-dependent risk of recurrence in treated patients was 17% at 12 months and 25% at 24 months (untreated, 41 and 51%). However, the difference between the two treatment groups tended to disappear when the end-point of treatment was the chance of initiating a 2-yr remission. The cumulative probability of long-term remission tended to overlap in the two treatment groups by the second-year of follow-up *(figure 1)*. This finding can be interpreted as a consequence of the treatment delay in patients randomized to be initially untreated, who actually started treatment at the time of first relapse. When adjusting for the difference in time at treatment initiation, the probability of prolonged seizure remission was almost identical in both treatment arms *(figure 1)*.

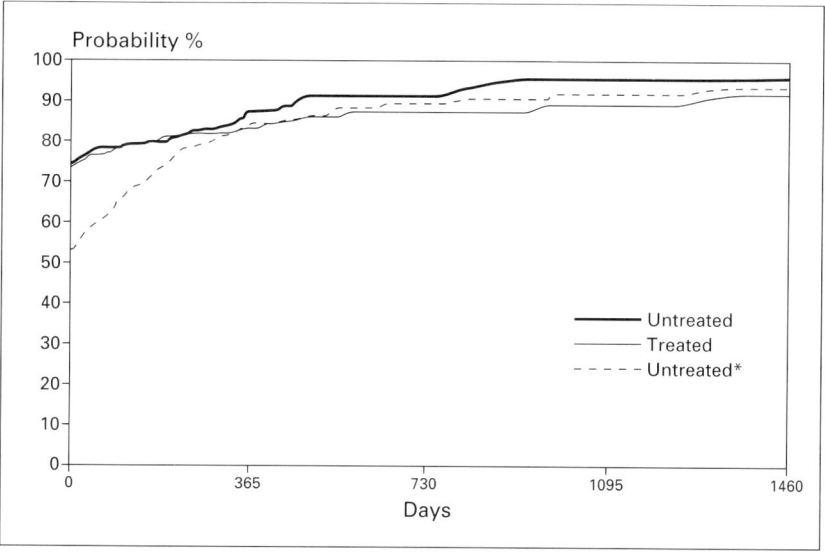

Figure 1. Cumulative time-dependent probability of initiating a period of 1 year seizure free according to whether an antiepileptic drug was given after the first seizure. * Considers as entry time the time of treatment initiation (see Patients and methods for details).

The results of these trials tend to confirm the observational reports that the long-term prognosis of the first seizure is substantially unaffected by immediate treatment. However, the comparative effects of the treatment of the first seizure and the treatment of the relapse on the chance of long-term *permanent* remission (ie, off drugs) have not yet been assessed.

Mortality after a first seizure

There are few reports on the death risk of patients with a first epileptic seizure. In one population-based study reporting one-year mortality in a sample of children and adults with a first epileptic seizure in Gironde, France, the overall standardized mortality ratio (SMR) was 9.3 (95% CI 7.9-10.9) [26]. The SMR for unprovoked seizures was 4.1 (95% CI 2.5-6.2). Mortality was increased in patients with remote symptomatic seizures (SMR 6.5; 95% CI 3.8-10.5), provoked seizures (SMR 10.1; 95% CI 8.1-12.4), and seizures secondary to progressive neurological conditions (SMR 19.8; 95% CI 14.0-27.3). By contrast, there were no deaths among patients with idiopathic seizures and mortality was not increased in patients with cryptogenic seizures (SMR 1.6; 95% CI 0.4-4.1). In an adult

Swedish population-based cohort, the SMR in patients with a newly diagnosed unprovoked seizure was 2.5 (95% CI 1.2-3.2), with a first peak (SMR 7.3; 95% CI 4.4-12.1) during the first two years after diagnosis and a second peak (SMR 5.4; 95% CI 2.7-11.2) at years 9-11 [29]. These figures were comparable with those from other population-based studies, reporting an SMR which ranged from 2.3 to 3.3 [30,31]. Mortality risk was higher with remote symptomatic etiology and age younger than 60. Consistent with other studies [30,31], the Swedish study reported the highest mortality risk in the younger age groups and a progressive decrease of the SMR with age.

The cohort of patients enrolled in the pragmatic trial on the treatment of the first seizure was followed for a total of 3,098 person-years [FIRST Group, unpublished]. There were 15 deaths (3.6%). SMR peaked at 10-29 years (8.1; 95% CI 2.1-23.6) and at 30-39 years (9.6; 95% CI 1.2-34.7). SMR was 2.2 (95% CI 0.3-7.9) by one year of follow-up, 3.7 (95% CI 0.5-13.4) by two years, and 2.1 by 3-5 years (95% CI 0.7-4.9).

In a retrospective U.S population-based cohort study, the 30-day mortality of a first episode of status epilepticus was 19% [27]. In this population, 89% of deaths occurred with nonfebrile acute symptomatic status epilepticus. In the same population, 40% of patients surviving the first 30 days after the seizure died within the ensuing 10 years [28]. The SMR was 2.8 (95% CI 2.1-3.5) and was significantly elevated in symptomatic status epilepticus. By contrast, patients with idiopathic/cryptogenic status epilepticus had no increased risk of death compared to the general population. Age, duration of status epilepticus, seizure type, and etiology contributed to mortality in the multivariate analysis.

Differences in the SMR across studies can be explained in part by the different populations at risk and by the study design and methodology, with special reference to the inclusion of provoked seizures and recurrent seizures. However, based on the published reports, documented seizure etiology is the single most important risk factor for the increased mortality in patients with a first epileptic seizure. The highest mortality risk in the youngest age groups can be interpreted in part in the light of the underlying epileptogenic conditions and of the lower number of competing causes of death.

In summary, about one third of patients with a first unprovoked seizure tend to recur at one year and about one half at two years. This contrasts with the significantly higher relapse rate after two (73%) or three unprovoked seizures (76%) [32]. Factors increasing the risk of relapse include documented etiology and abnormal EEG each of which, when present, tends to be associated with doubling of the risk of relapse. Partial seizures are also accompanied by an increased risk of relapse. Family history of epilepsy and timing of seizures may be also influential, although their role is as yet less clearly defined. There is still uncertainty on the role of other factors, including status epilepticus, post-ictal paresis, abnormal neurological and/or psychiatric signs, and prior provoked seizures, while age and sex do not seem to predict the risk of recurrence.

Treatment of the first seizure may reduce the short-term risk of recurrence, but it does not affect the long-term prognosis of epilepsy, ie the chance of achieving prolonged seizure remission. Mortality is higher in patients with a first seizure than the general population. A significant fraction of seizure-related mortality must be attributed to younger age and acute symptomatic seizures, including status epilepticus.

Based on the above findings, the prognosis of the first epileptic seizure is still far from defined for a number of reasons. In developing countries this is not a major issue because patients tend to arrive to medical observation after repeated seizures. The difficult diagnostic ascertainment and the reduced affluence of minor spells limits the value of the studies pooling convulsive seizures with nonconvulsive events. The time limits separating provoked from unprovoked seizures are as yet ill-defined and more standardized definitions are still required.

References

1. Commission on Epidemiology and Prognosis, International League Against Epilepsy: Guidelines for epidemiologic studies on epilepsy. *Epilepsia* 1993; 34: 592-6.
2. Chadwick D. Epilepsy. *J Neurol Neurosurg Psychiatry* 1994; 264-77.
3. Van Donselaar CA, Geerts AT, Schimsheimer RJ. Reliability of the diagnosis of a first seizure. *Neurology* 1989; 39: 267-71.
4. Berg AT, Shinnar S. The risk of seizure recurrence following a first unprovoked seizure: a quantitative review. *Neurology* 1991; 41: 965-72.
5. Beghi E, Ciccone A and The First Seizure Trial Group (FIRST). Recurrence after a first unprovoked seizure. Is it still a controversial issue? *Seizure* 1993; 2: 5-10.
6. Cleland PG, Mosquera I, Steward WP, Foster JB. Prognosis of isolated seizures in adult life. *Br Med J* 1981; 283: 1364.
7. Elwes RDC, Chesterman P, Reynolds EH. Prognosis after a first untreated tonic-clonic seizure. *Lancet* 1985; 2: 752-3.
8. Annegers JF, Shirts SB, Hauser WA, Kurland LT. Risk of recurrence after an initial unprovoked seizure. *Epilepsia* 1986; 27: 43-50.
9. Hopkins A, Garman A, Clarke C. The first seizure in adult life. *Lancet* 1988; 1: 721-6.
10. Boulloche I, Leloup P, Mallet E, Parain D, Tron P. Risk of recurrence after a single unprovoked generalized tonic-clonic seizure. *Dev Med Child Neurol* 1989; 31: 626-32.
11. Hauser WA, Rich SS, Annegers JF, Anderson VE. Seizure recurrence after a 1st unprovoked seizure: an extended follow-up. *Neurology* 1990; 40: 1163-70.
12. Hart YM, Sander JWAS, Johnson AL, Shorvon SD for the NGPSE. National General Practice Study of Epilepsy: recurrence after a first seizure. *Lancet* 1990; 336: 1271-4.
13. Shinnar S, Berg AT, Moshe SL, Petix M, Maytal J, Kang H, Goldensohn ES, Hauser WA. The risk of seizure recurrence after a first unprovoked afebrile seizure in childhood: an extended follow-up. *Pediatrics* 1996; 98: 216-25.
14. Martinovic Z, Jovic N. Seizure recurrence after a first generalized tonic-clonic seizure, in children, adolescents and young adults. *Seizure* 1997; 6: 461-5.
15. Ramos Lizana J, Cassinello Garcia E, Carrasco Marina LL, *et al*. Seizure recurrence after a first unprovoked seizure in childhood: a prospective study. *Epilepsia* 2000; 41: 1005-13.
16. Hui ACF, Tang A, Wong KS, Mok V, Kay R. Recurrence after a first ubtreated seizure in the Hong Kong Chinese population. *Epilepsia* 2001; 42: 94-7.
17. Camfield P, Camfield C, Dooley GM, *et al*. Epilepsy after a first unprovoked seizure in childhood. *Neurology* 1989; 39: 851-2.
18. Van Donselaar CA, Geerts AT, Schimsheimer RJ. Idiopathic first seizure in adult life: who should be treated? *Br Med J* 1991; 302: 620-3.
19. Collaborative Group for the Study of Epilepsy. Prognosis of epilepsy in newly referred patients: a multicenter prospective study. *Epilepsia* 1988; 29: 236-43.
20. Shinnar S, Berg AT, O'Dell C, *et al*. Predictors of multiple seizures in a cohort of children prospectively followed from the time of their first unprovoked seizure. *Ann Neurol* 2000; 48: 140-7.
21. MacDonald BK, Johnson AL, Goodridge DM, *et al*. Factors predicting prognosis of epilepsy after presentation with seizures. *Ann Neurol* 2000; 48: 833-41.
22. Camfield P, Camfield C, Dooley J, Smith E, Garner B. A randomized study of carbamazepine versus no medication after a first unprovoked seizure in childhood. *Neurology* 1989; 39: 851-2.
23. Gilad R, Lampl Y, Gabbay U, Eshel Y, Sarova-Pinhas I. Early treatment of a single generalized tonic-clonic seizure to prevent recurrence. *Arch Neurol* 1996; 53: 1149-52.
24. First Seizure Trial Group. Randomized clinical trial on the efficacy of antiepileptic drugs in reducing the risk of relapse after a first unprovoked tonic-clonic seizure. *Neurology* 1993; 43: 478-83.
25. Musicco M, Beghi E, Solari A, Viani F, for the First Seizure Trial Group (FIRST Group). Treatment of first tonic-clonic seizure does not improve the prognosis of epilepsy. *Neurology* 1997; 49: 991-8.
26. Loiseau J, Picot M-C, Loiseau P. Short-term mortality after a first epileptic seizure: a population-based study. *Epilepsia* 1999; 40: 1388-92.

27. Logroscino G, Hesdorffer DC, Cascino G, Annegers JF, Hauser WA. Short-term mortality after a first episode of status epilepticus. *Epilepsia* 1997; 38: 1344-9.
28. Logroscino G, Hesdorffer DC, Cascino GD, Annegers JF, Bagiella E, Hauser WA. Long-term mortality after a first episode of status epilepticus. *Neurology* 2002; 58: 537-41.
29. Lindsten H, Nystrom L, Forsgren L. Mortality risk in an adult cohort with a newly diagnosed unprovoked epileptic seizure: a population-based study. *Epilepsia* 2000; 41: 1469-73.
30. Hauser WA, Annegers JF, Elveback LR. Mortality in patients with epilepsy. *Epilepsia* 1980; 21: 399-412.
31. Cockerell OC, Johnson AL, Sander JWAS, Hart YM, Goodridge DM. Mortality from epilepsy: results from a prospective population-based study. *Lancet* 1994; 344: 918-21.
32. Hauser WA, Rich SS, Lee JR, Annegers JF, Anderson VE. Risk of recurrent seizures after two unprovoked seizures. *N Engl J Med* 1998; 338: 429-34.

Prognosis of epileptic syndromes: EPIGIR study

Jerôme Loiseau, Marie-Christine Picot and Pierre Loiseau

The epidemiologic research carried out in the last twenty years, whilst improving our knowledge of epileptic disorders, has provided results that are not easy to interpret [1, 2]. Epileptologic concepts change over time [3] and inclusion criteria and case classification vary from one study to another. For industrialized countries, annual incidence rates are estimated at anything from 26 to 70/100 000 for unprovoked seizures (single and recurrent) and from 24 to 53/100 000 for epilepsy (recurrent seizures) [4].

The aim of the present study was to evaluate the mortality and the risk of recurrence according to the epileptic syndromes in a prospective incidence survey of first seizures. This study also sought to evaluate how and to what extent the time dimension and the definitions can affect interpretation of the results of such a survey.

Methods

The data analyzed were obtained from a prospective incidence survey of first seizures [5] using the same methodology as in a Swiss cohort [6]. Eligible persons were all inhabitants of the Bordeaux area aged > 2 months who had a first epileptic seizure between March 1, 1984 and February 28, 1985. Unprovoked and provoked seizures were included. Febrile and neonatal seizures were excluded.

The catchment area was an administrative district of southwest France (Gironde) with little in- or out-migration. In a 1982 census, there were 1,128,164 residents. Most neurologists and neurophysiologists in the area agreed to participate in our prospectively data collection and to fill the questionnaires we sent, asking as usual for medical history, seizure description, neurologic examination and laboratory tests. Complementary surveys were made in the university hospital neurology departments and in some general hospitals.

A diagnostic review panel examined all information. Diagnoses were accepted only with compelling evidence (adequate history and/or EEG findings). We received questionnaire on 1 427 potential cases and progressively discarded 374 of those for the following reasons: misdiagnosis, existence of prior seizures, double registration, residence outside the Gironde.

Review of the medical records of the 1 053 patients retained for the study revealed a further 81 erroneous inclusions and 135 non-epileptic seizures (NES). Initial information was modified as additional material was obtained during the follow-up period by further questioning patients, family, and care providers, leading to some diagnostic modifications. A further 33 cases were reclassified as NES.

Finally, 804 individuals (482 males and 322 females) aged 2 months to 94 years were considered as having had an initial afebrile seizure during the inclusion period. Routine EEG was performed in 781 (97.1%) and CT scan in 481 (59.8%). In the group of unprovoked seizures, all but one patient had EEGs.

Patients had, as far as possible, been followed up for at least 5 years (1 year for provoked seizures), either by a neurologist or their general practitioner. Date and cause of death was obtained from the physician who recorded the death. No autopsy study was available.

Cases were categorized according to the International Classification of Epileptic Syndromes and Epilepsies (ICE), proposed in 1985 [7] and revised in 1989 [8] and later the ILAE Guidelines for Epidemiologic Studies [9].

In the present study, we reviewed and classified each case according to the Classification of Epileptic Syndromes [8]: firstly, on the strength of the clinical and paraclinical information available on inclusion (initial diagnosis), secondly, in the light of complementary data obtained during follow-up (modified diagnosis). When additional information on the status of the patient at inclusion became available, this led to modification of some cryptogenic syndromes into idiopathic or symptomatic syndromes. When an isolated seizure recurred, it was reclassified according to seizure type as cryptogenic localization-related syndrome (partial seizures) or undetermined epilepsy (apparently generalized or unclassified seizures). An initial acute symptomatic seizure followed within the inclusion period by a first unprovoked seizure was reclassified as symptomatic localization-related or cryptogenic/symptomatic generalized syndrome.

Alcohol-related seizures (seizures in persons with a history of chronic alcohol abuse, with no evidence of acute withdrawal or intoxication), seizures in patients with brain tumors or dementia were considered separately, because of difficulties in categorization (provoked or unprovoked seizures?).

A single seizure without any EEG or neuro-imaging abnormalities was considered as an "isolated seizure". Conversely, a single seizure with epileptiform EEG abnormalities or an epileptogenic lesion on neuro-imaging was considered as the first seizure of an epilepsy and so was classified as an epilepsy syndrome. A documented (by history, exam or imaging) cerebral insult was mandatory to place a patient in the category of "symptomatic localization-related syndrome". Focal (lateralized or localizing) EEG abnormalities (that did not conform to the criteria for the idiopathic category) without any documented cerebral insult yielded to classify a single seizure in the category of "cryptogenic localization-related syndrome". Patients in the category of "undetermined epilepsy" (syndrome 3.2) had apparently generalized seizures or seizures without unequivocal focal or generalized features and had neither EEG nor imaging specific findings.

The terms *idiopathic* and *cryptogenic* were used as defined in the International Classification of Epilepsies [8] and in the Guidelines for Epidemiologic Studies on Epilepsy [9].

The probability of recurrence of single unprovoked seizures has been estimated at 1 and 5 years by the method of Kaplan-Meier. The comparison of two or more groups of a pronostic factor was performed with the logrank test.

The SMR and the 95% CI were calculated, comparing the observed number of deaths among these subjects within the period (1 or 5 years) after the initial seizure with that expected based on the number of deaths observed in Gironde during 1985 (source: Institut

National Statistique Etudes Economiques). Stratification by gender and 5-year groups was used. SMR was determined for the whole cohort and according to the epileptic syndrome.

Results

Distribution of epileptic syndromes varied according to the time of the patients' evaluation and to the available data *(Table Ia)*. In 12 cases, a first acute symptomatic seizure at initial presentation was followed within the inclusion period by a first unprovoked seizure leading to reclassify them in the category of symptomatic localization-related syndrome (n = 10) or in that of cryptogenic/symptomatic generalized syndrome (n = 2).

The initial diagnosis was modified in 84 (17.7%) of the 475 cases of unprovoked seizures, 25 proving to be non-epileptic seizures (NES) and 11 provoked seizures. This modification was made mainly during the first year (89.3%) and was motivated by: reassessment of initial data in the light of subsequent information (n = 58), late appearance of abnormalities on EEG (n = 19) or CT scan (n = 1), onset of new seizure type (n = 6). Cryptogenic seizures were the category most often initially misclassified.

After modification of initial diagnosis in the light of complementary data obtained during follow-up on the patient's status at inclusion, 277 (34.5%) persons were considered as having a first provoked seizure (acute symptomatic), 439 (54.6%) as having a first unprovoked seizure (17 idiopathic, 104 symptomatic, and 42 cryptogenic localization-related

Table Ia. Distribution of epileptic syndromes according to the time of the evaluation for patients with a first seizure

Syndrome	Initial diagnosis	Modified initial diagnosis**	At 1 year follow-up***
1. Localization-related			
1.1. Idiopathic	19	17	17
1.2. Symptomatic	96	104	104
1.3. Cryptogenic	28	42	59***
2. Generalized			
2.1. Idiopathic	66	87	87
2.2. Cryptogenic or symptomatic	14	14	14
3. Undetermined whether focal or generalized			
3.2. Without unequivocal G/F features	21	11	23***
4. Special			
4.1. Acute symptomatic (provoked) seizures	266	277	277
4.2. Isolated seizures	206	164	135***
9. Unclassified (provoked or unprovoked seizures?)			
Alcohol related*	32	32	32
Cerebral tumors	39	39	39
Dementia	17	17	17
Overall	**804**	**804**	**804**

G/F: generalized or focal.
* Seizures in persons with a history of chronic alcohol abuse, with no evidence of acute withdrawal or intoxication.
** Rectification of initial diagnosis in the light of complementary data obtained during follow-up on the status of the patient at inclusion.
*** Isolated seizures in 29 patients recurred within the 1-year follow-up. According to the seizure type, they were reclassified in 17 cryptogenic localization-related epilepsies (partial seizures) and in 12 undetermined epilepsies (apparently generalized or unclassified seizures).

Table Ib. Distribution of unprovoked seizures according to the epileptic syndromes and recurrence before diagnosis

Syndrome	At inclusion*				
	All seizures	Single seizures		Recurrent seizures	
	n	n	%	n	%
1.1. Idiopathic localization-related	17	9	52.9	8	47.1
1.2. Symptomatic localization-related	104	90	86.5	14	13.5
1.3. Cryptogenic localization-related	42	5	11.9	37	88.1
2.1. Idiopathic generalized	87	58	66.7	29	33.3
2.2. Cryptogenic/symptomatic generalized	14	0	0	14	100
3.2. Undetermined epilepsies**	11	0	0	11	100
4.2. Isolated seizures	164	164	100	0	0
Overall	**439**	**326**	**74.3**	**113**	**25.7**

* Modified initial diagnosis in the light of complementary data obtained during follow-up on the status of the patient at inclusion.
** Without unequivocal generalized or focal features.

syndromes; 87 idiopathic and 14 cryptogenic or symptomatic generalized syndromes; 11 undetermined epilepsies; 164 isolated seizures), and 88 (10.9%) as having an unclassified syndrome (32 alcohol related, 39 cerebral tumors, 17 dementia).

Recurrence of 29 isolated seizures within the 1-year follow-up increased to 17 the number of cryptogenic localization-related syndromes and to 12 that of undetermined epilepsies.

To assess the predictive value of the syndromic classification on the risk of recurrence, we only considered the 326 patients with a single seizure at the time of inclusion. The distribution according to the epileptic syndromes of this group is reported in *Table Ib*.

The patient's status with regards to single seizure *versus* epilepsy (two or more seizures) varied according to the time of the evaluation. At inclusion, only 113 (25.7%) of the 439 patients who experienced unprovoked seizures had recurrent seizures *(Table Ib)*. At the end of the inclusion period, 172 (39.2%) fulfilled the diagnostic criteria for epilepsy (annual incidence per 100 000 persons: 15.3). The remaining 267 (60.8%) had only a single seizure. A specific epilepsy syndrome was assigned for 120 (annual incidence per 100 000 persons: 10.6) of these (7 idiopathic localization-related, 66 symptomatic localization-related, 2 cryptogenic localization-related, 45 idiopathic generalized) and 147 were classified as cases of isolated seizure.

Among the 326 patients with a single unprovoked seizure, the probability of recurrence was 31.8 at 1 year and 37.9 at 5 years *(Table IIa)*. The risk of recurrence was statistically different according to the epileptic syndromes. This risk was lower in those with isolated seizures. If we consider the distribution according to the syndromes before modification of the initial diagnosis, the comparison of the risk of recurrence was no longer significant *(Table IIb)*.

Mortality according to epileptic syndrome is presented in *Tables IIIa and b*. At 1 year, no patient with idiopathic etiology died, only 1 among 135 individuals with an isolated seizure was deceased and patients with cryptogenic seizures had a slightly increased mortality. Mortality was clearly increased for patients with remote symptomatic seizures and more in those with acute symptomatic seizures. Not surprisingly, it was greatest for epileptic events due to a progressive neurologic condition. In the subgroup of symptomatic localization-related syndrome, only seven of the 16 patients who died had recurrent seizures.

The number of deaths (n = 151) was different of the 149 previously reported [10] because in two of the 12 patients first included with an initial acute symptomatic seizure and then

Table IIa. Probability of recurrence (at 1 year and 5 years) of single unprovoked seizures (after modification of the initial diagnosis) according to the epileptic syndromes

Syndrome	Single unprovoked seizures at inclusion*				
	n	Probability of recurrence			
		At 1 year p<0.0001		At 5 years p<0.0001	
		Rate	95% CI	Rate	95% CI
1.1. Idiopathic localization-related	9	49.2	14.6-83.8	49.2	14.6-83.8
1.2. Symptomatic localization-related	90	45.4	34.6-56.2	-	-
1.3. Cryptogenic localization-related	5	75.0	32.6-117.4	100	0-100
2.1. Idiopathic generalized	58	43.1	30.4-55.8	58.7	46.0-71.4
4.2. Isolated seizures	164	18.5	12.4-24.6	27.9	20.8-35.0
Overall	**326**	**31.8**	26.6-37.0	**37.9****	31.5-44.3

* Rectified initial diagnosis in the light of complementary data obtained during follow-up on the status of the patient at inclusion.
** Without 90 cases of symptomatic localization-related syndrome.

Table IIb. Probability of recurrence (at 1 year and 5 years) of these 326 single unprovoked seizures before rectification of the initial diagnosis

Syndrome	Single unprovoked seizures at inclusion*				
	n	Probability of recurrence			
		At 1 year p=0.13		At 5 years p=0.38	
		Rate	95% CI	Rate	95% CI
1.1. Idiopathic localization-related	11	54.3	21.7-86.9	54.3	21.7-86.9
1.2. Symptomatic localization-related	73	39.6	27.9-51.3	-	-
1.3. Cryptogenic localization-related	0	-	-	-	-
2.1. Idiopathic generalized	38	26.3	12.3-40.3	47.5	31.6-63.4
4.2. Isolated seizures	195	28.2	21.8-34.6	37.8	30.8-44.8
Overall	**326****	**31.2**			

* Initial diagnosis before modification in the light of complementary data obtained during follow-up on the status of the patient at inclusion.
** Of wich nine patients with a first acute symptomatic seizure at initial presentation, then with a first unprovoked seizure occurred within the inclusion period.

who experienced a first unprovoked seizure during the inclusion period, the interval between seizure and death was < 1 year when considering the unprovoked seizure (> 1 year when considering the provoked seizure).

Cause of death also varied according to epileptic syndrome *(Tables IVa and b)*. At 1 year, it was seizure-related (5.9%), due to progression of underlying disease (63.6%), unrelated to seizure etiology (21.2%, including one suicide) and unknown because of insufficient information (9.3%). No possible SUDEP was found.

Table IIIa. Standardized mortality ratios according to epileptic syndrome for patients with a first epileptic seizure (1-year follow-up)

Syndrome	Number followed	By 1 year of follow-up			SMR	95% CI
		Lost	Deaths			
			Observed	Expected		
1. Localization-related						
1.1. Idiopathic	17	1	0	<0.1	0	-
1.2. Symptomatic	104	2	16	2.5	6.4	3.6-10.3
1.3. Cryptogenic	59	4	1	0.6	1.7	0.1-9.7
2. Generalized						
2.1. Idiopathic	87	0	0	0.1	0	-
2.2. Cryptogenic or symptomatic	14	0	1	<0.1	28.1	0.4-156.6
3. Undetermined whether focal or generalized						
3.2. Without unequivocal G/F features	23	0	2	0.1	18.5	2.1-66.7
4. Special						
4.1. Acute symptomatic (provoked) seizures	277	12	90	8.7	10.3	8.3-12.7
4.2. Isolated seizures	135	7	1	1.8	0.6	0.1-3.1
9. Unclassified (provoked or unprovoked?)						
Alcohol related*	32	5	3	0.4	7.7	1.6-22.6
Cerebral tumors	39	0	31	0.7	41.5	28.2-58.9
Dementia	17	0	6	1.1	5.4	2.0-11.7
Overall	**804**	**31**	**151**	**16.1**	**9.4**	**8.0-11.0**

G/F: generalized or focal.
* Seizures in persons with a history of chronic alcohol abuse, with no evidence of acute withdrawal or intoxication.

Table IIIb. Standardized mortality ratios according to epileptic syndrome for patients with a first unprovoked (idiopathic or cryptogenic) epileptic seizure (5-year follow-up)

Syndrome	Number followed	By 5 years of follow-up			SMR	95% CI
		Lost	Deaths			
			Observed	Expected		
1.1. Idiopathic localization-related	17	1	0	<0.1	0	-
1.3. Cryptogenic localization-related	65	9	2	0.6	3.3	0.4-12.1
2.1. Idiopathic generalized	87	5	2	0.1	19.6	2.2-70.9
3.2. Undetermined epilepsies*	31	8	3	0.2	15.5	3.1-45.4
4.2. Isolated seizures	121	21	6	1.7	3.6	1.3-7.8
Overall	**321**	**44**	**13**	**2.6**	**5.1**	**2.7-8.6**

* Without unequivocal generalized or focal features.
SMR of cryptogenic syndromes (CLR, UE, IS): 4.5 (95% CI: 2.2-8.0).

Conclusions

Definitions and clinical practice

"The importance of rigourous case definition in epidemiologic studies of seizure disorders and epilepsy cannot be overemphasized" [9]. However, definitions are still an issue. An

Table IVa. Causes of death according to epileptic syndrome for patients with a first epileptic seizure (1-year follow-up)

Syndrome	Number of deaths	Cause of death			
		During a seizure	Underlying disease	Unrelated to seizure	Unknown
1.1. Idiopathic localization-related	0	-	-	-	-
1.2. Symptomatic localization-related	16	1	1	13	1
1.3. Cryptogenic localization-related	1	1	0	0	0
2.1. Idiopathic generalized	0	-	-	-	-
2.2. Cryptogenic/symptomatic generalized	1	0	1	0	0
3.2. Undetermined (without unequivocal G/F features)	2	0	0	2	0
4.1. Acute symptomatic (provoked) seizures	90	7	57	15**	11
4.2. Isolated seizures	1	0	0	0	1
Alcohol related*	3	0	0	2	1
Cerebral tumors	31	0	31	0	0
Dementia	6	0	6	0	0
Overall	**151**	**9**	**96**	**32**	**14**

G/F: generalized or focal.
* Seizures in persons with a history of chronic alcohol abuse, with no evidence of acute withdrawal or intoxication.
** Of which one suicide.

Table IVb. Causes of death according to epileptic syndrome for patients with a first unprovoked epileptic seizure (5-year follow-up)

Syndrome	Number of deaths	Cause of death			
		During a seizure	Underlying disease	Unrelated to seizure	Unknown
1.1. Idiopathic localization-related	0	-	-	-	-
1.3. Cryptogenic localization-related	2	1	-	-	1
2.1. Idiopathic generalized	2	-	1	1	-
3.2. Undetermined (without unequivocal G/F features)	3	-	3	-	-
4.2. Isolated seizures	6	-	5	-	1
Overall	**13**	**1**	**9**	**1**	**2**

G/F: generalized or focal.

epilepsy syndrome is defined as an epileptic disorder characterized by a cluster of signs and symptoms customarily occurring together, *i.e.* by a constellation of clinical and laboratory information. Yet the number and type of clinical and laboratory tests performed in the study population are not standardized and reflect the clinical practice of treating physicians. In the Bordeaux [5], Rochester [11] and CAROLE [12] studies, the clinical description of seizures, EEG findings, imaging findings, and other laboratory data were used in the classification. However, MRI was not available for routine use in Rochester until 1984 and later in France, and not obtained at the time of diagnosis. Neuroimaging studies are generally not done in patients with unequivocal clinical and/or electrophysiologic findings suggesting a specific epileptic syndrome.

Difficulties of diagnosis at the time of the first visit

The epileptic nature of an initial paroxysmal event may, firstly, be difficult to confirm. Our 5.3% of false-positives are close to the 4% of NES reported by Braathen *et al.* [13].

Modifications were made principally during the first year. This delay is often determined, in practice, by the occurrence of a more clearly identifiable second seizure.

We adopted a syndromic approach. Seizure types are simply symptoms and give few indications regarding the possible paradoxical effect of certain antiepileptic drugs [14].

A precise diagnosis can be difficult at the time of the first visit. Our 12.4% of unprovoked seizures initially misclassified are similar to the 12% found by Arts *et al.* [15] after 2 years in 494 children. Shinnar *et al.* [16] reported that either etiology or syndrome classification or both were modified in 19% of 182 children followed for a mean 8.2 years after their second seizure. Among 613 children with newly diagnosed epilepsy, Berg *et al.* [17] found an evolution of the syndrome in 3.9% and a modification to the initial diagnosis in 9.8% after 2 years of prospective follow-up.

The reliability of an initial diagnosis varies according to the syndrome. In our study, cryptogenic seizures (syndromes 1.3, 3.2, 4.2) were more frequently misclassified than syndromes for which there are objective criteria. A syndromic diagnosis is based on clinical and paraclinical data. Picot *et al.* [18] have stressed that diagnostic certainty can be improved by using a semi-structured questionnaire. The diagnosis of idiopathic epilepsy which depends on specific electro-clinical correlations [9] can be complicated by the delayed appearance of EEG abnormalities (18 cases in our study, 1 in the fourth year). That of symptomatic epilepsy may require neuroimaging. Among 300 first-seizure patients, King *et al.* [19] diagnosed partial or generalized syndromes in only 47% with clinical information, *versus* 77% with EEG findings and 81% with MRI. Accurate syndromic classification depends on diagnostic techniques and these are conditioned by the health care system [20].

Reclassification is more frequent in a first-seizure survey than in one of newly diagnosed epilepsies. Isolated seizure are reclassified as soon as a second event occurs. As epilepsy has to begin with a first event, the distinction between a single seizure and the first seizure of an epilepsy depends both on recurrence risk factors and the duration of follow-up. In our study, single seizures classified as epilepsy recurred twice as often as isolated seizure and the entire single-seizure group decreased from 75% on inclusion to 45% at 5 years. A single seizure may not reccur at all with effective drug treatment.

The time dimension thus affects the validity of prospective incidence surveys in three ways: (i) a number of first seizures do not receive immediate medical attention (this question is under separate study); (ii) an epileptic event cannot always be initially diagnosed as such with certainty; (iii) the initial diagnosis is often modified in the light of subsequent information.

Most changes in our study were made during the first year of follow-up.

Pronostic factors for recurrence: Interest of syndromic classification

One of the hoped-for advantages of syndromic classification is that it will provide valuable information about prognosis from the time of diagnosis, without waiting for the outcome [20]. However, as Berg *et al.* [21] have stressed, this classification can be distorted by errors in case ascertainment or the application of classification criteria, as well as by a miscomprehension or an unawareness of the case history. An initial misclassification can also be the result of insufficiently sensitive ancillary tests or the late appearance of new signs linked to the evolution of the disease.

The type of seizures, the EEG and/or cerebral specific abnormalities are risk factors for recurrence. However, these characteristics are used to identify the type of syndrome.

A very important point is the role of an early treatment on the risk of recurrence. The difficulty to answer to this question is the confounding effect of the fact that there is a high tendency to treat patients who are more likely to recur. So, only randomized studies can provide a valid response.

Mortality after a first seizure

Aims of syndromic classification in mortality studies

Death may be seizure-related, and one may imagine that it depends on the seizure type, whatever its cause. Generalized seizures (primary or secondary) seem associated with increase in mortality, partial seizures not [22]. However in the syndromic classification, seizure type is taken into account only at the third level (*i.e.*, that of individual syndrome). When considering the first level (*i.e.*, that of major syndromic groups), as for instance localization-related epilepsies, simple, complex and secondarily generalized partial seizures are mixed. Similarly, when considering the second level (*i.e.*, that of syndromic subgroups), as for instance idiopathic generalized epilepsies, GTCS, absence and myoclonic seizures are together. In special syndromes (acute symptomatic as well as isolated seizures), patients may have partial or generalized seizures.

Role of the seizure type

Seizure-related deaths should be investigated according to the seizure type. For deaths due to the underlying condition, the etiology of seizures should be taken into account. All studies might be based on guidelines with precise consensus-obtained definitions. The major points are seizure-related deaths and deaths related to the underlying pathology.

References

1. Sander JWAS, Shorvon SD. Epidemiology of the epilepsies. *J Neurol, Neurosurg Psychiatry* 1996; 61: 433-43.
2. ILAE Commission Report. The epidemiology of the epilepsies: future directions. *Epilepsia* 1997; 38: 614-8.
3. Cockerell OC, Johnson AL, Sander JWAS, Shorvon SD. Prognosis of epilepsy: a review and further analysis of the first nine years of the British National General Practice Study of Epilepsy, a prospective population-based study. *Epilepsia* 1997; 38: 31-46.
4. Hauser WA. Incidence and prevalence. In: Engel J Jr, Pedley TA, eds. *Epilepsy: a comprehensive textbook*. Philadelphia: Lippincott-Raven, 1997: 47-57.
5. Loiseau J, Loiseau P, Guyot M, Duche B, Dartigues JF, Aublet B. Survey of seizure disorders in the French Southwest. I. Incidence of epileptic syndromes. *Epilepsia* 1990; 31: 391-6.
6. Jallon P, Goumaz M, Haengelli C, Morabia A. Incidence of first epileptic seizures in the canton of Geneva, Switzerland. *Epilepsia* 1997; 38: 547-52.
7. Commission on Classification and Terminology of the International League Against Epilepsy. Proposal for classification of epilepsies and epileptic syndromes. *Epilepsia* 1985; 26: 268-78.
8. Commission on Classification and Terminology of the International League Against Epilepsy. Proposal for revised classification of epilepsies and epileptic syndromes. *Epilepsia* 1989; 30: 389-99.
9. Commission on Epidemiology and Prognosis of the International League Against Epilepsy. Guidelines for epidemiologic studies on epilepsy. *Epilepsia* 1993; 34: 592-6.
10. Loiseau J, Picot MC, Loiseau P. Short-term mortality after a first epileptic seizure: a population-based study. *Epilepsia* 1999; 40: 1388-92.
11. Zarrelli M, Beghi E, Rocca WA, Hauser WA. Incidence of epileptic syndromes in Rochester, Minnesota: 1980-1984. *Epilepsia* 1999; 40: 1708-14.
12. Jallon P, Loiseau P, Loiseau J, on behalf of Group CAROLE (Coordination Active du Reseau Observatoire de l'Epilepsie). Newly diagnosed unprovoked epileptic seizures: presentation at diagnosis in CAROLE study. *Epilepsia* 2001; 42: 464-75.
13. Braathen G, Andersson T, Gylje H *et al.* Comparison between one and three years of treatment in un-

complicated childhood epilepsy: a prospective study. I. Outcome in different seizure types. *Epilepsia* 1996; 37: 822-32.
14. Perucca E, Gram L, Avanzini G, Dulac O. Antiepileptic drugs as cause of worsening of seizures. *Epilepsia* 1998; 39: 5-17.
15. Arts WF, Geerts A, Brouwer O, Peters A, Stroink H, van Donselaar C. Classification schemes in childhood epilepsy: reliability and causes of discrepancy. *Epilepsia* 1997; 38 (Suppl 3): 120.
16. Shinnar S, O'Dell C, Berg AT. Distribution of epilepsy syndromes in a cohort of children prospectively monitored from the time of their first unprovoked seizure. *Epilepsia* 1999; 40: 1378-83.
17. Berg AT, Shinnar S, Levy SR, Testa FM, Smith-Rapaport S, Beckerman B. How well can epilepsy syndromes be identified at diagnosis? A reassessment after two years of follow-up. *Epilepsia* 2000; 41: 1269-75.
18. Picot MC, Crespel A, Tricot M *et al*. Validity of diagnosis using the French translation of the semi-structured interview for seizure classification. *Epilepsia* 1999; 40: 1649-56.
19. King MA, Newton MR, Jackson GD *et al*. Epileptology of the first-seizure presentation: a clinical, electroencephalographic, and magnetic resonance imaging study of 300 consecutive patients. *Lancet* 1998; 352: 1007-11.
20. Berg AT, Shinnar S, Levy SR, Testa FM. Newly diagnosed epilepsy in children: presentation at diagnosis. *Epilepsia* 1999; 40: 445-52.
21. Berg AT, Levy SR, Testa FM, Shinnar S. Classification of childhood epilepsy syndromes in newly diagnosed epilepsy: interrater agreement and reasons for disagreement. *Epilepsia* 1999; 40: 439-44.
22. Hauser WA. Mortality in patients with epilepsy. *Epilepsia* 1997; 38 (Suppl. 3): 168.

Determining prognosis of epilepsy from a prevalence cohort
Estimated rate of spontaneous remissions during three decades

Elias Olafsson, Örn Olafsson and W. Allen Hauser

Introduction

To the individual presenting with epilepsy, the prognosis of symptoms and underlying disease is the most important question. Prognosis is important for determining treatment needs of the individual and also for health care authorities when determining allocation of resources.

It is only in the past two decades that researcher have started to address the issue of prognosis in epilepsy and in spite of several reports, many questions remain. Prospective incidence studies of epilepsy with long follow up, are the gold standard for determining prognosis. These studies are however rare and costly to conduct. Prevalence studies include information spanning long period of time and may be an alternative to incidence studies in providing information on prognosis. There are however many potential pitfalls when using prevalence studies to determine prognosis of epilepsy and several conditions have to be met before a prevalence study can be used in this way.

We present data showing how analysis of a prevalence cohort can give important information regarding the prognosis of epilepsy.

Material and methods

This study is based on a previously published [1] prevalence study from rural Iceland, where we identified all cases with epilepsy in a defined population. The population of the study area was around 90 000 on the prevalence day of December 31st, 1993 (c.f. 89 656 on December 1st 1993). The cases all met the inclusion criteria which were that the individual had had a seizure during the previous 12 months or was taking antiepileptic medications on the prevalence day. We have analyzed the data for individuals 20 years of age and younger at the time of the diagnosis to determine: duration of illness on the prevalence day, etiology and seizure type.

This study determines the number of individuals diagnosed with epilepsy during a 31 year period preceding the prevalence day. The study is limited to individuals where survival for 30 years is to be expected, i.e. those who were young (< 21 years of age) and without associated brain disease at the time of diagnosis. The basic assumption is then that when a uniform incidence of cases is not observed during the study period then the *apparent reduction* in number of cases on the prevalence day is primarily due to *spontaneous remission* of the epilepsy.

We assume that the prevalence cohort meets the following criteria: a) There has not been a selective out-migration from the study area of individuals with epilepsy; b) There is not an excess in mortality among the groups studied; c) The relative contribution of the various etiologies and seizure types has remained the same throughout the 30 year period and are the same as in the incidence part of the prevalence cohort; d) The incidence of epilepsy has remained relatively unchanged during the 30 year period studied. This last criteria can be verified based on a previously published study which demonstrated that the incidence of epilepsy in Iceland in 1960 through 1964 [2, 3] was comparable to the incidence in 1993.

We have chosen to focus on four categories of individuals with epilepsy presenting at 20 years of age or younger, as follows: a) Epilepsy of unknown etiology; b) Partial epilepsy of unknown etiology; c) Primary generalized epilepsy, defined as generalized seizures with generalized epileptiform pattern on electroencephalography.

The previous prevalence study identified 428 individuals who met inclusion criteria for epilepsy on the prevalence day [1], and this includes 42 individuals who had first been diagnosed with epilepsy during the preceding 12 months and are an incidence cohort [3].

We assume that the population of the study area has remained the same proportion (34%) of the Icelandic population during the study period. We have calculated the "incidence" for those diagnosed in the respective time periods and still having "active epilepsy" on the prevalence day. The proportion of the population, < 21 years of age, has varied during the study period from 45% to 34% and we have incorporated that into the estimate.

The overall risk of mortality from any cause in this patient group is small. The highest risk would be for someone who was 20 years of age in 1963 or 4.8% for the entire period; 2% for an 11 year old in middle of the first time period (1967). We have not used this in generating the estimate and that has to be taken into account when interpreting the data, especially for the longest follow-up group.

Results

Spontaneous remission *(table 1)*

Epilepsy of unknown etiology N = 153

A relatively high number of cases was diagnosed from 1983 through 1992, and the rate of cases diagnosed during the 20 years prior to that is relatively stable. The incidence in this category during 1993 was 52.5 per 100 000 individuals and the corresponding number of cases from the three 10 year intervals was 47%, 23% and 16% of that number.

Table I. Deficiency of cases or "spontaneous remissions"

Year(s) of presentation	1993	1983-92	1973-82	1963-72
Population (estimated) 1)	89 656	844 424	758 191	674 743
Proportion of 20 yoa and younger in population	0.34	0.36	0.4	0.45
Estimated number of 20 yoa and younger	30 483	303 993	303 276	303 634
Years from diagnosis – range	< 1	1 to 10	11 to 20	21 to 30
All idiopathic, ≤ 20 yoa 2)				
Number	16	75	37	25
Cases per 100.000	52.5	24.7	12.2	8.2
Proportion still with active epilepsy 2)	100%	47%	23%	16%
Partial idiopathic, ≤ 20 yoa				
Number	6	25	11	9
Cases per 100.000	19.7	8.2	3.6	3.0
Percentage of "all" cases	100%	42%	18%	15%
Primary generalized, ≤ 20 yoa				
Number	7	24	16	9
Cases per 100.000	23.0	7.9	5.3	3.0
Percentage of "all" cases	100%	34%	23%	13%
Generalized idiopathic, ≤ 20 yoa 3), 4)				
Number	3	26	9	7
Cases per 100.000	9.8	8.6	3	2.3
Percentage of "all" cases	100%	87%	30%	23%

Yoa: years of age.
1) 34% of the total (average) population of Iceland during each 10 year period.
2) Proportion of individuals who are considered to still have "active epilepsy" on the prevalence day.
3) Including one individual with unknown seizure category.
4) All had generalized tonic clonic seizures (GTC); one had GTC and myoclonic seizures; nine (20%) had focal epileptiform changes on EEG.

Partial epilepsy of unknown etiology N = 51

Considerable drop off in cases observed during the first 10 years but the number of individuals diagnosed prior to 10 years seem to remain relatively unchanged. The incidence of partial epilepsy of unknown etiology in the incidence cohort was 19.7 per 100 000 person years, and we estimate that approximately 58% go into spontaneously remission during the first 11 years after onset of epilepsy.

Primary generalized epilepsy N = 56

The incidence in this category during 1993 was 23.0 per 100 000 individuals and a sharp drop off in number indicates that 66% go into spontaneous remission during the first 11 years, followed by smaller but considerable numbers in the next two decades from diagnosis.

Generalized idiopathic epilepsy N = 45

The incidence in this category during 1993 was 9.8 per 100 000 individuals. A relatively small number of spontaneous remissions is seen during the first ten years or 13% followed by a drop to 30% of that expected during the second decade after diagnosis.

No remission

An average of 62% (85/137) of individuals with epilepsy of unknown etiology who were 20 years of age or younger at the time of diagnosis did have at least one seizure during the 12 month period preceding the prevalence day. The number for those diagnosed during the preceding 30 years was as follows, according to year of diagnosis: 1963-72: 64% (16/25); 1973-82: 65% (24/37), 1983-92: 60% (45/75).

Discussion

A considerable drop out of cases is apparent when incidence rate is compared with prevalence rate for epilepsy [5]. We compare the prevalence rate of 480 per 100 000 [1] with the incidence rate in this cohort (47 per 100 000 population) [3] and knowing that the incidence rate, for young people, has remained stable [2] during the 30 year observation period. This major discrepancy in the number of cases can best be explained by *spontaneous remissions* of a good proportion of cases that must have presented with epilepsy during the observation period but are not found as such on the prevalence day.

A strength of this study is that it is population based and this approach gives us information that spans 30 years. We have not previously seen a prevalence study used to assess the prognosis of epilepsy in this way, and we feel this may be a useful approach to obtaining long term information on the prognosis of the various types of epilepsy. However other potential explanations for the apparent loss of cases must be carefully evaluated.

The inclusion criteria for the patients in the prevalence study, were similar to those recommended by the ILAE commission on epidemiological studies [6] except in the current study, individuals were included if they had had seizure during the one year preceding the prevalence day, as compared with five years recommended by the Commission.

The main approach of this study was to look at individuals with epilepsy of unknown etiology and who were young at the time of diagnosis. In this group the mortality is not expected to be increased during the period of observation, based on a previously published study from Iceland [4], which found that when followed for 30 years after diagnosis, there was no increase in mortality for this group.

We found that primary generalized epilepsies of young people with no known cause for their seizures (i.e. idiopathic seizure with generalized spike wave on EEG) are apparently associated with a very high spontaneous remission rate or 64% during the first 10 years, and additionally 9% and 10% remit up to 20 and 30 years from diagnosis respectively. The remission rate for partial epilepsy of unknown etiology is very similar.

Little is known about what predicts poor prognosis in young people with epilepsy of unknown etiology, and no particular seizure type or EEG abnormality seems to carry with it a particularly bad prognosis. Exception may be a study from Rochester, Minnesota [7], which found that partial epilepsies are more likely to recur after a first unprovoked seizure than seizures of unknown etiology as a whole.

The number of cases in the incidence group for both generalized idiopathic epilepsy, is quite small and the drop in cases between the first and the second decade may possibly give a better measure of the biologic behavior of this particular category.

The main weakness of this study is the assumption that the population has remained stable concerning in and out migration of with regard to presence of epilepsy of unknown etiology in young people. We believe that e.g. parents with handicapped children with seizure disorder tend to move out of the rural areas and to the more populated areas, but there is no good evidence that this also applies to seizure disorders without associated brain disease. We believe that this assumption is valid and that the results of this study give an accurate estimate of the prognosis of epilepsy of unknown etiology in young individuals.

Our results indicate that spontaneous remission is to be expected in around half of young individuals with epilepsy of unknown etiology, during the first 10 years after diagnosis. Further remission occurs and 30 years after diagnosis only around 20% are expected to be still having seizures or require medications. We believe that this approach is useful and gives valuable information, but further studies are needed.

References

1. Olafsson E, Hauser WA. Prevalence of epilepsy in rural Iceland: a population-based study. *Epilepsia* 1999; 40: 1529-34.
2. Gudmundsson G. Epilepsy in Iceland, a clinical and epidemiologic investigation. *Acta Neurol Scand* 1966; 43 (Suppl 25): 1-124.
3. Olafsson E, Hauser WA, Ludvigsson P, Gudmundsson G. Incidence of epilepsy in rural Iceland. *Epilepsia* 1996; 37: 951-5.
4. Olafsson E, Hauser WA, Gudmundsson G. Long-term survival of people with unprovoked seizures: a population-based study. *Epilepsia* 1998; 39: 89-92.
5. Sander JWAS. Some aspects of prognosis in the epilepsies: a review. *Epilepsia* 1993; 34: 1007-16.
6. Commission on epidemiology and prognosis; International League Against Epilepsy. Guidelines for epidemiologic studies on epilepsy. *Epilepsia* 1993; 34; 592-6.
7. Annegers JF, Shirts SB, Hauser WA, Kurland LT. Risk of recurrence after an initial unprovoked seizure. *Epilepsia* 1986; 27: 43-50.

Long term prognosis of first epileptic seizures: EPIGEN study

Pierre Jallon, Jean Sébastien Landry

Several studies on the incidence rate of the first epileptic seizures have been performed. Their results are however conflicting with reported incidence rate between 61 and 129 cases per 100 000 people [1]. Differences in the results may derive from methodological bias including sample population, inclusion criteria, analysis of etiological factors and specific clinical and instrumental criteria to define an epileptic seizure and its cause. Moreover, they do not independently consider the outcome of provoked or/and unprovoked first epileptic seizures in a large population. In the canton of Geneva (Switzerland), the systematic practice of performing an EEG in all the cases in which an epileptic seizure is probable led us, ten years ago, to collect all cases of suspected first unprovoked or provoked epileptic seizure from all the EEG laboratories in the canton. The diagnosis was based on clinical data obtained from the patient chart at the time of the EEG. All patients have had, by definition, a routine EEG performed several hours to 8 days after the seizure.

Applying these criteria, we found an incidence rate of 69.8 [2], similar to that reported in a French cohort where the same methodology was used [3].

In order to evaluate the natural evolution of a first epileptic seizure we have recently examined the clinical and EEG data of same population reevaluated ten years after the first evaluation. We have (re-) classified all the cases following the ILAE classification of epileptic syndromes and the ILAE classification of risk factors [4, 5].

The aim of the present study is to evaluate the mortality risk, the recurrence rate of a first provoked or non provoked epileptic seizure and the factors implicated in the death and recurrence risk.

Methods

Between June 1, 1990 and May 31 1991, all the patients referred for a first suspected epileptic seizure to the two hospitals of the county of Geneva and local private neurologists were included in a prospective study.

Inclusion criteria were: 1) residence in Geneva at the time of the first provoked or unprovoked seizure; 2) age at the study entry more than one month and 3) clinical and EEG performed at the first evaluation.

Excluded were children with neonatal convulsions or febrile seizures and those with a clinical and EEG evaluation excluding an epileptic seizure.

According to a census taken in 1991, in the Geneva canton (one of the 23 cantons of the Swiss confederation) the canton's total population was 384 657: 183 119 males (47.6%) and 201 538 females. Resident aliens at the time of the study represented 36.5% of the population.

Investigations with CT scan and MRI were performed in 70% and 20% of our patients respectively.

Specific epileptic syndromes, were defined on clear clinical and EEG data, according to the ILAE classification of epileptic syndromes. Only patients with specific EEG abnormalities such as paroxysmal focal or generalized abnormalities have been classified as a specific syndrome. Patients with a first epileptic seizure but with normal or non specific EEG or/and focal slow waves have been classified under the heading of *"special syndrome": either considered as an isolated seizure* or in *relation with an acute condition*. Therefore, this last group represents a large majority (92%) of our patients.

For the analysis of the risk factors, we referred to the guidelines of the ILAE Commission of epidemiology and prognosis of epileptic seizures and epilepsies [5].

Results

Baseline evaluation: (EPIGEN 1)

During the year of study 403 patients were referred. After reviewing all the file records, 94 cases were excluded either because the diagnosis of epileptic seizure remained unclear or because at the time of the seizure the patient was not living in the canton of Geneva. Twelve children have presented febrile convulsions. Therefore, two hundred and seventy six patients have been included in the study. The incidence of all first epileptic seizure, provoked and unprovoked during the 1-year period was 71.7 per 100 000. The age-adjusted incidence as compared with that in the US population was **69.8 in 100 000** (1991). The age-adjusted incidence was higher among males (88.5) than among women (56.5) *(table I)*. The age-specific incidence showed a bimodal case distribution *(figure 1)* with a relative low level in children, a peak in the group aged 20-29 – more marked in the male population – and an impressive increase in the elderly population which begins more early and is greater in the male population.

Epileptic seizures

One hundred and forty seven seizures have been classified as tonico-clonic seizures (53.2%), three as absences, one as myoclonic jerks and one as tonic seizure. Eighty six (31.2%) have been classified as partial seizures – 60.5% of these were secondarily generalized. Nineteen were undetermined and only 4 could not be classified. Finally we observed 15 cases of status epilepticus – eight of these were non convulsive status.

Table I. Age and sex distribution of incident cases in Geneva county

Age	Cases Males	Incidence Males	Cases Females	Incidence Females	Total cases	Incidence
0-9	10	49.4	9	46.5	19	**53.7**
10-19	12	56.2	5	24.2	17	**40.5**
20-29	28	96.1	19	61.6	47	**78.4**
30-39	22	72.9	9	28.6	31	**50**
40-49	30	101	5	15.6	35	**56.7**
50-59	15	63	16	62.5	31	**64**
60-69	17	108.7	13	69.3	30	**87.2**
70-79	16	190.4	19	143.9	35	**110.7**
> 80	12	282	19	178.1	31	**207.7**
	162	**88.5**	**114**	**56.6**	**276**	**71.7**

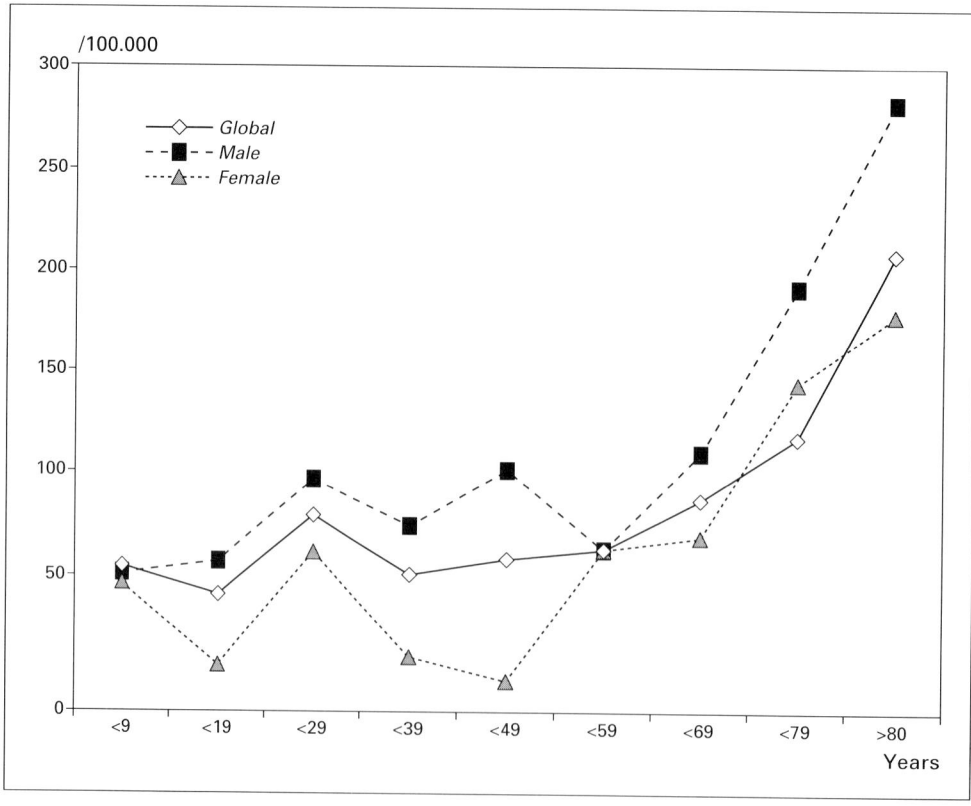

Figure 1. Age and sex distribution of incidence cases in the Geneva cohort.

Epileptic syndromes

Only four patients have been classified as a partial epilepsy (four epilepsies with rolandic spikes). Seventeen cases were classified as a generalized epilepsy (three absence-epilepsy of childhood and 14 "awakening grand mal"). The large majority of our patients has therefore been classified as special syndrome – either *isolated* seizure (155) or acute symptomatic seizures (100).

Etiology

Table II shows data on seizure etiology following the ILAE classification of risk factors. One hundred cases have been classified as provoked seizures, yielding an incidence rate of 26/100 000 (36.2%). The most important cause of provoked seizures was related to alcohol consumption (35%), other toxic substances (13%) and acute cerebro-vascular accidents (CVAs) (14%). One hundred and seventy six cases were classified as unprovoked seizures or epilepsies (45.7/100 000). They were associated with a static condition in 60 cases – 55% of them are in relation with a CVA –, and with a progressive condition in 33 cases – 51.5% were related to an infectious disease (HIV). The greater incidence of HIV infection found in the Geneva canton between 1990 and 1994 explains the high incidence rate observed among the middle adult *(figure 2)*. Eighty three cases were considered as of unknown cause *(table II)*.

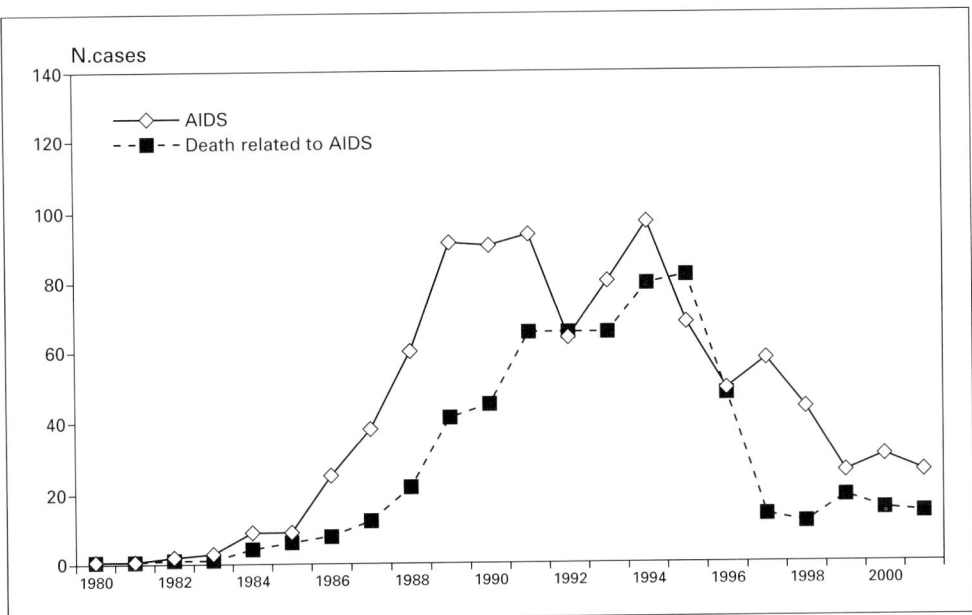

Figure 2. Number of AIDS and death related to AIDS observed in the Geneva county.

Table II. Distribution of etiology and epileptic syndromes in the initial cohort

	Males	Females	Total	Incidence
Provoked seizures	61	39	100	26
Unprovoked (Static condition)	39	21	60	15.6
Unprovoked (Progressive condition)	21	12	33	8.6
Unknown etiology	41	42	83	21.6
Total	**162**	**114**	**276**	**71.7**

Follow-up (EPIGEN 2)

The 276 newly diagnosed patients constituting the initial cohort were tentatively followed up to the end of 2001 or until the date of death if death occurred before the end of 2001. One hundred and eleven died (40.2%) and 63 were loss to the follow-up – the majority had returned in their origin country. Compared to followed patients, the group lost to the follow-up did not differ in terms of age, age at the first seizure, and EEG and neuro-imaging findings. Thus, ten years later, it was possible to have a contact with 102 patients.

Mortality

At the end of the follow-up, 111 patients had died (40.2%). Sixty of 162 males (37%) and 51 of 114 (44.7%) females.

The standardized mortality ratio (SMR) was calculated by dividing the observed number of deaths by the expected number of death in patients who have been followed correctly (213 patients). The 95% confidence interval (95% CI) was calculated, assuming a Poisson distribution for the observed number of deaths.

The total cohort mortality was significantly increased with a standardized mortality ratio (SMR) of 7 (95% CI: 6.2-8.4). The increase in mortality was similar in males (SMR: 6.6; 95% CI: 5-8.5) and females (SMR: 7.7; 95% CI: 5.7-10.2).

According to age, we found a very high SMR (47.9; 95% CI 23.9-85.7) in the group of patients aged 30-39 yrs – probably in relation with complications of HIV infection (13 patients upon 17 died). Conversely SMR decreases with age *(table III)*.

We can observe that the deaths occurred predominantly in the first years of follow-up *(figure 3)*.

The factors found to be associated with increased mortality were the etiology, and the age of patients at the time of diagnosis.

Death occurred in 41% of patients with provoked seizures. In patients with a progressive condition, death occurred in 69.7% (74% was in relation with a HIV infection). Finally in patients with unknown etiology death occurred in 19.3%. No patients with a partial or generalized idiopathic epilepsy died.

Following the etiologic classification, the SMR was more elevated in patients with unprovoked seizures in relation with a progressive condition (SMR = 11.5; 95% CI: 7.2-17.2), compared to patients with a static condition (SMR: 8.6; 95%CI: 5.8-12.3) and with an unknown etiology, (SMR: 3.8; 95% CI: 2.1-6.1) *(table IV)*.

Unfortunately, it was not possible to obtain from the authorities the causes of death.

Table III. All-cause mortality by age-group

Age	N patients followed	Expected deaths	Observed deaths	SMR	95% CI
< 30	50	0.29	2	6.98	0.8-25.2
30-39	21	0.23	11	47.9	23.9-85.7
40-49	30	0.58	8	13.7	5.8-26.9
50-59	23	0.98	14	14.3	7.7-24
60-69	28	2.78	19	6.8	4.2-10.6
70-79	32	7.9	23	2.9	1.8-4.3
> 80	29	28.2	34	1.2	0.8-1.7
Total	**213**	**15.9**	**111**	**7**	***6.2-8.4***

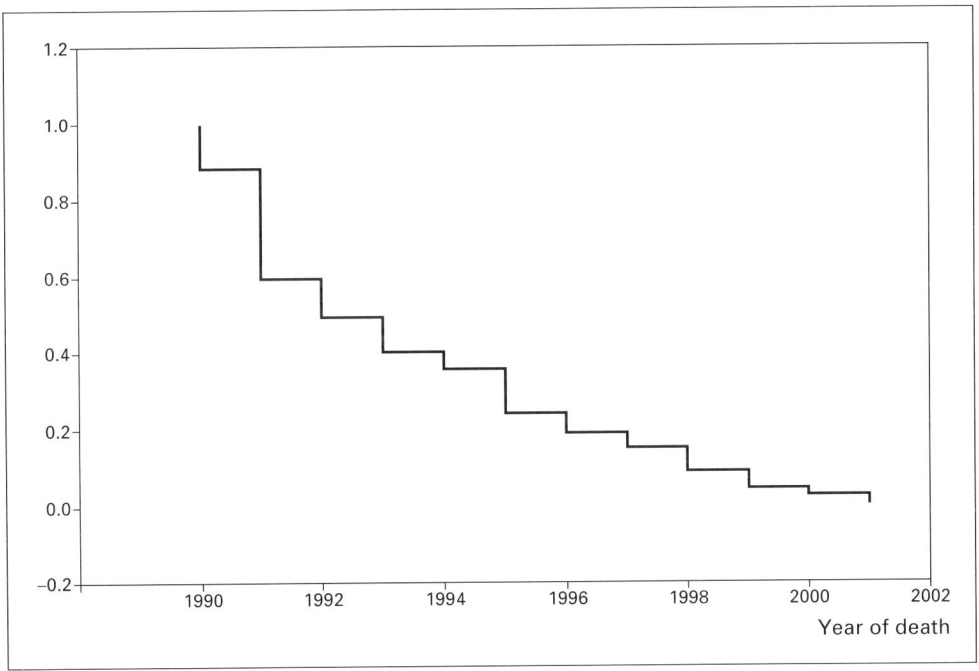

Figure 3. Occurrence of deaths in the followed patients.

Recurrence

Thirty-three patients (32.3%) of the 102 patients that achieved a ten years follow-up have had a relapse. The majority of patients has relapsed early: 44% in the first year and 70% in the first three years after the diagnosis *(figure 4)*.

Twenty one patients have changed of epileptic syndrome. Ninety two per cent of classified seizures were primarily classified in the group "special syndromes" (255 patients), 155 with an isolated seizure and 100 with a seizure in relation with an acute condition. Ninety of these 255 patients achieved the ten years follow-up period. A relapse occurred in 18 patients

Table IV. Death in epileptic patients by etiology at diagnosis

Etiology	N. patients followed	Expected deaths	Observed deaths	SMR	95% CI
Provoked seizures	80	6	41	6.8	4.9-9.2
Unprovoked seizures	133	9.9	70	7	5.5-8.9
Unprovoked static condition	49	3.6	31	8.6	5.8-12.3
Unprovoked seizures Progressive condition	27	2	23	11.5	7.2-17.2
Unprovoked seizures Unknown etiology	57	4.2	16	3.8	2.1-6.1
Total	**213**	**15.9**	**111**	**7**	**6.2-8.4**

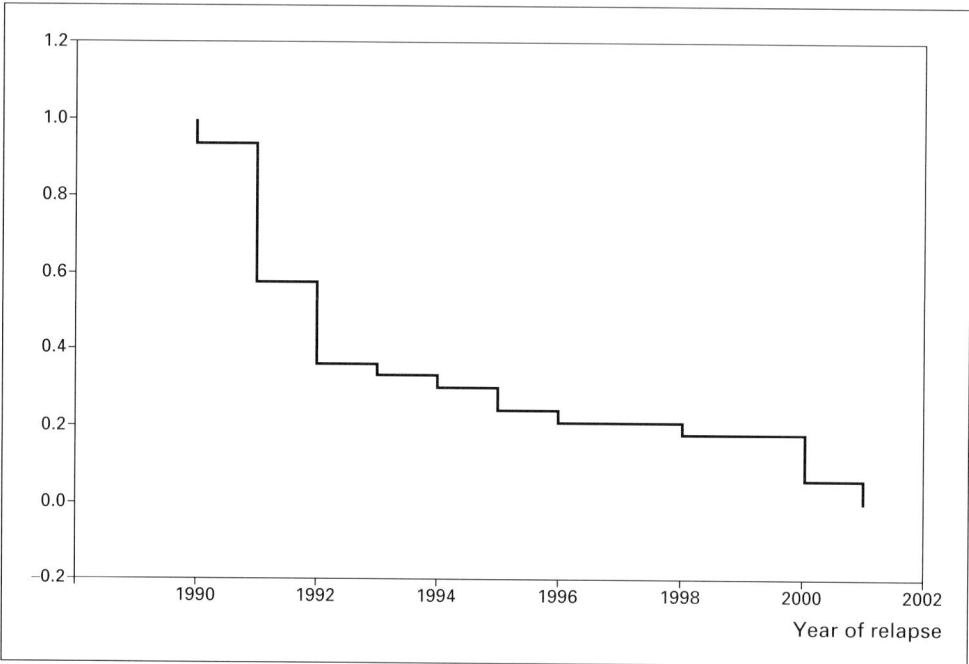

Figure 4. Occurrence of relapse in the patients followed.

of the first group: 15 have become partial epilepsies, three generalized epilepsies. Seven were secondarily classified as undetermined epilepsies. Patients with partial or generalized epilepsies at diagnosis did not change.

Following the etiologic classification, in the 33 patients who had relapsed: 10 patients have had a provoked seizures, and 7 of them have moved on another etiologic classification (4 with stable condition and 3 unknown etiology). Five patients with seizures in relation with a stable condition did not change. Only one of 3 patients with seizure in relation with a progressive condition has moved on the group of epilepsy in relation with a stable condition. In patients with seizure of unknown etiology (15 patients) 12 remained in the same group and three changed (2 as epilepsy in relation with a stable condition and one with epilepsy in relation with a progressive condition).

When we consider the risk factors for recurrence, statistical analysis showed that age at the first seizure (p < 0.01), absence of therapy at the first observation (p < 0.001) and presence of focal EEG abnormalities (p < 0.001) were the most significant factors. We also noted that the presence of a progressive condition in the group of unprovoked seizures favorized recurrence, even though not significantly.

Pharmacoresistance

At the end of the study, 19 patients (18,6%) still have seizures and were under treatment with the following distribution:

	Partial Epilepsies	*Generalized epilepsies*	*Undetermined epilepsies*	*Special syndromes*	*Total*
Unprovoked epilepsies, static condition	4	2	–	1	7
Unprovoked epilepsies, progressive condition	1	–	1	–	2
Unprovoked epilepsies, unknown etiology	4	2	4	–	10
Total	9	4	5	1	19

Discussion

- The incidence rate of first provoked and unprovoked seizures in EPIGEN is lower than that estimated by Hauser and Hersdorffer [6] in the Rochester study (69.8 *vs* 72.9 to 86.9) but similar to that reported by Loiseau *et al.* [3] (69.5) who used the same methodology for case ascertainment. However, this rate is surely underestimated because a number of seizures are not taken in charge by neurologists, or are misdiagnosed or/and not diagnosed [7].
- The very high incidence in the elderly people has been noted in many previous studies in industrialized countries. The decreasing incidence rate reported in children in our study has also been reported in industrialized countries and is probably in relation with health prevention measures.
- We noted a high incidence rate in the 30 years adult population – clearly related to cerebral complications of the HIV infection.
- We know that epilepsy and epileptic syndrome are not always synonymous. An epileptic syndrome is an epileptic disorder characterized by a cluster of symptoms occurring *together*. Epilepsy is defined by the occurrence of at least two unprovoked seizures whereas an epileptic syndrome may be individualized after a single event. For this reason we decided to strictly follow the recommendations of ILAE Commission of epidemiology and prognosis: "diagnosis of epilepsy is essentially based on a bona fide of epileptic seizures... An abnormal EEG (with epileptiform abnormalities) after an isolated seizure could suggest classification of a seizure as epilepsy". Thus, in our group, only 21 patients who presented with a first seizure met the criteria that permitted them to be assigned to an epileptic syndrome. All the other cases (255) were classified as a "special syndrome" *even when the EEG showed focal slow waves and /or when the neuro-imaging was abnormal.*
- The use of ILAE guidelines for epidemiological studies was straightforward. They are particularly useful in studies of initial seizures in which the diagnosis of an epileptic syndrome is disappointing.

- One hundred and eleven patients died. The crude all cause SMR for our study was calculated as 7 (95% CI 6.3-8.4). It was similar in patients with provoked seizures (SMR: 6.8) and unprovoked seizures (SMR: 7) and significantly higher in patients with unprovoked seizures in relation with a progressive condition (SMR: 11.5). The SMR's according to age was markedly higher in the 30-39 years group SMR: 47.9). This high SMR is clearly in relation with a cerebral complication of the HIV infection. According to the gender, SMR was higher in the female population than in the male population. (SMR: 7.7 *vs* 6.6). No etiologic factor can explain this difference.

- During the ten years of follow-up, in the population who survived and have been correctly followed (102 patients) 33 patients have relapsed. Twenty one have a change of epileptic syndrome, the majority moving from "special syndrome" to a specific epileptic syndrome.

- The most important factors inducing a greater risk for recurrence were the age at the first seizure *(figure 5)*, the presence of a progressive condition in the group of unprovoked seizures, and an EEG with focal abnormalities *(figure 6)*. Interestingly, patients with abnormal neuroimaging (with lesion) had less relapse. The majority of these patients have had a CVA, which could explain a selection bias. Another interesting finding was the effect of therapy at the first observation. Patients with a clear epileptic syndrome or patients with a high risk of recurrence have been immediately treated, but this treatment did not seem to influence the long term recurrence risk *(figure 7)*.

- At the end of the study, 19 patients have still seizures and are under treatment, which represent a 18.6% of pharmacoresistance. The majority of these patients have a partial epilepsy, with unprovoked seizures either in relation with a static condition or of unknown etiology. This pharmacoresistency of partial epilepsies is well known.

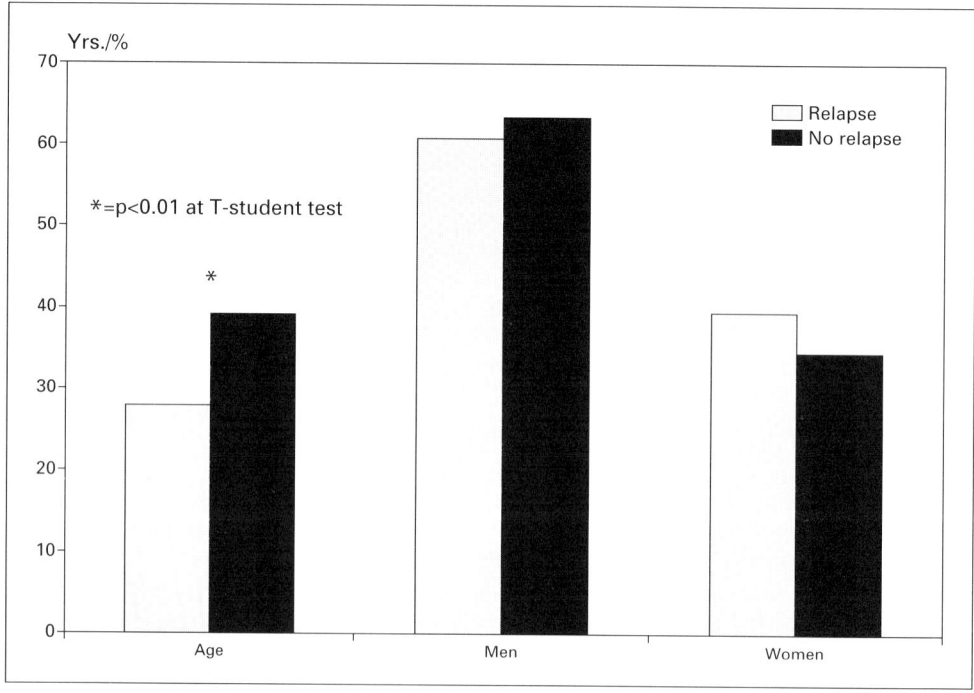

Figure 5. Age and sex differences between patients with and without relapse.

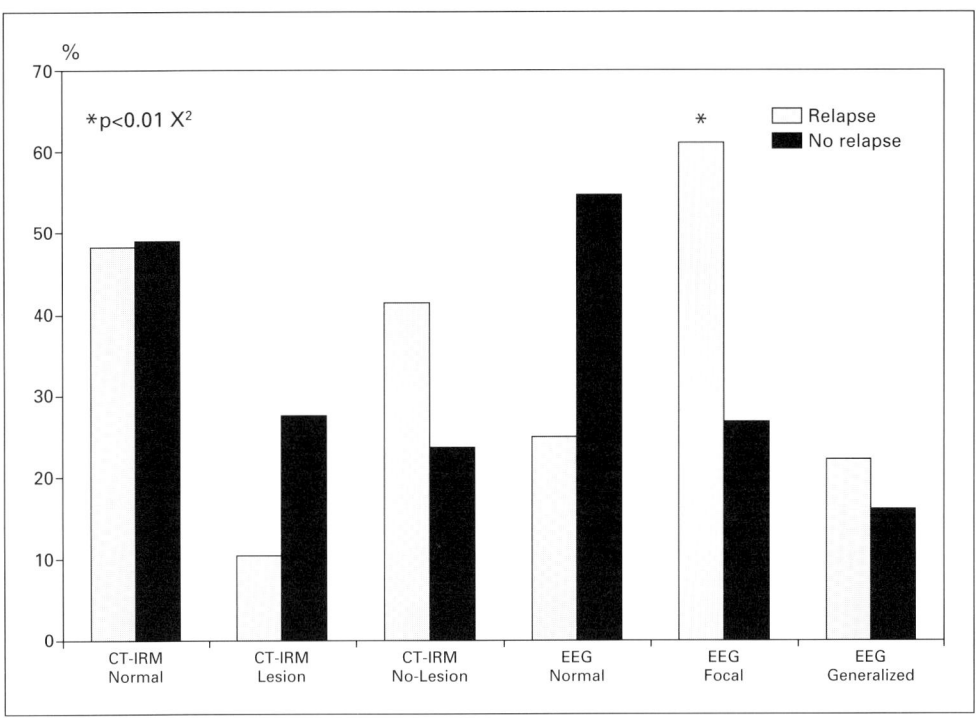

Figure 6. Investigations in patients with and without relapse.
* p < 0.01 X^2

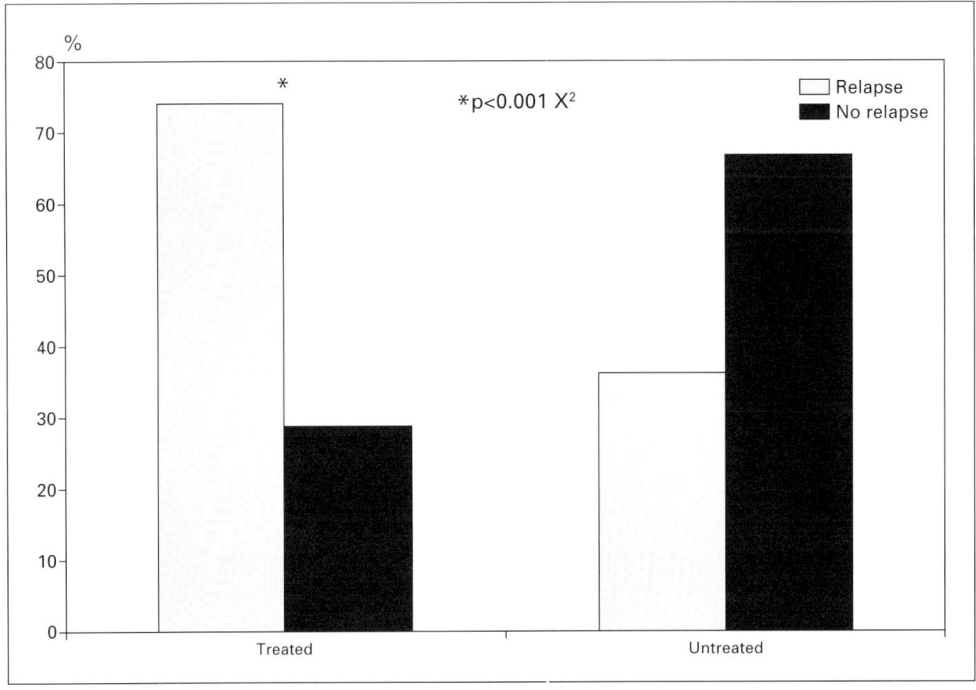

Figure 7. Treatment at the first observation in patients with and without relapse.
* p < 0.001 X^2

References

1. Jallon P. Epidemiology of epilepsies. *Handbook of Clinical Neurology.* H. Meinardi, ed.; 1999, Elsevier Science, Amsterdam. Vol. 72: The Epilepsies, Part I.
2. Jallon P, Goumaz M, Haenggeli T, Morabia A. Incidence rate of first epileptic seizures in Geneva county. *Epilepsia* 1997; 38: 547-52.
3. Loiseau J, Loiseau P, Guyot M, Duché B, Dartigues JF, Aublet B. Survey of Epileptic Disorders in Southwest France: Incidence of epileptic syndromes. *Epilepsia* 1990; 31: 391-6.
4. Commission on Classification and Terminology of the International League Against Epilepsy. Proposal for Revised Classification of Epilepsies and Epileptic Syndromes. *Epilepsia* 1989; 30: 389-99.
5. Commission on Epidemiology and Prognosis of the International League against Epilepsy. Guidelines for epidemiologic studies on epilepsy. *Epilepsia* 1993; 34: 592-6.
6. Hauser WA, Hesdorffer DH. *Epilepsy: frequency, causes and consequences.* Demos Press, New York; 1990.
7. Jallon P, Loiseau P, Loiseau J. On behalf of groupe CAROLE (coordination Active du Reseau Observatoire de l'Epilepsie. Newly diagnosed unprovoked epileptic seizures: presentation at diagnosis in CAROLE study. *Epilepsia* 2001; 42: 464-75.

Prognosis of epilepsy: The Rochester Studies

Allen Hauser

Background

The ambitious Rochester Project [1] established a record linkage system for all diagnoses for residents of Rochester Minnesota. The core was the unit record system developed by Plummer for the Mayo Clinic at the turn of the century. This linked all medical data from inpatient, outpatient, emergency room contacts and home visits by physicians and other health professionals at the Mayo Clinic into a single record. Plummer also developed a phonetic diagnostic indexing system that effectively allowed record retrieval by diagnosis. Joseph Berkson streamlined this system by bringing in Mc Bee cards to facilitate retrieval by diagnostic categories. Dr Kurland expanded this diagnostic system to include most other medical practitioners in the area (some resisted), as well as other medical facilities in the region where residents of the community were likely to seek health care. Through the use of the indexing system of the Rochester Project, if was possible to identify all local residents with a specific diagnosis such as epilepsy. To assure full identification of all cases with a particular diagnosis, a broad list of diagnostic categories were screened and all charts reviewed. For epilepsy, this included categories such as loss of consciousness, syncope, and faints. There were 516 diagnostic incidence cases of epilepsy identified over the 33-year period of the study but over 3000 records with a possible diagnosis of interest were screened to identify these cases and many additional special diagnostic categories were also reviewed [1].

Definitions

A critical part of the study was to establish definitions. Epilepsy was defined as recurrent (two or more) unprovoked seizures. Single seizures and what are now termed acute symptomatic seizures were not considered epilepsy although these cases were abstracted and enumerated. Strict definitions were developed for an etiologic classification in what may have been self-fulfilling, these definitions have been born out in cohort studies to be valid in terms of risk. Cases not meeting these definitions were classified as "without identified cause", a category including present day "Idiopathic" and "Cryptogenic" cases. Seizures were classified by seizure type based upon the ILAE recommendations from 1970 based upon the detailed description of seizure semiology in the medical records. Even though final recorded diagnostic terminology had changed over the period of the study, it was possible to reclassify cases to meet at that time contemporary criteria. I also included categories for what are now considered syndromes including JME, West Syndrome, Benign Rolandic Epilepsy, and Lennox Gastaut syndrome. There were several categories of prevalence presented to allow comparison with other contemporary studies, and remission was evaluated using several definitions. Cases were considered to be in remission if individuals were seizure free for 5 years although for reasons of power, subgroup analysis was done using a 2-year definition of seizure freedom.

Study methodology

All cases records were personally reviewed and clinical and laboratory data were abstracted. Although detailed EEG information was abstracted, EEG findings were not used to modify the classifications based upon clinical description. This was done to allow comparisons with other field studies where EEG was not available.

Letters were sent out to all cases identified, followed by a personal telephone interview which I conducted. Over 90% of living incidence and prevalence cases were personally interviewed, and I spoke with the families of many of those deceased at the time of follow-up.

Incidence and prevalence

Incidence was determined for the entire study period and for 4 time intervals. Prevalence was determined for several definitions for 4 prevalence days. Both incidence and prevalence were higher than that reported for contemporary studies in developed countries despite what appeared to be more restrictive criteria for inclusion, but case ascertainment methods were more complete probably explaining the differences. The now typical "U" shaped pattern of age specific incidence was identified *(figure 1)*. While these were the data most were interested in, the establishment of an incidence cohort to allow prognostic studies was in my opining the most valuable part of the case identification effort.

There was a suggestion of time trend findings to be confirmed in subsequent studies. Despite probable under ascertainment of cases in the first decade, incidence seemed to fall in children. At the same time incidence increased over time in the elderly. These time trends were later confirmed in the expanded cohort [2].

Studies of remission

Initial studies: 1968

The most striking findings in terms of prognosis related to the high proportion of cases going into remission. A number of definitions were used to try to understand the frequency

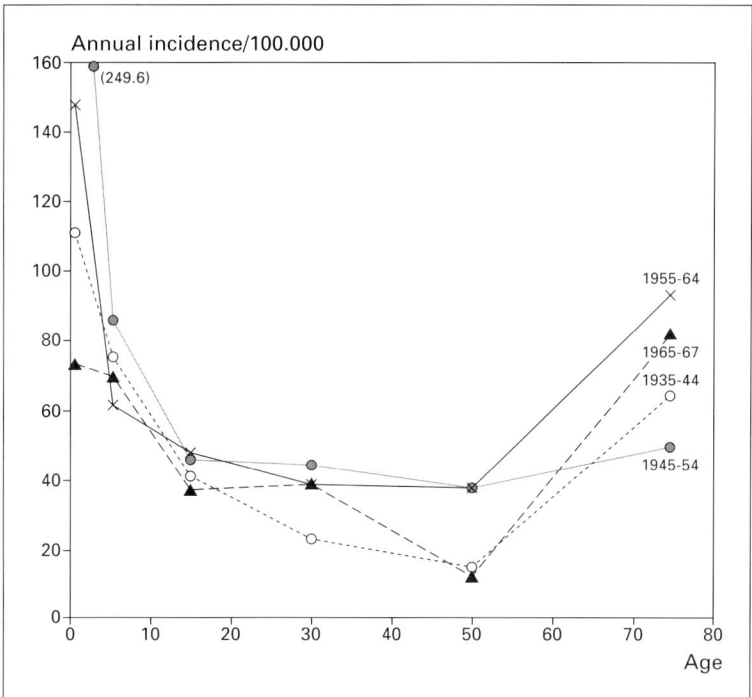

Figure 1. Incidence of epilepsy in Rochester Minnesota 1935-1967.

of people going into remission and many subgroup analyzes were presented [2]. These definitions were purposely conservative because of the dramatic discrepancy between these findings and the data from contemporary clinic based studies such as the comprehensive review and report of Rodin [3]. Data was based upon personal interview with patients or patient's family. Using actuarial methods, we found that by 5 years after diagnosis, 29% of all cases were seizure free *(figure 2)*. That proportion increased to 40% at 10 years after diagnosis and 55% by 20 year after diagnosis. Remission was highest in children, in those with absence seizures, and was better in those with presumed complex partial seizures (presumed temporal lobe seizures) than in those with simple partial seizures or motor seizure felt to originate in other areas. Even those with myoclonic seizures a subgroup generally assumed to have an exceedingly poor prognosis had a substantial proportion of cases going into remission. Interestingly, remission was similar in those with unknown cause and those with a presumed etiology.

Subsequent studies of remission

Several additional papers have been papers for the data set on this topic although several differences exist between the methods used for the initial publication and later publications. The data set was expanded to include a longer duration of incidence case identification. Analytic methods have been better developed, and multivariable techniques have been used. The later studies also differ methodologically from the initial report in that follow-up was truncated upon migration from the geographic area likely to be covered by the record linkage system. This eliminated the need to do follow-up by phone, an expensive process, but does raise questions regarding potential biases. Remission was even higher when analysis was restricted to those who remained local residents.

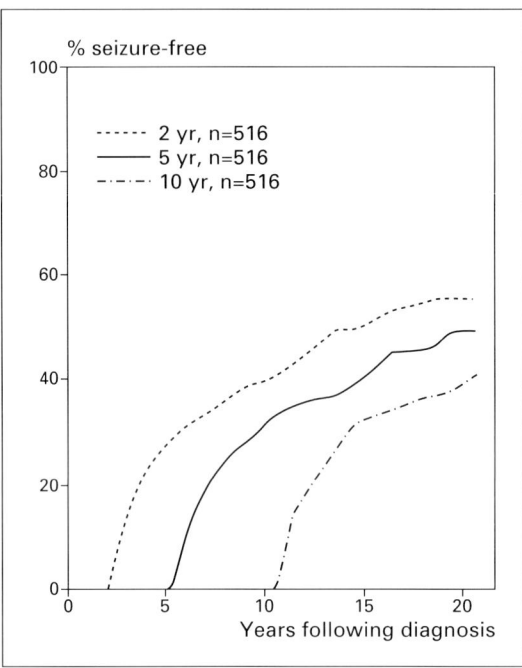

Figure 2. Remission of epilepsy by various definitions, Rochester Minnesota.

In our next publication we limited the analyses to a 5-year seizure free definition of remission [4]. We found that the overall prognosis was even better than reported earlier. We concentrated on the group of cases with unknown cause and again found that children were more likely to go into remission than adults, that those with generalized seizures were more likely to go into remission than those with partial seizures, and that the majority of those going into remission were able to successfully discontinue medication. We evaluated the risk of relapse after 5-year remission. Relapse was about 1% per year for the first 10 years after fulfilling remission criteria and fell to 5% per year after that time.

In a follow-up analysis of this came cohort, Steven Schaeffer did an elegant multivariate analysis [5]. Controlling for other factors, young after of onset (under age 15) was an independent predictor of remission. Having any generalized seizure and having a generalized spike and wave EEG pattern were both predictions of continuing seizures.

Studies of mortality

Initial studies

Relative survivorship was determined for the entire group, and separately for the cohort identified between 1935 and 44, and for the cohort identified after 1945. Age/gender, time period specific comparisons were made although the breakdown was not as sophisticated as in later analyses. For the entire cohort we found a relative survivorship of 90% at 5 years following diagnosis and 80% subsequently *(figure 3)*. The more detailed analysis dealt with the 430 cases diagnosed after 1945. The median follow-up was only 10 years. Most of the excess mortality occurred in the first 5 years after diagnosis. Mortality was

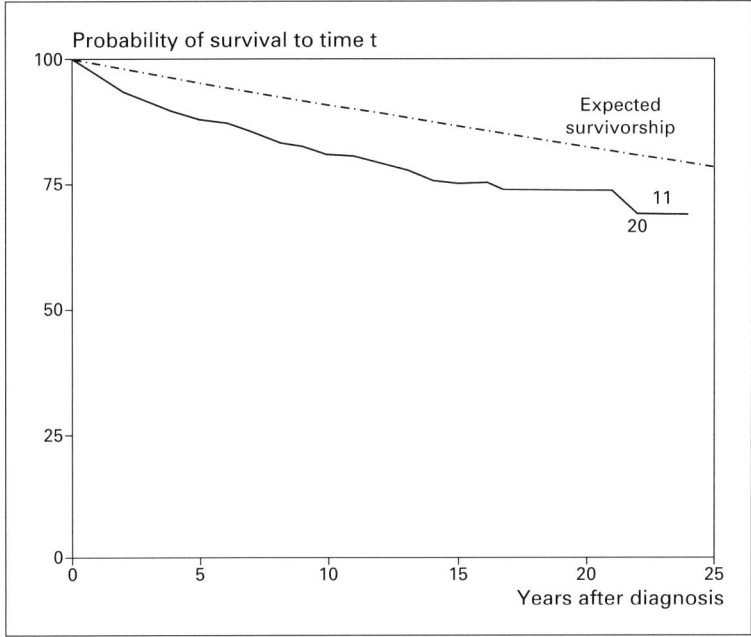

Figure 3. Relative survival of people with epilepsy of unknown cause. Rochester Minnesota, 1935-67.

greater for men than women and not unexpectedly was greater for those with epilepsy associated with a presumed etiology. Survivorship was pour for those under age 1 at diagnosis and effectively the same as expected for those age 1 through 19. Relative survivorship was unchanged for those with absence seizures and for those with complex partial seizures. Data was also presented for EEG categories and differences were as expected given presumed correlations with pathology.

I did provide standardized mortality ratios (SMR) in the paper although at that time I did not feel this was the optimal method of comparison. For all cases of epilepsy, the SMR was 2.9 in the first 5 years, 2.2 in the second five years after diagnosis and 1.9 between 10 and 15 years after diagnosis.

Follow-up studies on mortality

After expanding the incidence data set through 1975, we again evaluated mortality using standardized mortality ratios for all comparisons [6]. The SMR was elevated for all comparisons may within etiologic subgroups although this increase was only for the first 5 years for those with epilepsy of unknown cause, and was greatest for those with epilepsy with a presumed cause. Among those with epilepsy of unknown cause, mortality was not increased for women, an observation later confirmed in mortality studies in Iceland [7, 8]. A late increase in mortality (after 20 year following diagnosis) was observed raising the question of a late effect from epilepsy or possibly from antiseizure medication. We also evaluated cause specific mortality. An increase in mortality associated with accidents, vascular disease, and with pulmonary causes of death was noted. There was also an increase in mortality attributable to malignancies although this that persisted after death associated with CNS neoplasms was excluded from the analysis. There was no evidence for an excess of suicide.

When those with idiopathic epilepsy were examined alone, there was still a significant excess of deaths attributed to neoplasm, vascular disease and accidents.

The capriciousness of diagnoses included on death certificates caused concern about the reliability of these findings on cause specific mortality. Because of this several studies were undertaken to evaluate specific disease co-morbidity. These studies differed significantly from the SMR mortality studies in that the incidence of specific disease in the epilepsy cohort was compared to the incidence of these same conditions in the populations of Rochester. Specific estimates could be made because studies of the incidence in the general population of Rochester for a contemporary time period had been performed. We were about to review the cohort using the same definition to determine specific levels of risk. Our earliest attempt to address co-morbidity was related to cardiovascular risks in people with epilepsy. There was a suggestion that antiseizure medications could be protective from coronary deaths because of their anti-arrhythmic properties. We evaluated myocardial infarctions and cardiac deaths in the epilepsy cohort and found a 50% excess of myocardial infarctions but no excess risk of death from coronary artery disease [9]. In a later analysis, we further evaluated mortality, finding a dramatic excess among children with neurodeficit. This finding has subsequently been confirmed in other studies [10]. We found an excess risk for heart disease deaths primarily in the adult population. We found a 50% increase in risk for ischemic heart disease (IHD) in cases with no known cause of epilepsy and a 2-fold increase in the symptomatic cases. This increase seemed primarily related to IHD in those with epilepsy attributed to cerebrovascular disease. We found a 2-fold increase in Sudden Death. This was again limited to the symptomatic cases and seemed to occur in the elder with epilepsy due to stroke. We did not find an increase in risk for sudden death in those with idiopathic epilepsy. We found no relation between long-term medication use and sudden death or other cardiac symptoms. In a later analysis limited to those at highest risk for SUDEP (age 20-40) a 10-fold increase in risk was reported.

We also evaluated with risk for cancer in the cohort, making comparisons with rates of cancer in the general population of Rochester. The risk for brain tumors was increased 22 fold in those with epilepsy of unknown cause, but there was no increase in risk for other cancers. These findings are contrary to most studies including our own that made comparisons through mortality statistics [11]. We assumed that the increase risk for brain tumors was related to the underlying cause of the epilepsy rather than the induction in some way by seizures or by long-term antiseizure drug risk.

Other outcomes

A number of studies were done addressing pregnancy complications and outcomes. We found that women with epilepsy had a reduced number of children, but only in periods of high birth rates in the general population and primarily for person-years of follow-up prior to diagnosis [12]. Fertility was reduced for men for all time periods, and for intervals after diagnosis. We suggested the effects in males might be due to antiseizure medication. In these studies we had inexact comparisons of births in the general populations. A better-designed study of this question was performed in Iceland. In this study we failed to find any reduction in number of offspring born to men or to women with epilepsy when compared with the general population [13]. This was true in both high and low fertility periods in the general population.

We also perform several other studies of related to reproduction. We did not find an excess of pregnancy wastage [14]. We confirmed an increase risk for oral contraceptive failure in women taking antiseizure medication. We also confirmed an increased risk for congenital malformations among women taking antiseizure medication [15, 16].

We found that the offspring of women with epilepsy were more likely to have a child with epilepsy than the offspring of men with epilepsy. This observation remains unexplained despite some 20 years of study of this topic by Dr Ruth Ottman. The studies to explain this phenomenon have led to the identification of the gene for partial epilepsy with auditory features [17].

There are theoretical reasons for people with epilepsy to be at increased risk for fractures. We evaluated this risk in the incidence cohort. There was an increase in risk for spinal compression fractures among people with epilepsy but no evidence for an increase in risk for fractures at other sites when compared with the risk in the general population of Rochester [18].

Studies of special groups

Febrile seizures

Extensive information on the frequency, characteristics and prognosis of febrile seizures was presented in the paper published in 1975 [2]. This data received little attention and I suspect few read to the end of the paper. One third of the cases had recurrent febrile seizures of those with recurrence, more than half had a third episode. Only 2.3% of the cohort subsequently developed epilepsy. Subsequent studies further defined features associated with increased risk for epilepsy [19].

Acute symptomatic seizures

The risk for unprovoked seizures following acute symptomatic seizures has been evaluated. There was an increased risk for unprovoked seizures and epilepsy in those with acute symptomatic seizures associated with acute CNS pathology such as head injury or stroke; there is no increase in risk associated with acute symptomatic seizures associated with acute metabolic conditions such as hyponatremia or eclampsia [20].

Status epilepticus

In recent years we have determined the frequency status epilepticus (seizures of greater than 30 minutes duration) and prognosis of those suffering from this condition [21-24]. The prognosis was good for those with unprovoked seizures with status.

Single unprovoked seizures

We attempted to evaluate seizure recurrence in people reported to be seen at their first seizure [25]. While findings are similar to other studies of this topic done prospectively, it is my feeling that recurrence risk was overestimated doe to likely misclassification of cases because of incomplete histories. This was the case in studies in the Bronx and in Minneapolis [26, 27].

Summary

The studies of the convulsive disorders in Rochester Minnesota have provided insights into the frequency and prognosis of epilepsy. Even though the population is small, the detailed medical records available have provided reliable information while controversial at times has largely proved correct in subsequent prospective studies. The availability of incidence studies of other conditions in the community facilitated our ability to evaluate a number of potential co-morbid conditions. These and other epidemiologic studies have changed the opinions of prognosis of the epilepsies and have contributed to the modification of the clinical approach to people with epilepsy. The studies highlight the need for well-characterized cohorts in whom long-term follow-up can be established.

References

1. Hauser WA, Kurland LT. The epidemiology of epilepsy in Rochester, Minnesota, 1935-1967. *Epilepsia* 1975; 16: 1-66.
2. Annegers JF, Hauser WA, Lee JR, Rocca WA. Secular trends and birth cohort effects in unprovoked seizures: Rochester, Minnesota 1935-1984. *Epilepsia* 1995; 36: 575-9.
3. Rodin EA. Prognosis of patients with epilepsy. Charles C. Thomas, Springfield, Ill, 1968.
4. Annegers JF, Hauser WA, Elveback LR. Remission of seizures and relapse in patients with epilepsy. *Epilepsia* 1979; 20: 729-37.
5. Shafer S, Hauser WA, Annegers JF, Klass DW. EEG and other early predictors of later epilepsy remission: a community study. *Epilepsia* 1988; 29: 590-600.
6. Hauser WA, Annegers JF, Elveback LR. Mortality in patients with epilepsy. *Epilepsia* 1980; 21: 399-412.
7. Olafsson E, Hauser WA, Gudmundsson G. Long-term survival of people with unprovoked seizures. *Epilepsia* 1998; 39: 89-92.
8. Rafnsson V, Olafsson E, Hauser WA, Gudmundsson G. Cause-Specific Mortality in Adults with Unprovoked seizures. *Neuroepidemiology* 2001; 20: 232-6.
9. Annegers JF, Elveback LR, Labarthe DR, Hauser WA. Ischemic heart disease in patients with epilepsy. *Epilepsia* 1976; 17: 11-4.
10. Annegers JF, Hauser WA, Shirts S. Heart disease mortality and morbidity in patients with epilepsy. *Epilepsia* 1984; 25: 699-704.
11. Shirts SB, Annegers, JF, Hauser WA, Kurland LT. Cancer incidence in a cohort of patients with seizure disorders. *J Natl Canc Inst* 1986; 77: 83-7.
12. Webber MP, Hauser WA, Ottman R, Annegers JF. Fertility in persons with epilepsy: 1935-1974. *Epilepsia* 1986; 27: 746-52.
13. Olafsson E, Hallgrimsson JT, Hauser WA, Ludvigsson P, Gudmundsson G. Pregnancies of women with epilepsy: a population based study in Iceland. *Epilepsia* 1998; 39: 887-92.
14. Annegers JF, Baumgartner KB, Hauser WA, Kurland LT. Epilepsy, antiepileptic drugs, and the risk of spontaneous abortion. *Epilepsia* 1988; 29: 451-8.
15. Annegers JF, Hauser WA, Elveback LR, Kurland LT. Do anticonvulsants have a teratogenic effect? *Arch Neurol* 1974; 31: 364-73.
16. Annegers JF, Hauser WA, Elveback LR, Anderson VE, Kurland LT. Congenital malformations and seizure disorders in the offspring of parents with epilepsy. *Int J Epidemiol* 1978; 7: 241-7.
17. Kalachikov S, Evgrafov O, Ross B, Winawer M, Barker-Cummings C, Boneschi FM, Choi C, Morozov P, Das K, Teplitskaya E, Yu A, Cayanis E, Penchaszadeh G, Kottmann AH, Pedley TA, Hauser WA, Ottman R, Gilliam TC. Mutations in LGI1 cause autosomal-dominant partial epilepsy with auditory features. *Nat Genet* 2002; 30: 335-41.
18. Annegers JF, Melton, LJ, Sun CA, Hauser WA. Risk of age-related fractures in patients with unprovoked seizures. *Epilepsia* 1989; 30: 348-55.
19. Annegers JF, Hauser WA, Shirts SB, Kurland LT. Factors prognostic of unprovoked seizures after febrile convulsions. *N Engl J Med* 1987; 316: 493-8.

20. HesdorfferDC. Logroscino G. Cascino G. Annegers JF. Hauser WA. Risk of unprovoked seizure after acute symptomatic seizure: effect of status epilepticus. *Annals of Neurology* 1998; 44: 908-12.
21. Hesdorffer DC, Logroscino G, Cascino G, Annegers JF, Hauser WA. Incidence of status epilepticus in Rochester, Minnesota, 1965-84. *Neurology* 1998; 50: 735-41.
22. Cascino GD, Hesdorffer D, Logroscino G, Hauser WA. Morbidity of nonfebrile status epilepticus in Rochester, Minnesota, 1965-1984. *Epilepsia* 1998; 39: 829-32.
23. Logroscino G, Hesdorffer D, Cascino G, Hauser WA. Long-term mortality after a first episode of status epilepticus. *Neurology* 2002; 58: 537-41.
24. Logroscino G, Hesdorffer D, Cascino G, Annegers JF, Hauser WA. Short-term mortality after a first episode of status epilepticus: a retrospective cohort study in Rochester, Minnesota. *Epilepsia* 1997; 38: 1344-9.
25. Annegers JF, Shirts SB, Hauser WA, Kurland LT: Risk of recurrence after an initial unprovoked seizure. *Epilepsia* 1986; 27: 43-50.
26. Hauser WA, Anderson VE, Loewenson RB, McRoberts SM. Seizure recurrence following a first unprovoked seizures. *New Engl J Med* 1982; 307: 522-8.
27. Shinnar S, Berg AT, Moshe SL, Petix M, Maytal J, Kang H, Goldensohn ES, Hauser WA. The risk of seizure recurrence following a first unprovoked seizure in childhood: A prospective study. *Pediatrics* 1990; 85: 1076-85.

The prognosis of epilepsy in the national general practice study of epilepsy

Samden D. Lhatoo, Josemir W. Sander

Introduction

Of the various studies of the prognosis of the epilepsies, the National General Practice Study of Epilepsy (NGPSE) stands out as a unique resource in the understanding of this important aspect of seizure disorders [1-13]. Its main strength lies in its prospective design and large population base [4]. In addition, the long term follow up and the fact that it is now in its 18th year of data collection provide as comprehensive a picture of prognosis as has ever been possible in the UK. This chapter will concentrate on the remission and recurrence of seizure disorders as mortality, another essential facet in the description of prognosis, will be dealt with elsewhere.

Study design and methods

Methodological problems have beset many of the early studies of prognosis [14-16] and the NGPSE design has avoided many of the pitfalls that confound prognosis studies and their subsequent implications in clinical application. The elimination of the important bias of the over-representation of hospital based patients, and the incorporation of the temporal aspects of prognosis in patients with newly diagnosed epilepsy are of particular note. The unique system of general practice in the UK allowed a high degree of case ascertainment; the patient's general practitioner (GP) is usually the first medical professional to assess the patient, and where this is not the case, the GP is always informed of hospital presentations by the hospital specialist.

A sample size of 1 200 patients was chosen on pragmatic and scientific grounds as this was considered the maximum number of patients that could be recruited over four years from the 275 participating practices. Allowing for patients with febrile convulsions, this would also yield approximately 800 cases of newly diagnosed epilepsy. This number would be sufficient for the application of multivariate clustering techniques to develop and partially validate a classification scheme for seizures in general practice and would further allow estimation of yearly recurrence rates [4]. Cases were defined by the occurrence of one or more seizures, regardless of cause (including childhood febrile convulsions, single seizures and seizures associated with acute illnesses), and classified as definite epilepsy, probable epilepsy, febrile convulsions and not epilepsy. Patients with a suspected previous diagnosis of epilepsy and patients with neonatal seizures were excluded. Eventually, 564 patients with definite epilepsy, 228 patients with probable epilepsy and 220 patients with febrile seizures were enrolled in the study in the four years between 1984 and 1987. Patients were recruited from both rural and urban practices to reflect a balanced mix of cases. Classification was based on data obtained from the GP and from hospital specialists, and submitted to a diagnostic review panel six months after the index seizure, i.e. the seizure that resulted in registration with the study. In some cases, the index seizure did not necessarily equate with the first ever seizure, as these were patients who despite not having been diagnosed before, had prior seizures. Probable cases were defined as cases whose clinical presentation suggested a diagnosis of epilepsy but where the review panel felt that a certain diagnosis was not possible.

All patients were followed up prospectively from the time of diagnosis of the index seizure by a system of active follow up through specially designed annual forms completed by GPs who provided information on seizure status, medication, investigations and possible change of diagnosis, supplemented after five years by hospital enquiry. The Office for National Statistics flagged all patients and informed the study of any change of GP or deaths of patients.

Seizure classification was based on the International Classification of seizures [17] with adaptation for the fact that not all cases had an EEG. A further aetiological classification similar to that used in other large community based studies, to allow comparison [18], was stratified into the following groups:
1. Cryptogenic – no identified underlying cause or idiopathic;
2. Remote symptomatic – postnatal CNS lesions;
3. Acute symptomatic – seizures starting within 3 months of a CNS insult;
4. Seizures associated with congenital or perinatal neurological abnormality.

Those cases classified as symptomatic were further divided into aetiological groups:
1. Vascular – where there was clear evidence of vascular or embolic disease;
2. Tumour – either radiological evidence or an otherwise clear clinical picture of an expanding lesion;
3. Trauma – definite history of head injury with loss of consciousness of more than 1 hour;
4. Alcohol – where seizures occurred due to excessive intake, during withdrawal or due to excessive intake;
5. Post-infective – during or in the aftermath of a confirmed episode of encephalitis, bacterial meningitis or cerebral abscess. *Table I* represents the seizure type and aetiology of patients with definite epilepsy.

Recurrence after a first seizure

After two to four years of follow up, seizure recurrence after a first seizure was estimated at 6, 12, 24 and 36 months after the first ever seizure [5]. Patients with definite epilepsy were divided into four groups where group "A" represented analysis of all patients from

Table I. Seizure type and aetiology in patients with definite epilepsy

Parameter	No.	%	CI
Seizure type			
Generalised			
Tonic-Clonic	198	35	
Absence	6	1	
Mixed	14	2	
Others	3	< 1	
Total	221	39	
Partial			
Simple	15	3	
Complex	61	11	
Secondary generalised	151	27	
Mixed	65	12	
Total	292	52	
Unclassifiable	51	9	
Total	564	100	
Broad aetiology			
Idiopathic/cryptogenic	346	61	57, 65
Remote symptomatic	119	21	18, 25
Acute symptomatic	83	15	12, 18
Congenital neurological deficit	16	3	2, 4
Specific aetiology			
Idiopathic/cryptogenic	335[a]	59	55, 63
Vascular	90	16	13, 19
Tumour	38	7	5, 9
Alcohol	35	6	4, 8
Trauma	15	3	1, 4
Infection	9	2	1, 3
Other[b]	42	7	15, 60

CI = confidence interval.
[a] = Different from the "idiopathic" group in broad aetiology group, includes patients with congenital neurological deficits.
[b] = Includes metabolic, eclampsia, drugs.
Adapted from Cockerell et al. 1997 [3].

the first ever seizure, group "B" represented analysis from the index seizure, group "C" represented patients in whom the index seizure was also the first seizure and group "D" where the first seizure was within six months of the index seizure. The reason for stratification of this nature lay in the biases noted in previous studies of first seizures where estimates of recurrence have varied widely. The time from first seizure to study recruitment is crucial as longer time periods result in exclusion of patients who develop seizure recurrence before recruitment, thus artificially lowering recurrence rates in those that do not. In group "A", a second seizure occurred in 78% of patients within three years of the first seizure with very similar recurrence rates in group "D". In groups "B" and "C", recurrence rates were 56% and 46% respectively. The lower recurrence rates in group "C", where the index seizure was also the first seizure, emphasized the importance of identifying patients at the time of the first seizure.

The risk of seizure recurrence at three years in patients with definite epilepsy who had not had seizure recurrence by 6, 12 or 18 months was also calculated. This was 44% after a seizure free period of six months, 32% after a seizure free period of 12 months and 17% after a seizure free period of 18 months. It was estimated that the risk of recurrence after a first seizure (hazard rate) was 0.033 (95% confidence interval 0.030, 0.036) per week in the first 6 months after the first seizure, 0.007 (CI 0.005, 0.010) per week in 6-12 months and 0.004 (CI 0.003, 0.005) per week in the next 24 months. This pattern of maximum risk in the first few months was constant in all sub-analyses.

Table II shows recurrence rates for group "A" by aetiology, type of first seizure and age at first seizure. Recurrence rates were lowest in the aetiological group with alcohol related seizures. The recurrence rate was low in the acute symptomatic group but highest in the patients with congenital neurological deficits, as all had suffered recurrences by 12 months.

Only 15% of patients were treated with AEDs after the first seizure although eventually this number rose to more than 70%. The recurrence rate was lower in the treated group (38% [CI 27, 48] by 6 months; 50% [CI 40, 61] by 12 months; and 57% [46-68] by 36 months) than in the untreated group (64% [60-69] by 6 months; 70% [CI 66, 74] by 12 months and 81% [CI 77, 85] by 36 months).

Remission from seizures

Remission in the NGPSE was analysed after 9 years when median follow up was 7.1 years (25th, 75th centile; 5.7, 8.1) for the complete sample [3]. Only 33 patients were totally lost to follow up, emphasizing the completeness of follow up.

From the index seizure, 96% (95% CI 94,98) of the whole cohort (definite epilepsy and probable epilepsy) achieved a 1-years remission, 93% (CI 90,96) achieved a 2-year remission, 87% (CI 83,91) achieved a 3-year remission and 71% (CI 65,77) achieved a 5-year remission. From the first seizure, remission rates were slightly lower at 95% (CI 93,97) for 1-year, 90% (CI 87,93) for 2-year, 84% (CI 80,87) for 3-year and 67% (CI 62,72) for 5-year remission. When terminal remission (continuing remission at the time of analysis) from index seizure was analysed in patients with definite epilepsy alone, 84% (CI 78, 91) were in 1-year remission, 76% (CI 69,82) in 2-year remission, 68% (CI 62,74) in 3-year remission and 54% (CI 48,60) were in 5-year remission. The figures for the combined population of definite and probable epilepsy were slightly higher.

This suggested that the overall prognosis for epilepsy is good with the vast majority of patients enjoying long period of seizure freedom and well over half achieving continuing remission.

To allow for comparison with previous studies that had excluded single seizures or provoked seizures, analysis of the cohort without single seizures and acute symptomatic seizures was carried out. This showed that by 9 years, 82% (CI 76,87) had achieved 3-year remission and 60% (CI 52,68) had achieved a 5-year remission, suggesting that the effect of excluding these patients was only marginal and moreover justified the premise that there is little difference in pathophysiology between single and recurrent seizures.

During the follow up period, 161 patients (75 males, 86 females) died compared to 69 deaths from all causes that would have been expected in the standard population for England and Wales (SMR = 2.3 [CI 1.9, 2.7; p < 0.001]). In patients with definite epilepsy, the SMR was 3.0 (CI 2.5, 3.7). These figures were similar to a previous large study of mortality.

The effect of aetiology on remission

Patients with acute symptomatic epilepsy had the highest remission rates at 9 years, followed by idiopathic seizures and remote symptomatic seizures respectively *(table III)* [3]. The numbers of patients with congenital neurological deficits were too small for analysis. The current classification of epilepsy is considerably more discerning than the one used in

Table II. Actuarial percentage recurrences by aetiology, seizure type and age

	No of patients at risk after:				Actuarial % recurrence (95% CI) by:			
	0wk	26wk	52wk	104wk	26wk	52wk	104wk	156wk
Aetiology								
Acute symptomatic	83	50	41	31	33 (22, 43)	40 (29, 51)	41 (30, 52)	46 (34, 57)
Remote symptomatic	119	30	24	11	70 (62, 79)	75 (67, 83)	85 (77, 92)	85 (77, 92)
Idiopathic	345	129	99	63	62 (56, 67)	69 (64, 74)	78 (74, 83)	81 (77, 86)
Congenital neuro. deficit	16	2			88 (71, 100)	100		
Vascular	87	27	18	11	66 (56, 77)	73 (64, 83)	80 (71, 89)	82 (73, 92)
Tumour	34	3	2	2	83 (67, 99)	83 (67, 99)	83 (67, 99)	100
Alcohol	35	19	17	11	41 (25, 58)	48 (31, 65)	55 (37, 72)	55 (37, 72)
Cryptogenic	351	131	102	64	62 (57, 67)	69 (64, 74)	78 (73, 82)	81 (77, 85)
Seizure type (first)								
Tonic clonic	384	167	136	88	53 (48, 59)	60 (55, 65)	69 (64, 74)	72 (67, 77)
Partial	111	19	11	5	82 (75, 89)	89 (83, 95)	94 (90, 99)	94 (90, 99)
Age at first seizure (year)								
0–15	164	60	48	30	63 (56, 71)	70 (63, 77)	79 (73, 85)	83 (77, 89)
16–39	180	71	58	39	58 (51, 65)	63 (56, 70)	69 (62, 76)	73 (66, 80)
40–59	93	44	37	23	49 (39, 59)	55 (45, 65)	68 (58, 78)	69 (59, 79)
≥ 60	127	36	21	13	67 (59, 76)	79 (71, 87)	83 (76, 90)	83 (76, 90)

From Hart et al. 1990 [5].

Table III. 3-year and 5-year remission at 3, 5, 7 and 9 years after follow-up according to aetiology

Aetiology	Years from follow up			
	3	5	7	9
3 year remission (%)				
Idiopathic	41 (36, 47)	68 (63, 74)	78 (73, 83)	86 (81, 92)
Remote symptomatic	38 (26, 49)	59 (47, 71)	69 (57, 80)	75 (62, 87)
Acute symptomatic	70 (59, 82)	83 (73, 92)	91 (83, 98)	93 (85, 100)
5 year remission				
Idiopathic		37 (31, 42)	58 (52, 64)	69 (60, 77)
Remote symptomatic		34 (21, 46)	54 (40, 67)	61 (46, 75)
Acute symptomatic		68 (56, 80)	78 (67, 89)	78 (67, 89)

Adapted from Cockerell *et al.* (1997) [3].

this and previous studies of prognosis and the results therefore have to be interpreted in the light of this. For example, patients with idiopathic epilepsy include those with idiopathic or primary generalised epilepsy as well as those with cryptogenic epilepsy where investigations were negative in discerning a structural cause for the epilepsy. The similarity in remission rates in the idiopathic and remote symptomatic groups probably suggests the heterogeneity of conditions causing epilepsy in these two groups rather than homogeneity in prognosis. The better prognosis for recurrence in the acute symptomatic group reflects the provoking factors that would be expected in this group.

The effect of age on remission

Patients were stratified by age at index seizure into age < 16 years, 16-39 years, 40-60 years and > 60 years [3]. The age distribution of patients with definite epilepsy is shown in *table IV*. The 3-year cumulative remission rates at 9 years for each of these groups were 96% (CI 89,-) 82% (CI 76,88), 90% (CI 82,88) and 85% (CI 73,96) respectively. 5-year remission rates were lower at 57%, (CI 48,66), 73% (CI 62,84), 84% (CI 68, 99) and 61% (CI 45, 76) respectively. When 3 year terminal remission rates were considered at 9 years for the same groups, these were 66% (CI 56, 76), 67% (CI 57, 76), 75% (CI 62, 89) and 68% (52, 83) respectively. 5-year terminal remission rates were 46% (CI 36, 56), 55% (CI 46, 64), 66% (CI 52, 80) and 60% (CI 46, 75%) respectively. Age at index seizure appeared to have a statistically significant effect on cumulative remission rates ($p = 0.007$), with the youngest age group having the worst prognosis and those aged 60 years having the best prognosis. Although children could have been said to expect a better prognosis, this has not been borne out in some population-based studies, and in the NGPSE, the effect of age was small. Indeed it appeared to have no significant effect on terminal remission rates. This may in part relate to the 9-year period of follow up, which may be short as far as many childhood epilepsies are concerned. The effect of epilepsy due to congenital neurological deficits may also be significant.

The effect of seizure type on remission

Patients with partial seizures had a smaller chance of remission than those with generalised seizures [3]. 80% (CI 73, 87) of partial onset seizure patients achieved 3- year remission compared to 91% (CI 84, 97) with generalised onset, which may reflect a greater proportion of lesional epilepsy in the former group and a greater proportion of primary generalised epilepsy in the latter. 5-year remission rates were similarly lesser for partial seizures (63% [CI 54, 72]) than generalised seizures (71% [CI 60, 82]).

Table IV. The age distribution of patients with definite epilepsy in the NGPSE

Age (yr)	No.	%
0-4	39	7
5-9	51	9
10-14	49	9
15-19	66	12
20-29	74	13
30-39	62	11
40-49	35	6
50-59	52	9
60-69	63	11
70-79	43	8
80-89	23	4
> 90	7	1
Total	564	
Median (25th, 75th centile)	32 (15, 28)	

CI = confidence interval.
From Cockerell et al. 1997 [3].

Factors predicting prognosis

The Cox proportional hazards regression model was used to analyse the factors associated with 1, 2, 3 and 5 years remission [10]. The eight characteristics used to test for prognostic importance were sex, age at first seizure, number of seizures before index seizure, number of seizures in the first six months after the index seizure, aetiology, classification, seizure type at index seizure and interval from first seizure to index seizure.

In those with onset of seizures at the age of 5 years and older, univariate analysis indicated that the chances of achieving seizure remission decreased with increasing numbers of seizures (before the index seizure and between the index seizure and 6 months) whilst it increased in patients with acute symptomatic seizures. Stepwise selection confirmed the overall importance of the number of seizures in the first 6 months after the index seizure for all four-remission periods ($p < 0.001$). Indeed, this was the only predictor significant at $p = 0.05$ for 1 year and 2 years of remission. For 3 years and 5 years of remission, two other indicators of initial seizure occurrence, namely, the numbers of seizures before the index seizure ($p = 0.006$ and $p = 0.025$) and numbers of seizures in excess of 10 before the index seizure ($p = 0.018$ and $p = 0.016$), were also selected. The number of seizures in the first 6 months after the index seizure on univariate analysis in the whole sample gave hazard ratios of 0.62 (CI 0.55, 0.70) for 1 year of remission, 0.61 (CI 0.53, 0.70) for 2 years of remission, 0.62 (CI 0.53, 0.71) for 3 years of remission, and 0.59 (CI 0.49, 0.71) for 5 years of remission (all $p \leq 0.001$). Restriction of these analyses to patients with definite seizures only or to patients who fulfilled the usual criteria for epilepsy (at least 2 seizures) and exclusion of those with acute symptomatic seizures did not alter these findings.

Factors such as seizure type and aetiology appear not to be important, unless as variables associated with the single most important prognostic factor – the number of seizures occurring in the first 6 months after presentation in patients aged 5 or over. If a patient has 10 seizures in the first 6 months, there is a 51% chance of achieving a 1-year remission by 2 years compared with a 78% chance if the patient only experienced 2 seizures in the same interval. Similarly the chances for 5-year remission by 8 years are 30% and 55% (table V).

There were no significant differences for chances of remission between generalised or partial seizures.

Table V. The chance of achieving 1-year or 5 year remission over time as a function of the number of seizures between the index seizure and 6 months

	Percentage achieving 1-yr remission				Percentage achieving 5-yr remission			
Number of seizures between Index seizure and 6 months	Index only	2	5	10	Index only	2	5	10
Years from 6 months after index seizure								
1	56	44	31	24				
2	87	77	61	50				
3	94	87	74	62				
4	96	91	79	67				
5	97	93	82	71	46	35	23	16
6	98	94	85	74	61	48	33	24
7	98	94	85	74	65	52	36	27
8	98	94	85	74	70	56	40	30
9	98	94	85	74	80	67	49	38

From MacDonald et al. 2000 [10].

Conclusion

The NGPSE provides important information on the prognosis of the epilepsies. Its prospective design renders this particularly valuable, as seizure disorders are mostly dynamic and subject to many continuing factors that influence remission and recurrence. Further data, currently being compiled, will provide further insights into the long-term prognosis of the epilepsies.

References

1. Cockerell OC, Johnson AL, Sander JW, Hart YM, Goodridge DM, Shorvon SD. Mortality from epilepsy: results from a prospective population-based study. *Lancet* 1994; 344: 918-21.
2. Cockerell OC, Johnson AL, Sander JW, Hart YM, Shorvon SD. Remission of epilepsy: results from the National General Practice Study of Epilepsy. *Lancet* 1995; 346: 140-4.
3. Cockerell OC, Johnson AL, Sander JW, Shorvon SD. Prognosis of epilepsy: a review and further analysis of the first nine years of the British National General Practice Study of Epilepsy, a prospective population-based study. *Epilepsia* 1997; 38: 31-46.
4. Hart YM, Sander JW, Shorvon SD. National General Practice Study of Epilepsy and Epileptic seizures: Objectives and study methodology. *Neuroepidemiology* 1989; 8: 221-7.
5. Hart YM, Sander JW, Johnson AL, Shorvon SD. National General Practice Study of Epilepsy: recurrence after a first seizure. *Lancet* 1990; 336: 1271-4.
6. Lhatoo SD, Sander JW, Shorvon SD. The dynamics of drug treatment in epilepsy: an observational study in an unselected population based cohort with newly diagnosed epilepsy followed prospectively over 11-14 years. *J Neurol Neurosurg Psychiatry* 2001; 71: 632-7.
7. Lhatoo SD, Langan Y, MacDonald BK, Zeidan S, Sander JW. Sudden unexpected death: a rare event in a large community based prospective cohort with newly diagnosed epilepsy and high remission [7]. *J Neurol Neurosurg Psychiatry* 1999; 66: 692-3.
8. Lhatoo SD, Johnson AL, Goodridge DM, MacDonald BK, Sander JW, Shorvon SD. Mortality in epilepsy in the first 11 to 14 years after diagnosis: Multivariate analysis of a long-term, prospective, population-based cohort. *Ann Neurol* 2001; 49: 336-44.
9. MacDonald BK, Johnson AL, Sander JW, Shorvon SD. Febrile convulsions in 220 children - neurological sequelae at 12 years follow-up. *Eur Neurol* 1999; 41: 179-86.

10. MacDonald BK, Johnson AL, Goodridge DM, Cockerell OC, Sander JW, Shorvon SD. Factors prediciting prognosis of epilepsy after presentation with seizures. *Ann Neurol* 2000; 48: 833-41.
11. Manford M, Hart YM, Sander JW, Shorvon SD. The National General Practice Study of Epilepsy. The syndromic classification of the International League Against Epilepsy applied to epilepsy in a general population. *Arch Neurol* 1992; 49: 801-8.
12. Manford M, Hart YM, Sander JW, Shorvon SD. National General Practice Study of Epilepsy (NGPSE): partial seizure patterns in a general population. *Neurology* 1992; 42: 1911-7.
13. Sander JW, Hart YM, Johnson AL, Shorvon SD. National General Practice Study of Epilepsy: newly diagnosed epileptic seizures in a general population. *Lancet* 1990; 336: 1267-71.
14. Sander JW. Some aspects of prognosis in the epilepsies: a review. *Epilepsia* 1993; 34: 1007-16.
15. Sander JW, Sillanpaa M. Natural history and prognosis. In: Engel J, Pedley TA, eds. Epilepsy, Philadelphia: Lippincott-Raven, 1997: 69-86.
16. Shorvon SD. The temporal aspects of prognosis in epilepsy. *J Neurol Neurosurg Psychiatry* 1984; 47: 1157-65.
17. Commission on Classification and Terminology of the ILAE. Proposal for revised clinical and electroencephalographic classification of epileptic seizures. *Epilepsia* 1981; 22: 489-501.
18. Hauser WA, Andersen VE, Loewenson RB, McRoberts SM. Seizure recurrence after a first unprovoked seizure. *N Engl J Med* 1982; 307: 522-8.

Prognosis of epilepsy based on epidemiological studies from Västerbotten, northern Sweden

Lars Forsgren

Introduction

In 1983 an initiative came from Ethiopia to perform neuroepidemiological studies in a rural part of the country. Review of the neuroepidemiological literature at that time revealed the scarcity of population-based neuroepidemiological studies, and this also applied to epilepsy. Several population-based studies had been published from Rochester in Minnesota, the United States, with only a few studies from other parts of the world. In order to provide additional comparative data for the planned epidemiological studies in Ethiopia, a number of epidemiological studies of epilepsy were initiated to be carried out in the county of Västerbotten in northern Sweden *(figure 1)*. These initial studies were later followed by additional studies, as well as follow-up of the cohorts first identified.

Västerbotten County is located between latitudes 64 and 66 degrees, just south to the Arctic Circle. The county has an area of 55 428 square kilometres, which is 1.3 times the size of Switzerland, or 1.5 times the size of Belgium. The overall population density of the county is low, 4.4 inhabitants per square kilometre, with a total population between 245 000 to 250 000 during the periods of investigation. The eastern coastal area has a considerably higher population density than the rest of the county, especially the southeastern area where the largest city, Umeå, is located. Umeå has a university and a university hospital. In one of the incidence studies, the catchment area was the southeastern part of the county, with an adult population of about 100 000.

The population is culturally rather homogenous. The population is fairly stable, but due high unemployment in the inland area there is a migration to the coastal area of the county and to southern Sweden.

During the last years several epidemiological studies with prognostic information have been published from Västerbotten County.

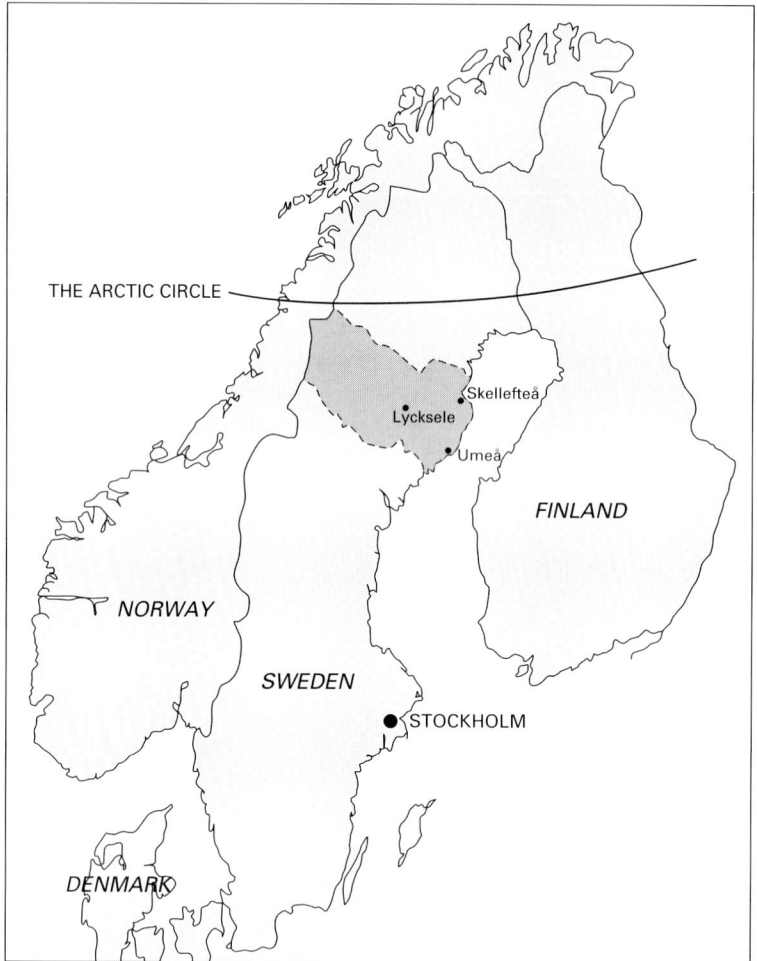

Figure 1. Map of Scandinavia and Finland with the investigation area hatched.

Incidence study 1985-87

Study population, definitions, sources for identification and investigations

This is a prospective population-based incidence study of children [1] and adults 17 years and older [2] with a first diagnosis of one or more unprovoked epileptic seizures. Seizures were categorized as unprovoked if they occurred without an identifiable causative metabolic or structural abnormality, the same definition as used by Hauser *et al.* [3]. Cases were identified during a period of 20 months (Nov. 1985 to June 1987). The catchment area was the whole county of Västerbotten. Cases were identified through multiple sources. All nurses and doctors in the county who were anticipated to come in contact with seizures in the study area were repeatedly during the investigation period requested to report or refer all patients with a newly diagnosed or suspected seizure disorder. Another source for identification was through the department of clinical neurophysiology where all EEGs in the county are evaluated. In adults one or several EEG investigations were performed in 96% of adult cases identified, with the patient awake and/or asleep. Investigations with computerized tomography (CT) and magnetic resonance imaging (MRI) were performed in 97% and 42% of patients respectively. In children EEG was recorded in all, and CT was performed in 44% and MRI in 6%.

For all cases below age 75 years two age- and sex matched referents from the county were identified for case-referent studies.

Result

Altogether 66 children (neonatal seizures excluded) and 107 adults were identified corresponding to a rate of initial diagnosis (first attendance rate) of 79 and 34/100 000 for children and adults respectively [1, 2]. In adults, epileptiform activity was recorded on the EEG in 28%, either during wakefulness or sleep, or both. Unspecific abnormalities only were found in 51% [4]. In patients investigated with both CT and MRI results were concordant in 87% of examinations [4].

The adults in this cohort with newly diagnosed unprovoked seizures identified during 1985-87 was followed up for 10 years to assess the prognosis regarding mortality, seizure remission, seizure recurrence, psycho-social aspects and leisure-time activity.

Follow-up study of 1985-87 incidence cohort – mortality

The 107 newly diagnosed patients constituting the 1985-87 cohort were followed up to the end of 1996 or until the date of death if death occurred before the end of 1996 [5]. At the end of follow-up 24 of 61 males and 15 of 46 females had died compared with the expected 9.0 males and 6.6 females in the general population. The total cohort mortality was significantly increased with a standardized mortality ratio (SMR) of 2.5 (95% confidence interval [CI] 1.2-3.2). The increase in mortality was found both in males (SMR 2.7, 95% CI 1.8-3.9) and females (SMR 2.3, 95% CI 1.4-3.7).

Mortality was significantly increased during the first 2 years following diagnosis with an SMR of 7.3 (95% CI 1.4-3.7) the first year, and an SMR of 3.6 (95% CI 1.6-8.1) the second year. A late increase in mortality with an SMR of 5.4 (95% CI 2.7-11.2) was also found at years 9-11 *(figure 2)*.

Factors found to be associated with increased mortality were aetiology, seizure type and age at diagnosis. Patients with remote symptomatic cause had an SMR of 3.3 (95% CI 2.4-4.5) and the significantly increased mortality was found in both males (SMR 3.8) and females (SMR 2.6). Mortality was not increased in patients with idiopathic epilepsy (SMR 1.1, 95% CI 0.5-2.4). Patients with partial seizures had a significantly increased risk for death, found both in males (SMR 2.1, 95% CI 1.2-3.6) and females (SMR 2.1, 95% CI 1.2-3.7). In patients with generalized tonic-clonic seizures the risk for death was only significantly increased in males (SMR 3.9, 95% CI 2.3-6.8). The highest SMR was found in ages below 60 years (SMR around 10), lower in ages 60-79 years (SMR 2.4) and not significantly increased in ages 80 years and above (SMR 1.3, 95% CI 0.7-2.4). The excess mortality was higher in patients 60 years and older, 39 per 1 000, than in patients below age 60, 21 per 1 000.

Death was due to myocardial infarction and cerebrovascular disease in 6 cases each, to glioma in 5 cases, to myocardial insufficiency and pneumonia in 4 cases each, to tumours outside the nervous system and alcohol-related homicide in 2 cases each, and to other causes in 10 cases. When cause-specific mortality was analysed the following causes were

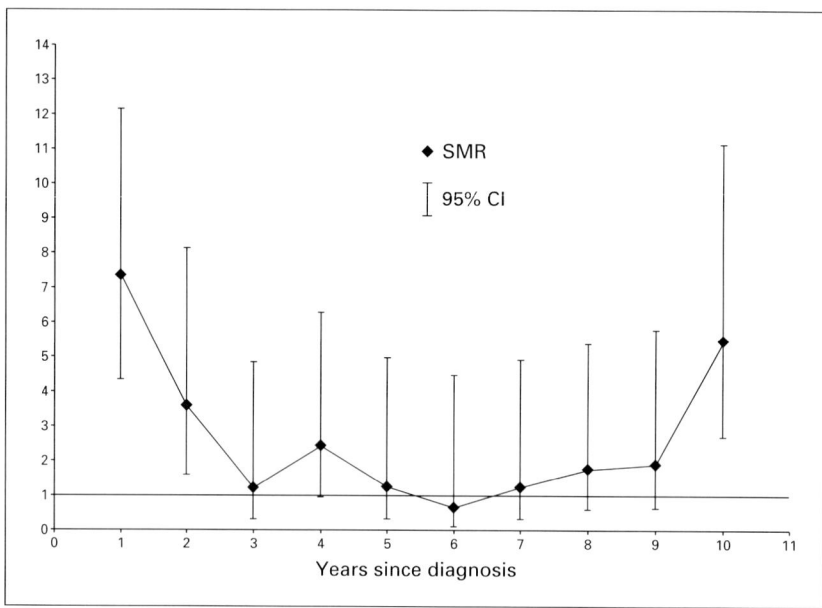

Figure 2. Mortality risk in a prospectively identified cohort with newly diagnosed unprovoked epileptic seizures. Shown are SMR (symbols) and 95% confidence intervals (lines) during 10 years of follow-up. Reprinted from Epilepsia, Vol 41, Lindsten H, Nyström L, Forsgren L, Mortality risk in an adult cohort with a newly diagnosed unprovoked epileptic seizure: a population-based study, Pages 1469-73, Copyright 2000, with permission from Blackwell Publishing.

found to significantly increase the mortality risk: cerebrovascular disease with an SMR of 4.2 (95% CI 2.2-8.0), tumours (including CNS-tumours) with an SMR of 3.4 (95% CI 1.9-5.8), and myocardial insufficiency with an SMR of 1.8 (95% CI 1.2-3.0).

Follow-up study of 1985-87 incidence cohort – seizure remission

This study also includes all 107 newly diagnosed patients constituting the 1985-87 cohort and who were followed up to the end of 1996 or until the date of death if death occurred before the end of 1996 [6]. Time to achieve remission was estimated using the life-table method and the Kaplan-Meier method. The log-rank test was used to compare survival curves. Altogether 89 patients had more than 1 unprovoked seizure and thus fulfilled the criteria for epilepsy. In 81 of these patients antiepileptic drug (AED) treatment was started, either at the time of diagnosis of epilepsy (76 patients) or at the time of the first seizure following diagnosis. AED treatment was changed in 31 patients during follow-up, either to another monotherapy (12 patients) or to add-on therapy (8 patients) or to another monotherapy followed by add-on therapy (3 patients). No patient received more than 2 AEDs. Treatment was stopped in 21 patients, successfully in 19 while 2 restarted treatment because of seizure recurrence. None of the patients with a single seizure received AED treatment.

From the date of index seizure (unprovoked seizure leading the patient to seek medical contact and be diagnosed irrespective of whether this was first, second or later seizure) the cumulative 1-year remission rate was 73% (95% CI 63-83), and 68% (95% CI 57-79) when calculated from the date of epilepsy diagnosis. The corresponding cumulative 3-year remission rates were 70% (95% CI 60-80) and 64% (95% CI 53-75) respectively.

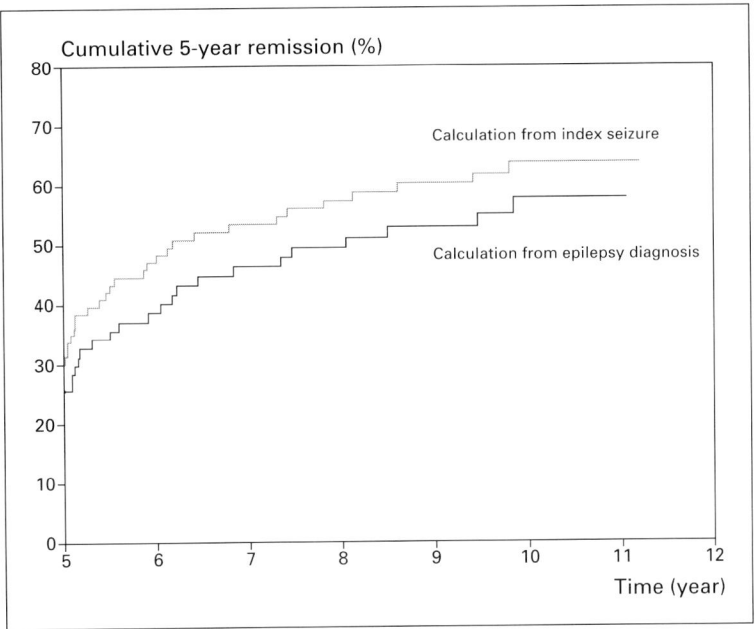

Figure 3. Overall cumulative 5-year remission of seizures after the index seizure and epilepsy diagnosis in an adult population-based cohort with a newly diagnosed unprovoked epileptic seizure.
Reprinted from Epilepsia, Vol 42, Lindsten H, Stenlund H, Forsgren L, Remission of seizures in a population-based adult cohort with a newly diagnosed unprovoked epileptic seizure, Pages 1025-30, Copyright 2001, with permission from Blackwell Publishing.

The rate for longer cumulative remission, 5 years or more, was 64% (95% CI 53-75) calculated from date of the index seizure, and 58% (95% CI 45-71) calculated from the date of epilepsy diagnosis *(figure 3)*. The cumulative 1- and 5-year remission rate calculated from the date of epilepsy diagnosis did not differ substantially when patients with tumours were excluded, 68% (95% CI 57-79) and 57% (95% CI 44-70) respectively.

In patients with 1-year remission, the probability to ever attain a 5-year remission did not differ with respect to when the 1-year remission was achieved, i.e. after the first, second or later year of follow-up. Around 70% of patients with 1-year remission, even when occurring several years following the onset of epilepsy, will eventually attain a 5-year remission. However, the likelihood of achieving 1-year remission (and thus the chance to later attain 5-year remission) of low if 1-year remission is not achieved during the first 3 years following epilepsy diagnosis. Thus, most patients with refractory seizures can be identified within a few years from the diagnosis of epilepsy.

Being seizure free during the year following start of AED treatment is a significant predictor for achieving 5-year remission. All patients being seizure free during the first year of AED treatment achieved a 5-year remission while the rate was only 27% for patients with 1 or more seizure during the first year of AED treatment (p < 0.01).

Age at index seizure, number of seizures before index seizure, aetiology, seizure type and EEG at inclusion were not predictors for achieving 1- and 5-year remission although EEG showed a tendency to be a predictor for 5-year remission (focal spikes or generalised spike-wave activity vs. normal or non-specific slowing; p = 0.06).

Follow-up study of 1985-87 incidence cohort – seizure recurrence

The study population and follow-up was identical to the study of seizure remission (above). As in the study of seizure remission, seizures were classified as remote symptomatic or idiopathic according to the definitions in the ILAE guidelines [7]. One exception from the ILAE guidelines was that CNS tumours were classified as remote symptomatic, irrespective of whether seizures were the presenting symptom or not. Time to recurrence was estimated using the life table method and the Kaplan-Meier method. The log-rank test was used to compare survival curves. Significant variables from the univariate analyses were also investigated with multivariate analysis using the Cox regression model.

Recurrence rates from the index seizure (see definition above) were 41% (95% CI 32-50) and 57% (95% CI 47-67) at 1 and 2 years respectively following the index seizure [8]. At 750 days after the index seizure, the recurrence was 58% (95% CI 49-68). After 750 days no new recurrences occurred. Although most recurrences occurred during the first year from index seizure, there was no statistical difference between the first and second year (recurrence risk ratio first vs. second year; 1.66 [95% CI 0.92-2.99]).

The recurrence risk was significantly higher for patients with remote symptomatic seizures than for the idiopathic group with unknown aetiology, p = 0.007. The cumulative recurrence rate for the idiopathic group at 1 year was 29% (95% CI 15-43%). The rates for 2 years and 750 days were 43% (95% CI 28-58) and 46% (95% CI 31-61) respectively. For the remote symptomatic group the recurrence rate was 49% (95% CI 36-62) at year 1 and 67% (95% CI 55-79) for 2 years and 750 days *(figure 4)*.

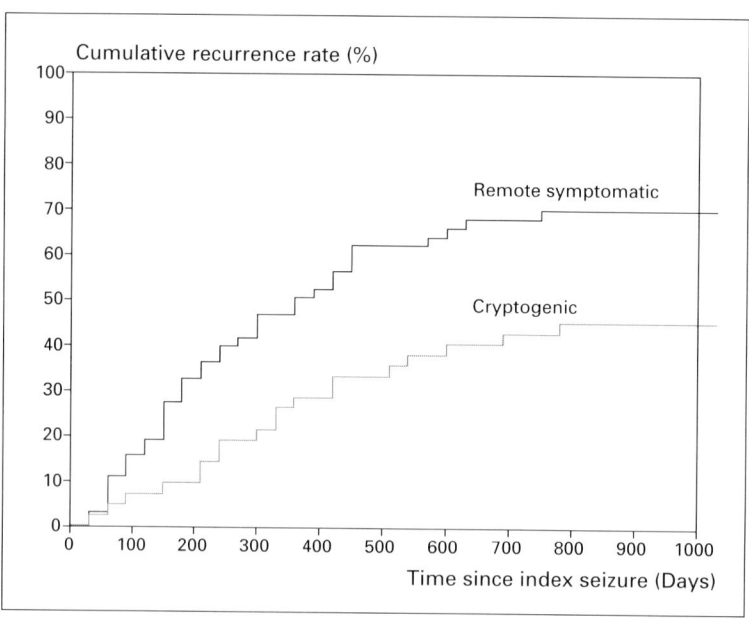

Figure 4. Cumulative recurrence rates by aetiology in an adult population-based cohort with a newly diagnosed unprovoked seizure.
Reprinted from Acta Neurol Scand, Vol 104, Lindsten H, Stenlund H, Forsgren L, Seizure recurrence in adults after a newly diagnosed unprovoked epileptic seizure, Pages 202-07, Copyright 2001, with permission from Blackwell Munksgaard.

Two or more seizures before the index seizure predicted seizure recurrence (p = 0.007) while one seizure before the index seizure was not predictive. Patients treated with AEDs experienced recurrence significantly more often than untreated patients (p = 0.001).

The following variables were found not to be statistically significant predictors for seizure recurrence: gender, age at index seizure, index seizure type, index seizure occurring during wakefulness or sleep, time from index seizure to diagnostic evaluation, and EEG. Multivariate analysis of factors found to be significant at univariate analysis, with therapy excluded, found aetiology and number of seizures before index seizure to remain as significant predictors for seizure recurrence, p = 0.007 for both variables.

Higher recurrence risk for the AED treated group should not be interpreted as AEDs having a proconvulsive effect. Patients were selected or not selected for treatment based on clinical evaluation where those believed to be at high risk for seizure recurrence were started on antiepileptic treatment.

Follow-up study of 1985-87 incidence cohort – socio-economic prognosis

In August 1997 the 1985-87 cohort was followed-up regarding socio-economic data [9]. At that time 67 patients and 107 referents were still alive. Four severely mentally retarded patients living in institutions were excluded. Information on vocational status, source of income and education was collected from patients through a questionnaire with additional telephone interview in cases that did not respond or gave incomplete answers on the questionnaire. Data on income were provided by the local social insurance. Data on sickness periods, temporary disability pensions and disability pensions were provided by local social insurance offices, or by the National Social Insurance Board.

The questionnaire part of the study included 62 patients (1 refusal) and 93 referents (4 refusals and 7 that could not be contacted). Income data from 1984 (prior to onset of epilepsy), income, sickness periods and incapacity rate (the sum of days of sickness periods, and days receiving temporary disability pension or disability pension) data from 1986, 1990, and 1996 and diagnosis data from 1990 and 1996 were compared. Data regarding vocational status, source of income, and education were also compared for years 1986-90, 1990-93, 1994-96, and 1997.

Patients had lower income than referents during the whole period of investigation, i.e. from 1-2 years before seizure onset and during the entire period of follow-up. This difference can, at least partly, be explained by longer sickness periods and a higher frequency of disability pensions among patients. However, the relative growth of income was similar between patients and referents during follow-up. Within the patient group, a significantly lower income was found during the latter part of follow-up in patients seizure free < 1 year compared with patients seizure free > 1 year.

Analysis of the underlying diagnosis responsible for incapacity rate between 1990 and 1996 found epilepsy to contribute to 10% of overall incapacity rate among patients. The contribution of epilepsy to the overall incapacity rate differed considerably depending on seizure history, and was much higher in patients seizure free < 1 year, 17-56%, than in patients seizure free > 1 year, 0-5%. In patients seizure free < 1 year, incapacity related to epilepsy increased and incapacity not related to epilepsy decreased during follow-up.

Employment rates did not evolve negatively after seizure onset and were close to employment rates of referents during follow-up. No difference was found between patients and referents regarding education.

Follow-up study of 1985-87 incidence cohort – leisure time activity

The same group that was followed up for investigation of the socio-economic prognosis was also followed up to the latter part of 1997, concerning leisure time activity [10]. Information was collected through questionnaires, and when necessary, complemented through telephone interview. Patients and referents were questioned about various leisure time variables, e.g. participating in sports or physical activities, outdoor life, club organized activities, theatre, cinema, travelling abroad. An overall activity index was also calculated for every responder, based on the number of leisure time activities a person was active in. Furthermore, the variables marital status and holding a driver's license were also investigated.

Patients were less physically active than referents during the whole period of follow-up. The proportion of patients with low physical activity became larger during follow-up while no change was found in referents. During the latter part of follow-up, 1994-97, the difference between patients and referents was statistically significant. During 1997 patients travelled significantly less often abroad than referents. During the initial period of follow-up, 1986-93, patients seizure free > 1 year participated significantly more often in hobbies than patients seizure free < 1 year.

The overall activity index was higher for referents than for patients during the entire follow-up period, and the difference was statistically significant for 1997.

There was no difference between patients and referents regarding marital status and driver's licence.

Although significant differences were found between patients and referents for some of the variables investigated, it should be noted that a large fraction of patients belonged to the active group. For example, more than half of the patients were in the physically active group during the whole period of follow-up. Furthermore, no difference was found for most variables investigated. Thus, patients and doctors should have an optimistic view of the possibility for most patients with onset of epilepsy to live an active life during the coming 10 years following diagnosis. This is hardly surprising considering the good prognosis for many with new onset epilepsy. At the end of follow-up time of the present study, almost half of the patients did not longer fulfil the ILAE criteria for active epilepsy [7].

Follow-up study of 1985-87 incidence cohort – febrile convulsions

In addition to the studies of unprovoked seizures, a population-based study on children with a first febrile convulsion (FC) was also performed in the same study area and with the same method for identification as for patients with unprovoked seizures [11]. A total of 128 children with a first FC were identified. Out of these, 115 children participated in a case-referent study concerning genetic and social risk factors where two referents per case were selected from the general population, matched for age and sex. The questionnaire used in that study was answered by 103 cases and 193 referents [12]. These responders were followed up with a new questionnaire (and when necessary complemented by telephone interview) during 1993, 6-7 years after the first FC [13]. When appropriate, answers were crosschecked against information in the medical records.

The cases had their first FC at a median age of 18 months, their second FC at 24 months and their third at 26 months. FC recurred in 42% of the FC cohort, and 3.8% of the children in the referent cohort experienced FC during follow-up. Single or recurrent afebrile seizures occurred in 4.3% and epilepsy in 3.3% of the FC cohort, while no afebrile seizures occurred in the referent cohort. The risk of having a sibling with FC was three times higher in the FC cohort (95% CI 1.3-6.2), while there was no difference between the cohorts in the risk of siblings developing afebrile seizures. Except for two children (with mental retardation not aetiologically linked to FC) in the FC cohort all children attended normal school and none needed remedial instruction. Thus, there were no indications that FCs had a major negative influence on the cognitive development as measured by the age of school start or by the need for remedial instructions.

The influence of epilepsy on mortality in mental retardation

All patients with mental retardation (MR) living in Västerbotten on December 31, 1985 were identified and characterised in different aspects, e.g. aetiology and concurrent diseases, with an emphasis on epilepsy [14]. MR was defined as I.Q. < 70 present before age 18 years. The severity of MR was classified as mild (IQ 50-55 to 70), moderate (35-40 to 50-55), severe (20-25 to 35-40) and profound (less than 20-25). A diagnosis of epilepsy was given to cases with recurrent unprovoked seizures. Only persons with active epilepsy were included, i.e. those where the last seizure had occurred in the last 5 years and/or the person were treated with AEDs on the prevalence day. Seizures were classified according to ILAE [15].

This prevalence cohort was followed up for 7 years, through 1992, to study the mortality pattern [16]. The cause of death pattern in Västerbotten, by 10-year age groups and sex, was used as a reference population for all causes. For cause-specific mortality the population of Sweden was used as a reference.

During an observation period of close to 10 000 person-years, 124 of 1 478 persons with MR died. This was significantly greater than that expected from death rates in the general population with an SMR of 2.0 (95% CI 1.7-2.3), higher in females (SMR 2.6; 95% CI 2.0-3.3) than in males (SMR 1.6; 95% CI 1.2-2.0). Mortality increased with increasing degree of MR. In cases with mild and moderate MR the SMR was 1.5-1.8 (95% CI 1.1-2.0/2.7). In severe MR the SMR was 2.0 (95% CI 1.5-2.6) and in profound MR 8.1 (95% CI 5.6-12).

Compared to cases with only MR, mortality was higher in cases with both MR and epilepsy where SMR was 5.0 (95% CI 3.3-7.5). The highest mortality was found in cases with MR and additional epilepsy and cerebral palsy (CP) where the SMR was 5.8 (95% CI 3.4-9.8).

Mortality was significantly increased in cases below age 60 years, but not in the elderly. The most conspicuous mortality was found in children and adolescents (0-19 years) with an SMR of 5.1 (95% CI 1.8-14) in cases with only MR. In cases with MR and epilepsy in the same age group, the SMR was 40 (95% CI 24-67), and 52 (95% CI 30-90) in cases with CP in addition to MR and epilepsy. Mortality was also significantly increased in adults in ages 20-59 years, but less pronounced than in the youngest age group. The SMR was 3.8 (95% CI 2.8-5.0) in cases with only MR, 5.0 (95% CI 2.9-8.7) in cases with additional epilepsy, and 8.0 (95% CI 4.1-16) in cases with additional epilepsy and CP. The combination of MR, epilepsy and the most severe form of CP, with tetraplegia, resulted in a SMR of 12 (95% CI 6.6-21).

Analysis of mortality by seizure type in cases with MR and epilepsy showed mortality to be increased for all seizure types. SMR was 3.7 (95% CI 1.0-14) in cases with partial seizures that did not generalise, and 5.0 (95% CI 2.3-11) in cases with partial seizures that occasionally generalised. Mortality was much increased in cases where seizures always were clinically generalised from the onset of the seizure, with an SMR of 8.1 (95% CI 5.7-12).

Mortality was affected by seizure frequency. In patients who had been seizure free the year preceding the prevalence date, mortality was not significantly increased (SMR 2.0; 95% CI 0.9-4.7). In cases with 1-50 seizures during the preceding year mortality was significantly increased with an SMR of 4.7 (95% CI 2.8-7.9). The highest mortality was found in cases with weekly or more seizures (> 50 seizures per year) where SMR was 17 (95% CI 11-27).

Comparison of the underlying cause of death (as listed on death certificates) between the study population and the general population found congenital malformations, neurological diseases, mental disorders, and respiratory diseases to be significantly more common causes of death in the study population.

In patients with MR and epilepsy who died, the death certificates reported epilepsy as the underlying cause of death in 1 of 30 cases. In another 6 cases epilepsy was listed as a contributing cause of death. In 5 of these cases the epilepsy diagnosis could be verified. Despite an association between seizure type and mortality and seizure frequency and mortality, death was rarely a direct effect of seizures. Examination of medical files, death certificates and necropsy reports (performed in 11 cases) of the 30 deaths of cases with epilepsy, found 2 deaths to be probably seizure related – 1 case with brain contusion and subdural haematoma after a fall probably caused by a seizure; 1 case found dead in bed and with no known cause of death. The remaining 28 deaths were not directly seizure related.

This may indicate that seizure frequency and severity in patients with MR are variables that in most cases can be regarded as markers of the severity of the underlying etiology that contribute to mortality, and less often as events directly responsible for death.

Other studies

As stated in the beginning of this chapter, the basic ideas for the studies in Västerbotten matured during the planning phase of neuroepidemiological studies in rural Ethiopia. It is therefore appropriate to mention that the neuroepidemiological project in Ethiopia was implemented and resulted in one thesis and several publications. A prevalence study of active epilepsy, with cases identified through house-to-house survey, found a rate 5.2 per 1000 [17]. In this study 73% of identified patients were investigated by EEG, a frequency unique for a rural study of epilepsy in Africa. In a later incidence study of epilepsy in the same study area, mortality was discussed in relation to the prevalence and incidence rates found [18]. It was found that annual crude death rate was doubled in the epilepsy population compared to the general population in the study area, 32/1000 vs. 16/1000. This difference becomes even larger when age has been standardized for showing a SMR of 2.9.

One of aims of the population-based studies of epilepsy and febrile convulsions in Västerbotten was to identify risk factors for epilepsy and febrile convulsions through case-referent methodology. A hypothetical model of major factors of importance for occurrence of epileptic seizures and epilepsy *(figure 5)* was presented in a paper where, among other things, depression was found to be associated with the occurrence of epilepsy [19]. The association of depression with an increased risk for unprovoked seizures has subsequently been reported [20].

In a recent study of children with a first unprovoked seizure, a number of pre- and perinatal factors were assessed in a case-referent study [21]. In the multivariate analysis the following risk factors were identified: vaginal bleeding, gestational age, Caesarean section and smoking during pregnancy. Caesarean section should not be considered as a risk factor in itself but more a result of present or threatening disorders in the mother or fetus. Despite these results, in the majority of cases no pre- and/or perinatal risk factors were identified, in alignment with earlier results [22].

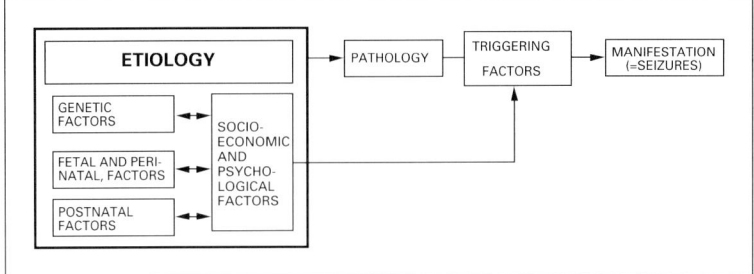

Figure 5. A hypothetical model of major factors of importance for occurrence of epileptic seizures and epilepsy.
Reprinted from Epilepsy Res, Vol 6, Forsgren L, Nyström L, An incident case-referent study of epileptic seizures in adults, Pages 66-81, Copyright 1990, with permission from Elsevier Science.

The future

Between 1992-95 another prospective study was performed to identify cases with new onset unprovoked seizures [23]. Altogether 160 adults were identified corresponding to a rate of initial diagnosis (first attendance rate) of 56 per 100 000. Two age- and sex matched referents were identified for each case. This cohort will be followed up in the coming years with respect to seizure prognosis and mortality and other variables. A paper on possible aetiological factors for the occurrence of unprovoked seizures will soon be submitted.

The cohort with MR and epilepsy will be studied again with respect to mortality. Follow-up time will be doubled in this study compared to the previous study and additional statistical analyses will be performed to try to disentangle the relative contributions of MR and epilepsy to the increased mortality.

References

1. Sidenvall R, Forsgren L, Blomquist HK, Heijbel J. A community-based prospective incidence study of epileptic seizures in children. *Acta Paediatr* 1993; 82: 60-5.
2. Forsgren L. Prospective incidence study and clinical characterization of seizures in newly referred adults. *Epilepsia* 1990; 31: 292-301.
3. Hauser WA, Anderson VE, Loewenson RB, McRoberts SM. Seizure recurrence after a first unprovoked seizure. *N Engl J Med* 1982; 307: 522-8.
4. Forsgren L, Fagerlund M, Zetterlund B. Electroencephalographic and neuroradiological findings in adults with newly diagnosed unprovoked seizures. *Eur Neurol* 1991; 31: 61-7.
5. Lindsten H, Nyström L, Forsgren L. Mortality risk in an adult cohort with a newly diagnosed unprovoked epileptic seizure: a population-based study. *Epilepsia* 2000; 41: 1469-73.
6. Lindsten H, Stenlund H, Forsgren L. Remission of seizures in a population-based adult cohort with a newly diagnosed unprovoked epileptic seizure. *Epilepsia* 2001; 42: 1025-30.
7. Commission on Classification and Terminology of the International League Against Epilepsy. Guidelines for epidemiologic studies on epilepsy. *Epilepsia* 1993; 34: 592-6.
8. Lindsten H, Stenlund H, Forsgren L. Seizure recurrence in adults after a newly diagnosed unprovoked epileptic seizure. *Acta Neurol Scand* 2001; 104: 202-7.
9. Lindsten H, Stenlund H, Edlund C, Forsgren L. Socioeconomic prognosis after a newly diagnosed unprovoked epileptic seizure in adult age. A population-based case-referent study. *Epilepsia* 2002; 43: 1239-50.
10. Lindsten H, Stenlund H, Forsgren L. Leisure time activity after a newly diagnosed unprovoked epileptic seizure in adult age. A population-based case-referent study. *Acta Neurol Scand* 2002; 106: in press.

11. Forsgren L, Sidenvall R, Blomquist HK, Heijbel J. A prospective incidence study of febrile convulsions. *Acta Paediatr Scand* 1990; 79: 550-7.
12. Forsgren L, Sidenvall R, Blomquist HK, Heijbel J, Nyström L. An incident case-referent study of febrile convulsions in children: genetical and social aspects. *Neuropaediatrics* 1990; 21: 153-9.
13. Forsgren L, Heijbel J, Sidenvall R, Nyström L. A follow-up of an incident case-referent study of febrile convulsions seven years after the onset. *Seizure* 1997; 6: 21-6.
14. Forsgren L, Edvinsson S-O, Blomquist HK, Heijbel J, Sidenvall R. Epilepsy in a population of mentally retarded children and adults. *Epilepsy Res* 1990; 6: 234-48.
15. Commission on classification and terminology of the ILAE. Proposal for revised clinical and electroencephalographic classification of epileptic seizures. *Epilepsia* 1981; 22: 489-501.
16. Forsgren L, Edvinsson S-O, Blomquist H, Son K, Nyström L. The influence of epilepsy on mortality in mentally retarded patients. *Epilepsia* 1996; 37: 956-63.
17. Tekle-Haimanot R, Forsgren L, Abebe M, Gebre-Mariam A, Heijbel J, Holmgren G, Ekstedt J. Clinical and electroencephalographic characteristics of epilepsy in rural Ethiopia: a community based study. *Epilepsy Res* 1990; 7: 230-9.
18. Tekle-Haimanot R, Forsgren L, Ekstedt J. Incidence of epilepsy in rural central Ethiopia. *Epilepsia* 1997; 38: 541-6.
19. Forsgren L, Nyström L. An incident case-referent study of epileptic seizures in adults. *Epilepsy Res* 1990; 6: 66-81.
20. Hesdorffer DC, Hauser WA, Annegers JF, Cascino G. Major depression is a risk factor for seizures in older adults. *Ann Neurol* 2000; 47: 246-9.
21. Sidenvall R, Heijbel J, Blomquist H, Son K, Nyström L, Forsgren L. An incident case-referent study of non-neonatal epileptic seizures in children: pre- and perinatal risk factors. *Epilepsia* 2001; 42: 1261-5.
22. Nelson KB, Ellenberg JH. Antecedents of seizure disorders in early childhood. *Am J Dis Child* 1986; 140: 1053-61.
23. Forsgren L, Bucht G, Eriksson S, Bergmark L. Incidence and clinical characterization of unprovoked seizures in adults, a prospective population-based study. *Epilepsia* 1996; 37: 224-9.

The ecuadorian study of prognosis of epilepsy

Arturo Carpio *

Introduction

Remarkable and pioneering studies regarding descriptive epidemiology of epilepsy have been carried out in Ecuador [1, 2]. These population-based studies have proposed new methodological aspects to analyze epidemiology of epilepsy in developing countries [1]. According to these studies, the prevalence of epilepsy is about seven per 1 000, which is similar to the numbers reported in developed countries. Nevertheless, the reported incidence is much higher (around 140 per 100 000), in comparison to industrialized countries (40-70/100 000), which probably means the risks factors to develop epilepsy are different in socioeconomically deprived countries [2]. While studies from developed countries show a consistent pattern suggesting that the onset of epilepsy occurs at both extremes of life, rates from developing countries are highest in young and middle-aged adults [3], perhaps as a secondary manifestation of some prevalent diseases in these age-groups, such as infectious and parasitic diseases which are endemic in these countries. In the face of the above-mentioned descriptive studies, there are no observational prospective studies in developing countries to analyze prognosis of epilepsy. The Ecuadorian Study of Epilepsy is a prospective cohort study [4] designed to analyze the clinical manifestations and prognosis of seizures and newly diagnosed epilepsy in all age groups. To our knowledge, this is the first report to address the likelihood of seizure recurrence in a Latin American country

It has been suggested that epilepsy, in terms of etiology, risk factors, and prognosis, in developing countries is different from that in industrialized regions, but there are few studies of the natural history which allow comparisons [5]. In this context, we analyze in this report potential differences according to the available information.

---

* For the Ecuadorian Study group on Prognosis of Epilepsy, besides the author this group consists of Marcelo Placencia, Noemi Lisanti, Rafael Aguirre, Marcelo Román, Jorge Pesantez, and Carlos Barrionuevo. International Advisor: W. Allen Hauser. This study was financially supported by the "Consejo Nacional de Universidades y Escuelas Politécnicas del Ecuador (CONESUP)".

Cohort description

Three hundred forty newly-diagnosed epilepsy (recurrent unprovoked seizure) patients were recruited and followed-up from January, 1997, to December, 2000 at five hospitals in the three major cities of Ecuador: "Vicente Corral Moscoso" of Cuenca, "Teodoro Maldonado" of Guayaquil, "Baca Ortiz", "Eugenio Espejo" and "C. Andrade Marin" of Quito [4]. Patients from urban and rural areas were recruited. Additionally, 77 patients with single seizure due to neurocysticercosis (NC) seen at the "Vicente Corral Moscoso" of Cuenca were also analyzed separately.

Definitions

Epileptic seizures were classified by the neurologists' study group of every hospital according to the ILAE classification of seizures [6]. The epilepsy type or syndrome was classified according the ILAE classification [7] of epilepsy and epileptic symdromes (ICEES). The etiology was classified on the basis of the ILAE classification for epidemiological studies on epilepsy [8] and was categorized as remote symptomatic, cryptogenic, and idiopathic.

Patients

Eligibility for this study was restricted to the patients who at the time of the diagnoses had had recurrent (two or more) epileptic seizures, unprovoked by an immediate identified cause (newly diagnosed epilepsy). Multiple seizures occurring in a 24-h period were considered a single event. An episode of status epilepticus was considered a single event. Persons who had had only febrile seizures or only neonatal seizures were excluded. All patients received antiepileptic treatment at diagnoses. We excluded those with a first seizure more than 3 years prior to the index consultation or first medical contact for seizures more than 1 year prior to consultation.

Patients with single unprovoked seizure were also followed-up. These patients were included in the cohort in the event they presented a second seizure one week apart. Patients with acute symptomatic seizures were excluded from this cohort. A second cohort of patients of the "Vicente Corral Moscoso" Hospital of Cuenca with a first seizure (or more than one seizure in 24 hours) due to NC was also enrolled.

Follow-up

After enrollment, patients were followed-up by means of clinical interviews every two or three months. Those patients who did not return for clinical evaluation were contacted by telephone. Thirty patients were lost in follow-up. Three hundred ten patients were selected for final analysis. All patients received antiepileptic drugs according to the physician's decision.

Statistical analysis

Time to calculate recurrence was estimated using the life-table method and the Kaplan-Meier survival analysis [9]. Statistical significance was calculated using the Mantel method. Results are displayed as Kaplan-Meier survival curves with the cumulative probability of seizure recurrence plotted as a function of time after the second seizure. Univariate analysis for all risk factors and multivariable analysis were performed using the Cox proportional hazard model [10]. Distribution of variables among groups was analyzed by the chi square test. Differences were considered statistically significant at p < 0.05 (two tailed). The ethical committee of the University of Cuenca approved the study. Statistical analysis was done with the SPSS software.

Clinical features

Table I shows the clinical features of patients included in the cohort [4]. CT scans were performed on 245 patients, and EEG on 298. Mean age of the patients was 18 years old (SD 17). Males were more frequent (55.8%) than females. Children under 15 years old had a higher percentage (58.4%) than adults. Regarding seizure type, partial seizures were more frequent (51%) than generalized (44.8%). Regarding the etiology, 104 patients (33.5%) had symptomatic cause, 85 (27.4%) had cryptogenic, and 121 (39%) idiopathic. Forty-four patients (15.5%) had a family history (first degree of consanguinity) of epilepsy.

Table I. Characteristics of 310 patients with epilepsy

Feature	No. (%)	Recurrence	Chi-Square
Median age at diagnosis	18 years (SD 17, range, 0.1-82)		
Gender			NS
Male	173 (55.8)	42.4%	
Female	137 (44.2)	43.9%	
Age			NS
Children ($\leq$ 15 y.)	181 (58.4)	43.5%	
Adults	129 (41.6)	42.5%	
Seizure type			NS
Generalized	139 (44.8)	44.4%	
Partial	160 (51.6)	41.7%	
Unclassified	11 (3.5)	45.5%	
CT scan result			p < 0.05
Abnormal	109 (44.5)	51.4%	
Normal	136 (55.5)	35.3%	
EEG results			NS
Abnormal	215 (72.1)	45%	
Normal	83 (27.9)	37%	
Etiology			p < 0.05
Symptomatic	104 (33.5)	52.5%	
Cryptogenic	85 (27.4)	32.5%	
Idiopathic	121 (39.0)	42.5%	
Family history of epilepsy	44 (15.5%)	44.6%	N.S.

NS: Not significant.

Classification of epilepsy and epileptic syndromes

Classification of epilepsies is important in clinical practice and research because the etiology, treatment, and prognosis differ remarkably with the type of epilepsy [11]. This classification is widely accepted, and it is applied in clinical research as well as in daily clinical practice by epileptologists; however, some general neurologists and most practicing physicians still find it difficult to apply in many patients.

It is important to consider the differences between studies using prevalent cases of epilepsy and those which recruit newly-diagnosed epilepsy, especially when considering etiology.

In a design to analyze etiology, it is desirable to select incident cases instead of prevalent cases, because it is very difficult to distinguish potential etiology that preceded the disease from that which occurred after the disease developed, thus making it hard to differentiate between cause and effect. There is also a substantial difference in the distribution of syndromes in first seizures when compared with newly-diagnosed epilepsy groups. Certain seizure types characteristic of specific syndromes are less likely to call for medical attention at the time of an initial event. These include absence, myoclonic seizures, infantile spasms, and partial complex seizures, whereas generalized tonic-clonic seizures are most likely to come to medical attention.

Localization-related epilepsies

The frequency of localization-related epilepsies in newly-diagnosed epilepsy (58%) in the Ecuadorian cohort is more or less similar to that reported in developed countries [12], such as France (47%) *(table II)*. This similarity is more consistent when considering children *(table III)*: in the Ecuadorian study 48% of 181 children with incidence epilepsy had localization-related epilepsies, which is similar to studies [13-15] in the USA (59%), India (55%), and Finland (63%). However, there are differences among these groups when differentiating between symptomatic and cryptogenic seizures *(table III)*. This is probably due to the fact that criteria for classifying the symptomatic or cryptogenic localization-related epilepsies are subject to varying interpretations from one investigator to another, and are somewhat arbitrary because they depend on the extent of the diagnostic evaluation. The identification of cause (etiology) depends on the types of evaluation performed (e.g., imaging studies). The determination of localization may be largely determined by EEG evidence without any evidence of an identifiable underlying cause.

Prevalent cases series show a higher frequency of localization-related epilepsies [16, 17] in comparison with newly-diagnosed epilepsy patients. This trend is shown in prevalent studies from Sri Lanka (73%), India (63%) and Italy (63%). Additionally, these studies also show similar percentages. The frequency of idiopathic localization-related syndromes is low in all age groups, including children who account for only 1 to 6% of all prevalent cases in developing countries. 5% to 10% of such cases occur in developed countries *(tables II and III)*.

Table II. Distribution of epilepsies and epilepsy syndromes in patients with newly diagnosed unprovoked seizures (all age groups)*

	Carpio et al.[4] (Ecuador)		Manford et al.[22] (England)**		Jallon et al.[11] (France)	
	310	(%)	594	(%)	1 016	(%)
1. Localization-related	179	(58)	252	(42)	482	(47)
1.1 Idiopathic	10	(3)	7	(1)	48	(5)
1.2 Symptomatic	84	(27)	96	(16)	137	(13.5)
1.3 Cryptogenic	85	(27.5)	146	(24.5)	297	(29)
2. Generalized	93	(30)	66	(11)	343	(34)
2.1 Idiopathic	75	(24.2)	55	(9)	278	(27)
2.2 Cryptogenic or symptomatic	7	(2.3)	0	(0)	39	(4)
2.3 Symptomatic	11	(3.5)	11	(2)	26	(3)
Undetermined whether focal or generalized	38	(12)	190	(32)	177	(17)

* From reference 12, Carpio A, *et al.*
** Patients with special syndromes are excluded.

Table III. Distribution of epilepsies and epilepsy syndromes in children°

	Carpio et al.[8] (Ecuador)		Berg et al.[4] (USA)*		Sillanpa et al.[43] (Finland)**		Shah et al.[41] (India)**	
	181	(%)	613	(%)	245	(%)	1 742	(%)
1. Localization-related	86	(48)	359	(59)	95	(63)	954	(55)
1.1 Idiopathic	10	(6)	61	(10)	14	(9)	69	(4)
1.2 Symptomatic	29	(16)	195	(32)	75	(50)	466	(27)
1.3 Cryptogenic	47	(26)	103	(17)	6	(4)	419	(24)
2. Generalized	67	(37)	178	(29)	40	(27)	620	(36)
2.1 Idiopathic	52	(29)	126	(21)	33	(22)	252	(14)
2.2 Cryptogenic or symptomatic	7	(4)	43	(7)	7	(5)	159	(9)
2.3 Symptomatic	9	(5)	9	(1.5)			209	(12)
3. Undetermined whether focal or generalized	28	(15)	71	(12)	7	(4)	168	(10)

° From reference 12, Carpio A, et al.
* Newly diagnosed unprovoked seizures.
** Prevalent unprovoked seizures.

Generalized epilepsies

There is general agreement among studies about the criteria used to classify idiopathic syndromes. These syndromes are very specific and well defined with respect to several clinical factors, such as age at onset, seizure type, and specific EEG abnormalities (e.g., 3-Hz generalized spike and wave).

The frequency of generalized epilepsy is quite similar in studies including newly-diagnosed patients: the Ecuadorian study reported 30%, as against 34% in the study from France [11]. These studies also showed comparable numbers for the idiopathic, cryptogenic and symptomatic groups (table II). The distribution of generalized epilepsies and epilepsy syndromes in children are similar in studies from Ecuador (37%), the USA (29%), Finland (27%), and India (36%). Again, these studies are also comparable regarding the generalized idiopathic group (table III). The numbers of generalized idiopathic syndromes in the childhood series (table III) are fairly similar in the studies from Ecuador (29%), the USA (21%), and Finland (22%).

Most publications agree that childhood absence is the most frequent syndrome within the idiopathic group [18, 19]. Cryptogenic or symptomatic generalized epileptic syndrome accounts for 2.3% to 4.2% in both developing and developed countries. These low numbers are similar to the 1.7% reported in population-based studies [20]. The frequency of West syndrome, from 1.3 to 3.9% of all cases is also constant over the entire world. Similar low numbers account for Lennox-Gastaut syndrome. Symptomatic generalized epilepsies were reported in 3.5% of the Ecuadorian study [12], whereas an Indian study [16] reported 3%. Many studies [3, 11, 19, 21] reported a high frequency, from 10% to 12%, of "other idiopathic generalized epilepsies", confirming that it is difficult to include all patients in the current ICEES classification.

Epilepsies and epileptic syndromes undetermined whether focal or generalized

There is a broad variation, from 3% to 20%, among the reported frequencies of this category (tables II and III) both in prevalent and newly diagnosed patients. Again, this may be due to the inability of the ICEES classification to categorize some patients with epilepsy.

We agree with some authors as to the limited applicability of some specific diagnostic categories in the general population, as their recognition requires an experienced neurologist or epileptologist [22]. Nevertheless, we assume that the clinical pictures classified within these syndromic groups are also very important because of their prognosis and therapeutic specificity [18, 23, 24]. On the basis of the most recent publications worldwide, it is considered that the ILAE Classification of Epilepsies and Epileptic Syndromes is satisfactorily applicable to the large majority of cases observed at tertiary centers. However, classification of epilepsies in population-based surveys using syndromic classification is difficult because patients should be studied in comprehensive epilepsy centers equipped with high EEG and imaging technology. Obviously, this is difficult to obtain in developing countries [12].

Etiology

The ratio of idiopathic/cryptogenic (63.8%) to symptomatic epilepsy (36.2%) was similar to the studies from developed countries. However, there are differences in the causes of the symptomatic group *(figure 1)*. Perinatal brain damage (9%), neurocysticercosis (8.3%), other central nervous system infections (4.2%), stroke (4.8%), and head trauma (4.2%) were the most frequent disorders reported as causes of epilepsy. The Rochester study [25] reports that 65.5% of new cases were idiopathic; in the symptomatic group, the more frequent causes were vascular disease (10.9%), neurologic deficits present at birth (8%), brain trauma (5.5%), and neoplastic (4.1%). In the Ecuadorian cohort, when separating children under 15 years old (181 patients of the whole cohort), only 25% of the patients had symptomatic epilepsy, and 75% had idiopathic/cryptogenic epilepsy [12].

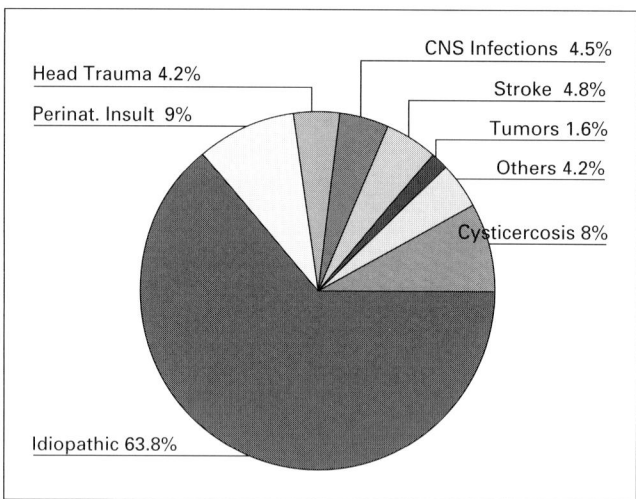

Figure 1. Etiology of epilepsy in 310 patients in Ecuador*.
* From reference 4, Carpio A, *et al.*

Newly-available information in developing countries shows that the proportion of idiopathic/cryptogenic (60-70%) to symptomatic epilepsy (30-40%) is similar to that reported in studies from developed countries [25, 26].

Remote symptomatic epilepsy increases with age, as has been documented by several studies: 18% in a cohort of children with newly-diagnosed epilepsy [13], 39% of the patients with unprovoked seizures in the French study [11], and 49% in a Swedish incidence survey in adults [24]. In the Ecuadorian study [4], when separated by age, 25% of children, and conversely, 53% of adults, had symptomatic epilepsy.

Prognosis of epilepsy

Risk of a third unprovoked seizure

Among the 310 recruited patients, 286 patients were followed-up for at least 6 months. Mean follow-up was 12 months (SD 11.6). Of the 286 patients, 43% had recurrent seizures during the follow-up. Estimated recurrence was 21% at six months, 29% at 12 months; 50% at 24 months, 68% at 36 months, and 79% at 48 months *(table IV)*. *Figure 2* shows Kaplan-Meier curves for all patients. In the univariate analysis there was not statistical difference among the groups shown in *table I*, except patients with abnormal results on CT scan (52% of recurrence), while 35% of patients had a normal CT scan ($p < 0.05$). Etiology was an independent predictor of recurrence in the multivariate analysis (in this analysis idiopathic and symptomatic were considered together): The recurrence in people with symptomatic epilepsy tended to occur sooner after the second seizure than was the case for those with idiopathic/cryptogenic epilepsy *(figure 3)*. Patients with idiopathic/cryptogenic epilepsy had less recurrence risk (38%) compared to patients with symptomatic epilepsy (52%) ($p < 0.05$). Estimated recurrence for patients with symptomatic epilepsy was 26% at six months, 34% at 12 months; 59% at 24 months, 81% at 36 months, and 90% at 48 months. Estimated recurrence for patients with idiopathic/cryptogenic epilepsy was 24% at six months, 27% at 12 months; 47% at 24 months, 60% at 36 months, and 72% at 48 months *(table IV)*. *Figure 4* shows probability of seizure recurrence as a function of CT scan results. Multivariate analysis did not show significant differences in recurrence risk by gender, age, family history of epilepsy, EEG results, or type of seizures.

Most studies regarding prognosis of seizures or epilepsy in adults [27-34] and children [35-40] in industrialized countries have examined the risk of recurrence following a first unprovoked seizure, which does not necessarily mean epilepsy, according to the ILAE definitions. Very few studies have reported the risk of recurrence after a second seizure [41, 42]. Most of the authors have reported that the majority of patients with epilepsy had a favorable long-term medical prognosis in terms of seizure remission or recurrence. Overall, about 1/3 (35%) of patients with a first seizure can be expected to have a second within the subsequent three to five years, although the risk varies from 23% to 71%, depending on clinical characteristics. About 3/4 of those with 2 or 3 unprovoked seizures

Table IV. Percentage of seizure recurrence after the second seizure in patients with epilepsy, according to etiology*

Follow-up	All patients	Symptomatic	Idiopathic**
	286°	99°	187°
Within 6 months	21%	26%	24%
Within 12 months	29%	34%	27%
Within 24 months	50%	59%	47%
Within 36 months	68%	81%	60%
Within 48 months	79%	90%	72%

* From reference 54, Carpio A, *et al.*
** P value < 0.05 for the difference between the groups.
° Number of patients.

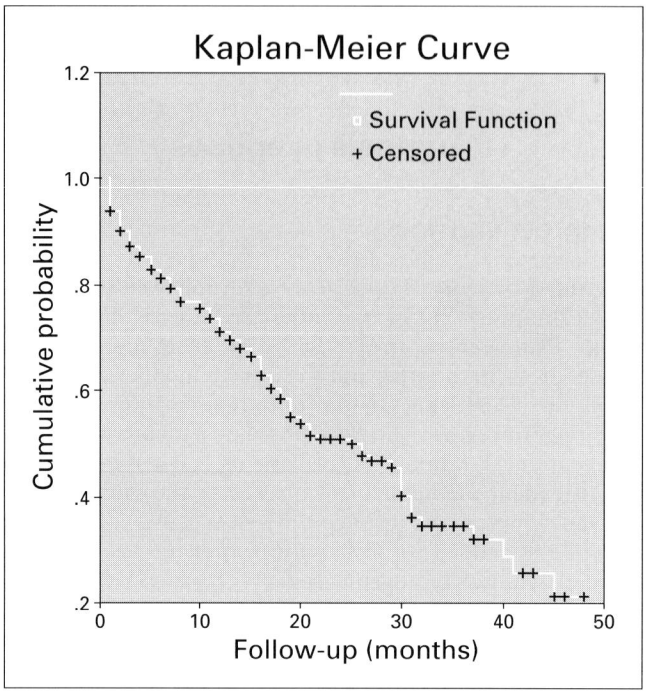

Figure 2. Probability of seizure recurrence in 289 patients with epilepsy*.
* From reference 4, Carpio A, *et al.*

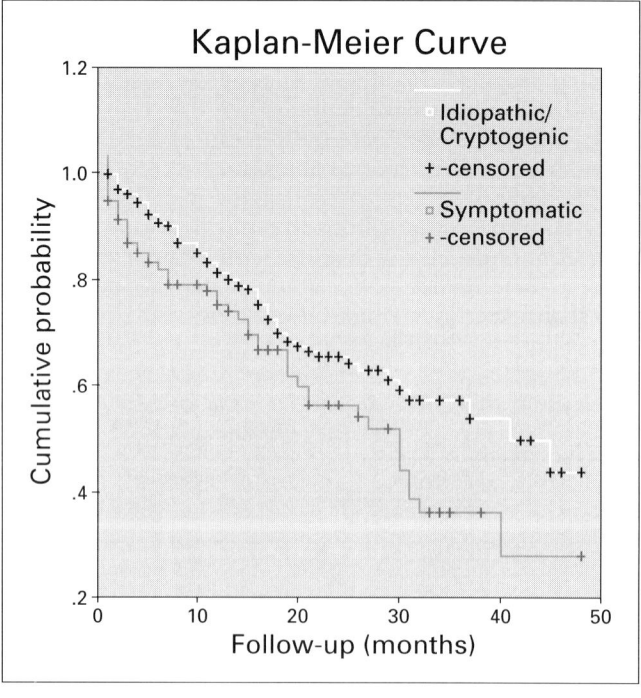

Figure 3. Probability of seizure recurrence in 289 patients with epilepsy as a function of etiology*.
* From reference 4, Carpio A, *et al.*

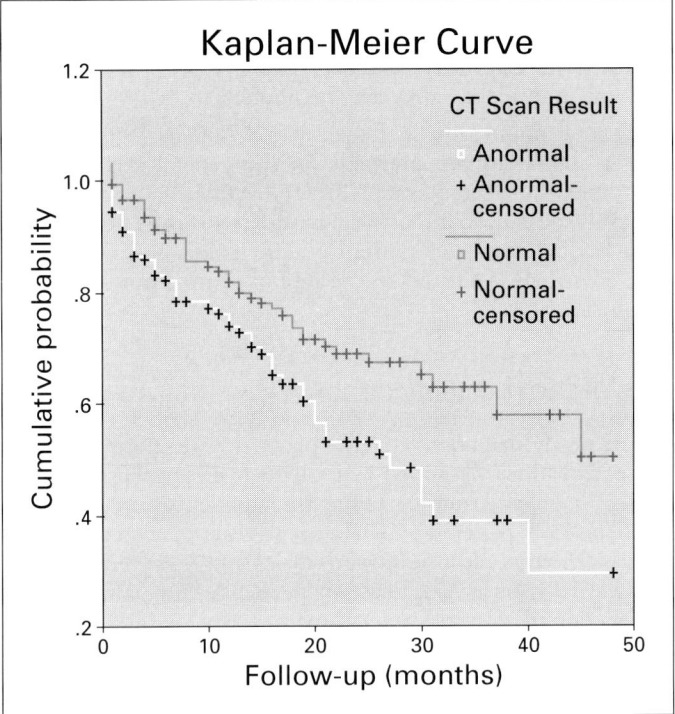

Figure 4. Probability of seizure recurrence in 289 patients with epilepsy as a function of CT scan result*.
* From reference 4, Carpio A, *et al.*

have further seizures within 4 years. Hauser *et al.* reported that the risk of a third unprovoked seizure was 73% after four years of follow-up [41]. In the study reported by Shinnar *et al.*, the cumulative risk of a third seizure was 71% at five years [42]. In the Ecuadorian cohort the risk of a third unprovoked seizure was 79% after four years of follow-up.

Unlike the relatively small risk of recurrence after a first unprovoked seizure (about 35%), there is a substantial risk of additional seizures among persons with two or more unprovoked seizures. The risk of a third unprovoked seizure is higher among those with remote symptomatic epilepsy (from 72% to 90%) than among those with idiopathic/cryptogenic epilepsy (from 64% to 72%), as shown in the above mentioned studies [4, 41, 42]. Etiology as a predictor factor of recurrence, as well as factors indicating a history of neurologic insult, such as imaging abnormalities, are fairly constant in most of the reported studies. The relatively low risk of further seizures among persons with a single unprovoked seizure [40] contrasts sharply with the higher risk after two or more unprovoked seizures, which supports the view that two unprovoked seizures are a necessary and sufficient criterion for the diagnosis of epilepsy [41, 42].

Mortality of epilepsy

In developed countries the overall mortality associated with epilepsy is two to three times that of the general population from other causes [43]. Mortality from epilepsy is difficult to assess in developing countries because incidence studies are difficult, death certificates are not very reliable, autopsies are also not easy to obtain, and the cause of death is not usually known with certainty. The overall autopsy rate is probably less than 5% in public hospitals and almost none in private hospitals. There is also a relative absence of reliable coroner's reports, and, if available, they are incomplete.

Mortality in the general population in Ecuador (8/1 000 in 1997, adjusted to the USA 2000 population) is similar to the mortality in the general population in a developed country, as for example, the United States (8.7/1 000 in 1997, adjusted to the USA 2000 population). However, the causes of mortality are different. Infectious and parasitic diseases remain one of the leading causes of mortality in Ecuador, and rate of death from these diseases combined is virtually identical to the rate of death from cardiovascular disease in the developed countries.

Characteristics of the mortality cohort

Four hundred twelve newly-diagnosed epilepsy patients were selected and followed-up from six main hospitals of Ecuador (We added 72 patients from another hospital to the previous cohort, using similar diagnosis criteria). Thirty-three patients were lost in follow-up. From the remaining patients 379 patients (1 137 patient-years of exposure), 42% were adults and 58% children (< 15 years old), 56% were males and 44% females. The mean age on entering the study was 18 years (± 17). Forty-six per cent of the patients had partial seizures, and 48.7% had generalized seizures. Sixty three per cent of the patients had idiopathic/cryptogenic etiology, and 37% had remote symptomatic etiology.

Standardized Mortality Ratio (SMR) was calculated by comparing the observed number of deaths in the epilepsy cohort with that expected in the Ecuadorian population, adjusting for age and time period. SUDEP rate in terms of patient-years of risk was also calculated.

All-cause mortality. During the follow-up period seven patients died. The crude all-cause SMR for the study group *(table V)* was calculated as 6.3. The SMRs by age specific groups at entry are summarized in *table V*. Seven deaths were reported, of which one patient had definite SUDEP (14.3%), two had probable SUDEP (28.6%), one had aspiration pneumonia (14.3%), two had seizure-related death (28.6%), and one had stroke (14.3%). The overall mortality rate was 6.1 in 1 000 patient-years at risk. The overall SUDEP rate was 2.6/1 000 patient-years.

Table V. All-cause mortality in patients with epilepsy[a]

Age	Patients with epilepsy	Expected Deaths*	Observed Deaths	SMR•
0-19	268	0.56	4	7.7
20-59	102	0.31	2	7.1
> 60	9	0.41	1	3.2
Total	379	1.28	7	6.3

[a] From reference 43, Carpio A, *et al.*
* Calculated by multiplying the number of person-years with epilepsy with the corresponding mortality rate of the Ecuadorian general population divided by 100.
• Observed number of deaths divided by expected number of deaths.

This study suggests that overall mortality for epilepsy in Ecuador is higher than that reported in the general population of a developed country [43]. A wide range of estimated SUDEP rates (< 1.5 to > 9 in 1 000 patient-years) has been published in recent cohort studies [44-49], depending on methods and the population under research. The SUDEP rate in our study (2.9/1 000 patient-years) is higher than that reported in the general population [e.g. 1.3 in Rochester, USA [45]] and as high as those reported in patients with severe epilepsy (3.8:1 000), in spite of the fact that our population corresponds to newly-diagnosed cases of epilepsy.

This cohort group is prone to selection bias because of completeness and accuracy of cause of death; however, it is diminished because follow-up is complete and more witness and clinical information is available. This study also has some limitations: we cannot compare rates of sudden death by seizure type, seizure etiology, age, or sex, due to the small numbers of our cohort. There was a high percentage of loss of patients in the cohort; therefore, it is possible that mortality may be even higher. An autopsy was performed on only one patient. The absolute number of SUDEP cases in this cohort is small. It does not allow internal comparisons. On the other hand, there are some advantages: Diagnosis of epilepsy is well documented, and definitions and analytic procedures are adjusted to ILAE recommendations. Although it is difficult to derive generalizations from this cohort, it represents an important sample from the six main hospitals of Ecuador.

Prognosis for seizure recurrence in patients with neurocysticercosis

Neurocysticercosis (NC) is the most frequent parasitic infestation of the central nervous system in the world [50]. Cysticercosis is endemic in some developing countries, but now is becoming a serious health problem in industrialized nations with high immigrant populations. NC is commonly associated with seizures, headache, and focal neurological deficits, and may lead to long-term neurologic sequelae such as epilepsy, hydrocephalus, and dementia. There is no doubt that acute symptomatic seizures are the main clinical manifestation of NC in those patients in whom a cysticercus is located in the brain parenchyma [51]. Based on prospective studies, the traditional idea that NC is the main cause of epilepsy in developing countries [50] can be questioned. Similarly, the view that epilepsy attributable to NC generally has an unfavorable course prognosis [52] contrasts with recent reports showing an overall favorable prognosis in terms of seizure control and seizure remission [53]. Although some authors have suggested that anticysticidal treatment is associated with reduced seizure recurrence [52] there are no hard data to support this from controlled clinical trials.

A prospective cohort study [54] was designed in order to determine the risk of seizure recurrence after a first seizure due to NC and to evaluate risk factors for seizures recurrence including the influence of antihelminthic treatment. We prospectively followed 77 patients with a first seizure and active or transitional NC for over 7 years (median 24 months). A diagnosis of NC was made based upon imaging studies [50]. Depending on the treating physician's preference some patients received albendazole, 15 mg/kg per day, for 8 days, (44 patients, group 1) and some did not (33 patients, group 2). All patients received steroids (Prednisolone 1 mg/kg per day for 8 days and then decreasing doses the following 8 days) and antiepileptic treatment (the routine practice in the VCM hospital for these patients is administration of phenytoin or carbamazepine).

Thirty-one patients (40.3%) experienced seizure recurrence. Kaplan-Meier estimated recurrence was 22% at 6 months, 32% at 12 months, 39% at 24 months, 49% at 48 and 84 months. Treatment with antihelminthics (albendazole) did not influence recurrence *(figure 5)*. On multivariable analysis, none of the following predicted recurrence: gender, presenting seizure type, classification of NC, localization of cysts, Todd paralysis, neurological deficits at presentation, EEG abnormalities. Only change in CT predicted recurrence: 22% in patients in whom cysts disappeared, 56% in patients with persistent cysts (p < 0.05). In this latter group, recurrence was associated with persistence of an active lesion. Of those with two seizures, risk of a third seizure was 52% within six years following the second seizure.

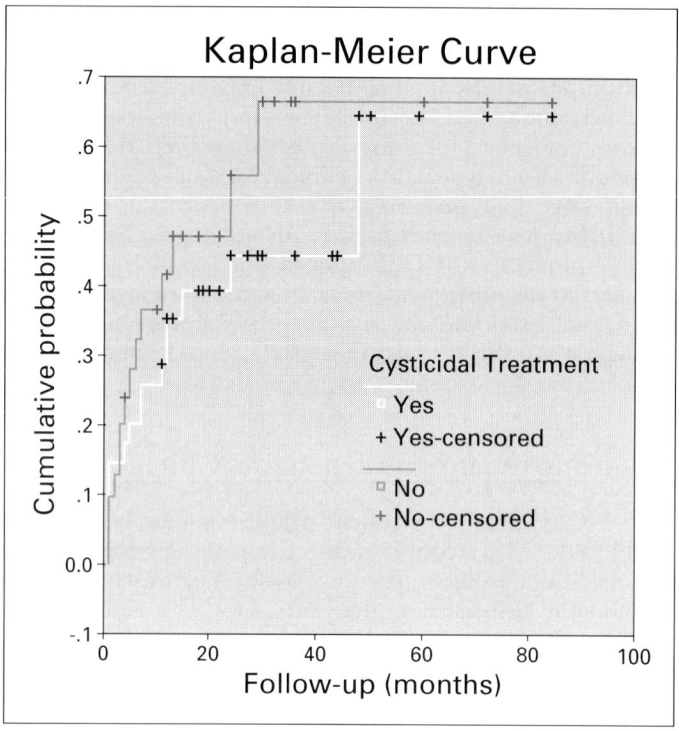

Figure 5. Probability of seizure recurrence after a first seizure in 77 patients with NC as function of cysticidal treatment*.
* From reference 54, Carpio A, *et al.*

Seizure recurrence is high following a first acute symptomatic seizure due to NC, but this seems related to persistence of active brain lesions. Recurrence risk is low and in keeping with seizure risk following other brain insults leading to a static encephalopathy in those in whom the NC lesion clears. NC patients should receive antiseizure medications until the acute lesion clears on CT. There is no correlation between treatment with antihelminthic agents and seizure recurrence

It seems that interpretation of risk of seizures after NC is difficult because of the failure to distinguish acute symptomatic seizures from epilepsy. This distinction must be considered in future studies of the effects of treatment on seizure recurrence in people with cysticercosis. These difficulties are increased in those patients who have mixed forms, including active, transitional, and calcified lesions. Further studies should be performed in order to estimate recurrence risk in those patients with probable unprovoked seizures due to calcifications alone, in comparison with patients with acute seizures due to transitional cysts. These should include a systematic assessment of treatment strategies. Meanwhile, people with acute NC should be treated with ASM until cyst resolution on CT.

Conclusions

- Prevalence of epilepsy in Ecuador is about seven per 1 000, which is similar to that reported in developed countries.
- Incidence of epilepsy in Ecuador is higher (around 140 per 100 000), in comparison to

industrialized countries (40-70/100 000), which probably means the risk factors to develop epilepsy are different in socioeconomically deprived countries.

- While studies from developed countries show a consistent pattern, which suggests that the onset of epilepsy occurs at both extremes of life, rates from Ecuador and other developing countries are highest in young and middle-aged adults, perhaps as a secondary manifestation of some prevalent diseases in these age-groups, such as infectious and parasitic diseases, which are endemic in poor countries.

- Classification of epilepsies using the syndromic classification involves difficulties because patients should be studied in comprehensive epilepsy center equipped with high EEG and imaging technology, which is difficult to achieve in developing countries; however, the utilization of the current ILAE's International Classification of Epileptic Syndromes and Epilepsies seems appropriate in order to make studies over the entire world comparable.

- The diagnostic categories defining the various age-related partial and generalized idiopathic epilepsies appear to be similar in developed and developing countries. The frequency of localization-related epilepsies in newly-diagnosed epilepsy is more or less similar among all the reported studies. This similarity is more consistent when considering children.

- There is also a general agreement among studies as to the criteria used to classify idiopathic syndromes. However, there are differences when differentiating symptomatic and cryptogenic seizures. This is probably due to the fact that criteria for classifying epilepsies are subject to different interpretations from one investigator to another, and somewhat arbitrary because they depend on the extent of the diagnostic evaluation.

- Our cohort, consisting of patients with newly-diagnosed patients, shows that the proportion of idiopathic/cryptogenic (64%) to symptomatic epilepsy (36%) is similar to that reported in studies from developed countries. However, there are differences among the symptomatic group, probably due to different risk factors (perinatal insults, CNS infections and parasitic diseases)

- The risk of seizure recurrence in people with newly-diagnosed epilepsy in Ecuador is similar to that reported in the industrialized countries.

- Our data suggest that roughly three quarters of those who have two unprovoked seizures will have further seizures within four years after the second seizure, which is very similar to the numbers reported by Hauser *et al.* in Rochester, Minnesota.

- There is an increased risk to recur seizures early in patients with symptomatic epilepsy and patients with abnormal CT scan in comparison with patients with idiopathic epilepsy and normal CT scans, respectively. These results are also comparable to those reported in industrialized nations.

- Despite differences in etiology in these disparate settings, the natural history of epilepsy seems universal.

- Although it is difficult to derive generalizations from this cohort, it represents an important sample from the six main hospitals of Ecuador.

- Epilepsy and neurocysticercosis are common diseases in developing countries. NC is not necessarily the main cause of epilepsy, as previously suggested, although it is one of the most frequent antecedents among patients with symptomatic epilepsy.

- NC patients also have a good prognosis in terms of remission of seizures. Anticysticercal treatment does not modify the risk of seizure recurrence.

- The mortality of epilepsy in Ecuador (SMR 6.3) is higher than that reported in developed countries. The SUDEP rate in our study is higher than that reported in the general population.

References

1. Placencia M, Sander JWAS, Shorvon SD, *et al.* Validation of a screening questionnaire for the detection of epileptic seizures in epidemiological studies. *Brain* 1992; 115: 783-94.
2. Placencia M, Shorvon SD, Paredes V, *et al.* Epileptic seizures in an andean region of Ecuador. Incidence an prevalence and regional variation. *Brain* 1992; 115: 771-82.
3. Carpio A, Bittencourt PRM. Epilepsy in the Tropics. In: Chopra JS, Sawney IMS (Eds.). Neurology in Tropics. New Delhi: B.I. Churchil-Livingstone Ltd, 1999: 527-32.
4. Carpio A, Hauser WA, Lisanti N, Aguirre R, Roman M, Pesantez M, Placencia M, *et al.* Prognosis of epilepsy in Ecuador: a preliminary report. *Epilepsia* 1999; 40 (Suppl 2): 110.
5. Bittencourt PR, Adamolekum B, Bharucha N, Carpio A, Cossio OH, *et al.* Epilepsy in the tropics: II. Clinical presentations, pathophysiology, immunologic diagnosis, economics, and therapy. *Epilepsia* 1996; 37: 1128-37.
6. Commission on Classification and Terminology of the International League Against Epilepsy: Proposal for revised clinical and electroencephalographic classification of seizures. *Epilepsia* 1981; 22: 489-501.
7. Commission on Classification and Terminology of the International League Against Epilepsy: proposal for revised classiffication of epilepsy and epileptic symdromes. *Epilepsia* 1989; 30: 389-99.
8. Commission on Epidemiology and Prognosis of the International League Against Epilepsy. Guidelines for Epidemiological Studies on Epilepsy. *Epilepsia* 1993; 35: 89-93.
9. Kaplan E, Meier P. Nonparametric estimation from incomplete observations. *J Am Stat Assoc* 1958; 53: 457-81.
10. Cox DR. Regression models and life-tables. *J R Stat Soc (B)* 1972; 34: 187-220.
11. Jallon P, Loiseau P, Loiseau J. Newly diagnosed unprovoked epileptic seizures: presentation at diagnosis in CAROLE study. Coordination Active du Reseau Observatoire Longitudinal de l'Epilepsie. *Epilepsia* 2001; 42: 464-75.
12. Carpio A. "Remote Symptomatic Epilepsies and Epileptic Syndromes"; In: Murthy JMK, Senanayake N (Eds.). Epilepsy in the Tropics. 2002, in press.
13. Berg AT, Shinnar S, Levy SR, Testa FM. Newly diagnosed epilepsy in children: presentation at diagnosis. *Epilepsia* 1999; 40: 445-52.
14. Shah KN, Rajadhyaksha S, Kanhere A, *et al.* Pattern and prevalence of epilepsies and epileptic syndromes in childhood in India. In Murthy JM. Epilepsy: The Indian Perspective. Hyderabad: Care Foundation. 1999: 35-60.
15. Sillanpaa M, Jalava M, Shinnar S. Epilepsy syndromes in patients with childhood-onset seizures in Finland. *Pediatr Neurol* 1999; 21: 533-7.
16. Murthy JM, Yangala R, Srinivas M. The syndromic classification of the International League Against Epilepsy: a hospital-based study from South India. *Epilepsia* 1998; 39: 48-54.
17. Senanayake N. Classification of epilepsies and epileptic syndromes using the 1989 International League Against Epilepsy Classification: a hospital-based study of 1 250 patients in a developing country. *Epilepsia* 1993; 34: 812-8.
18. Oka E, Istuda S, Outsuka I, Ohtahara S. Neuro-epidemiological study of childhood epilepsy by application of International Classification of epilepsies and epileptic syndromes (ILAE, 1989). *Epilepsia* 1995; 36: 658-61.
19. Shinnar S, O'Dell C, Berg AT. Distribution of epilepsy syndromes in a cohort of children prospectively monitored from the time of their first unprovoked seizure. *Epilepsia* 1999; 40: 1378-83.
20. Zarrelli MM, Beghi E, Rocca WA, Hauser WA. Incidence of epileptic syndromes in Rochester, Minnesota: 1980-1984. *Epilepsia* 1999; 40: 1708.
21. Waaler PE, Blom BH, Skeidsvoll H, Mykletun A. Prevalence, classification, and severity of epilepsy in children in western Norway. *Epilepsia* 2000; 41: 802-10.
22. Manford M, Hart YM, Sander JWAS, Shorvon SD. The National General Practice Study of Epilepsy: the syndromic classification of the International League Against Epilepsy applied to epilepsy in the general population. *Arch Neurol* 1992; 49: 801-8.
23. Sander JWA, Hart YM, Johnson AL, Shorvon SD. National general practice study of epilepsy. Newly diagnosed epileptic seizures in a general population. *Lancet* 1990; 336: 1267-71.
24. Forsgren L, Bucht G, Eriksson S, Bergmark L. Incidence and clinical characterization of unprovoked seizures in adults, a prospective population-based study. *Epilepsia* 1996; 37: 224-9.

25. Hauser WA, Annegers JF, Kurland LT. Incidence of Epilepsy and unprovoked seizures in Rochester, Minnesota: 1935-1984. *Epilepsia* 1993; 34: 453-68.
26. Carpio A. Epidemiology of Tropical Neurology in South America. In: Rose FC (Ed.). Recent Advances in Tropical Neurology. Amsterdam: Elsevier Sciences Publishers, 1995: 31-42.
27. Hauser WA, Rich SS, Annegers JF, Anderson VF. Seizure recurrence after a first unprovoked seizures: an extended follow-up. *Neurology* 1990; 40: 1163-70.
28. Hopkins A, Garman A, Clarke C. The first seizure in adult life. Value of clinical features, electroencephalography, and computerised tomographic scanning in prediction of seizures recurrence. *Lancet* 1988; 1: 721-6.
29. Cockerell OC, Johnson AL, Sander JW, Shorvon SD. Prognosis of epilepsy: a review and further analysis of the first nine years of the British National General Practice Study of Epilepsy, a prospective population-based study. *Epilepsia* 1997; 38: 31-46.
30. Semah F, Picot MC, Adam C, et al. Is the underlying cause of epilepsy a major prognostic factor for recurrence? *Neurology* 1998; 51: 1256-62.
31. Lindsten H, Stenlund H, Forsgren L. Remission of seizures in a population-based adult cohort with a newly diagnosed unprovoked epileptic seizure. *Epilepsia* 2001; 42: 1025-30.
32. MacDonald BK, Johnson AL, Goodridge DM, Cockerell OC, Sander JWAS, Shorvon SD. Factors predicting prognosis of epilepsy after presentation with seizures. *Ann Neurol* 2000; 48: 833-41.
33. Elwes RDC, Johnson AL, Shorvon SD, Reynolds EH. The prognosis for seizure control in newly diagnosed epilepsy. *N Engl J Med* 1994; 311: 944-7.
34. Hui ACF, Tang A, Wong KS, Mok V, Kay R. Recurrence after a first untreated seizure in the Hong Kong Chinese population. *Epilepsia* 2001; 42: 94-7.
35. Sillanpää M, Jalava M, Kaleva O, Shinnar S. Long-term prognosis of seizures with onset in childhood. *N Engl J Med* 1998; 338: 1715-22.
36. Arts WF, Geerts AT, Brouwer OF, Boudewyn Peters AC, Stroink H, et al. The early prognosis of epilepsy in childhood: the prediction of a poor outcome. The Dutch study of epilepsy in childhood. *Epilepsia* 1999; 40: 726-34.
37. Shinnar S, Berg AT, Moshé SL, et al. Risk of seizure recurrence after a first unprovoked afebrile seizure in childhood: an extended follow-up. *Pediatrics* 1996; 98: 216-25.
38. Camfield PR, Camfield CS, Dooley JM, et al. Epilepsy after a first unprovoked seizure in childhood. *Neurology* 1985; 35: 1657-60.
39. Carpay HA, Arts WFM, Geerts AT, Stroink H, Brouwer OF, Peters ACB, Van Donselaar CA. Epilepsy in childhood. An audit of clinical practice. *Arch Neurol* 1998; 55: 668-73.
40. Stroink H, Brouwer OF, Arts WF, Geerts AT, Peters AC, et al. The first unprovoked, untreated seizure in childhood: a hospital based study of the accuracy of the diagnosis, rate of recurrence, and long term outcome after recurrence. Dutch study of epilepsy in childhood. *J Neurol Neurosurg Psychiatry* 1998; 64: 595-600.
41. Hauser WA, Rich SS, Lee JR, Annegers JF, Anderson VE. Risk of recurrent seizures after two unprovoked seizures. *N Engl J Med* 1998; 338: 429-34.
42. Shinnar S, Berg AT, O'Dell C, et al. Predictors of multiple seizures in a cohort of children prospectively followed from the time of their first unprovoked seizures. *Ann Neurol* 2000; 48: 140-7.
43. Carpio A. Hauser WA, Lisanti N, Aguirre R, Roman M, Pesantez M, Barrionuevo C. Mortality of epilepsy in Ecuador. *Epilepsia* 2001; 42 (Suppl 2): 122.
44. O'Donoghue MF, Sander JWAS. The mortality associated with epilepsy, with particular reference to sudden unexpected death: a review. *Epilepsia* 1997; 38 (Suppl 11): S15-S19.
45. Hauser WA. Sudden unexpected death in patients with epilepsy: issues for further study. *Epilepsia* 1997; 38 (Suppl 11): S26-S29.
46. Leestma JE, Annegers JF, Brodie MJ, et al. Sudden unexpected death in epilepsy: observations from a large clinical development program. *Epilepsia* 1997; 38: 47-55.
47. Lindsten H, Nystrom L, Forsgren L. Mortality risk in an adult cohort with a newly diagnosed unprovoked epileptic seizure: a population-based study. *Epilepsia* 2000; 41: 1469-73.
48. King MA, Newton MR, Jackson GD, Fitt GJ, Mitchell LA, et al. Epileptology of the first-seizure presentation: a clinical, electroencephalographic, and magnetic resonance imaging study of 300 consecutive patients. *Lancet* 1998; 352: 1007-11.
49. Olafsson E, Hauser WA, Gudmundsson G. Long-term survival of people with unprovoked seizures: a population-based study. *Epilepsia* 1998; 39: 89-92.

50. Carpio A, Escobar A, Hauser WA. Cysticercosis and epilepsy: a critical review. *Epilepsia* 1998; 39: 1025-40.
51. Pal DK, Carpio A, Sander JWAS. Neurocysticercosis and Epilepsy. *J Neurol Neurosurg Psychiat* 2000; 68: 137-43.
52. Vázquez V, Sotelo J. The course of seizures after treatment for cerebral cysticercosis. *N Engl J Med* 1992; 327: 696-701.
53. Monteiro L, Nunes B, Mendonaca D, Lopes J. Spectrum of epilepsy in neurocysticercosis: a long-term follow-up of 143 patients. *Acta Neurol Scand* 1995; 92: 1, 33-40.
54. Carpio A, Hauser WA. Prognosis of first seizure in patients with neurocysticercosis. *Neurology* 2002 (in press).

The dutch study of epilepsy in childhood

Willem FM Arts*

Introduction

The Dutch Study of Epilepsy in Childhood is a prospective cohort study started in 1988. Its aims were to study various aspects of the prognosis of single seizures and epilepsy in childhood, explore the magnitude of the errors in the process of making the diagnosis of a single seizure or epilepsy, identify prognostically relevant variables with the intention to use them for the development of an individualised approach to treatment, and contribute to the discussion about the possible self-perpetuating nature of epileptic seizures.

Methods

During more than four years, all consecutive children, aged 1 month to 16 years, with a possible diagnosis of a single seizure or epilepsy from the University Hospitals in Rotterdam and Leiden as well as of the Juliana Children's Hospital and the Westeinde Hospital in The Hague, The Netherlands, were, after informed consent, recruited for the study and followed prospectively. Excluded were children with acute symptomatic seizures, children treated before with anti-epileptic drugs (AEDs) except for the treatment of neonatal seizures, and children whose referral was delayed for more than three months after the index seizure. Most children had been referred by their family physician (51%), the general paediatricians of the participating hospitals (25%) or came to the Emergency Room (16%). The estimated proportion of patients recruited was 75% of all children expected to develop epilepsy in the catchment area of the participating hospitals, based on an incidence rate of 40/100 000 per year.

---

* For the Dutch Study group on Epilepsy in Childhood. Besides the author, this group consists of O. Brouwer, B. Peters, H. Stroink, paediatric neurologists, C. van Donselaar, neurologist, A. Geerts, data manager and analyst, P. Schmitz, statistician. The study was financially supported by the Dutch National Epilepsy Fund.

The diagnosis of a seizure was made using predefined criteria, adapted from a Dutch study in adults [1]. A panel of three paediatric neurologists (excluding the treating paediatric neurologist) had to agree on the diagnosis after having received information about the event(s) from the letter to the family physician and a questionnaire completed by the recruiting paediatric neurologist. At that stage, the results of ancillary studies were not available to the panel. In the case of single events, disagreement between the members of the panel had to be solved by discussion. If the patient had had multiple events, the panel was also allowed to use the results of the EEG examination(s) in deciding on their nature.

Children with a clear diagnosis other than one or more seizures were not followed up. Children recruited after one or more unclear events were followed for one year to see whether any recurrence could shed more light on the nature of their events. After a single epileptic seizure, a child was followed for two years, unless after a recurrence, the diagnosis of epilepsy was made. All children with epilepsy (defined as two or more seizures) were followed for five years.

Epileptic seizures were classified by the panel according to the ILAE classification [2]. The epilepsy type was classified as partial or generalised with a subdivision as described by Aicardi [3]. After two years of follow-up, we reclassified the epilepsy type or syndrome according to the ILAE classification [4] that had been published after the start of our study. At that moment, we also checked whether the initial diagnosis of epilepsy had been correct. The aetiology was derived from the ILAE classification and was categorised as remote symptomatic (including mental retardation), cryptogenic and idiopathic [5, 6].

Possibly predictive variables were defined a priori and collected at intake and after six months of follow-up. All children had an EEG, supplemented with an EEG after partial sleep deprivation in those who had not shown epileptiform abnormalities in their standard EEG. Imaging studies were performed in all children, if necessary under general anaesthesia, unless the child had typical absences or if the treating paediatric neurologist did not consider it indicated. In most children, this was a CT scan, supplemented later by MRI if necessary.

After a single seizure, a child was not treated with an AED, unless the child had had a status epilepticus. After a single status, after one or more recurrences, or if the child had presented with multiple seizures, the treating paediatric neurologist was free to decide on prescribing treatment or not. He also selected the AED, but had to prescribe monotherapy with at least two first-line drugs successively before deciding on polytherapy.

After two and five years of follow-up, endpoints were determined using terminal seizure-free intervals (terminal remission, TR) as the main outcome criterion. A TR of less than six months after two years was defined as "poor", as was a TR of less than one year after five years.

Statistical analysis was done with SPSS. Univariate and multivariate stepwise backward analyses were performed to identify possibly relevant variables. For the analyses after five years, a modelling strategy was used [7]. The procedures followed were described more elaborately before [8-10].

Composition of the cohort

The cohort contains 881 children referred after one or more possibly epileptic events *(figure 1)*. After discussion in the panel, 121 children with a definite other diagnosis were excluded from follow-up. 224 Children were referred after a single event; 170 were considered to have had a definite seizure. Of these, 31 had been referred before the start of

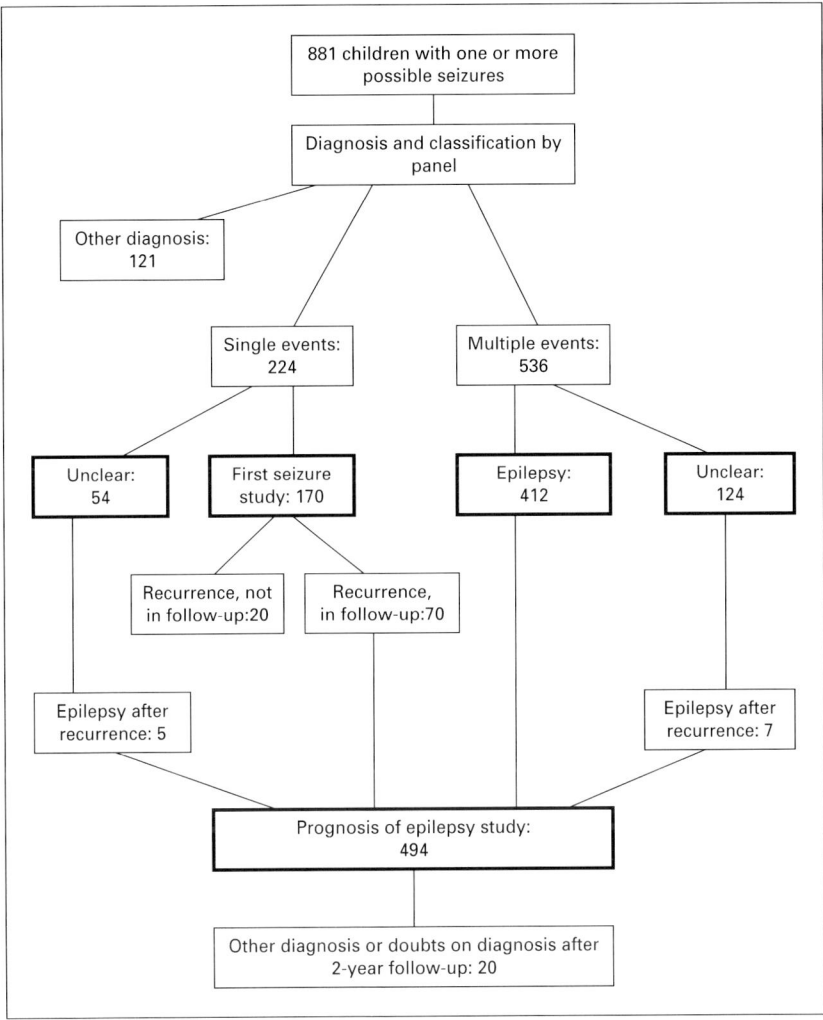

Figure 1. Flow chart of the DSEC cohort. Groups of children in accentuated squares have been followed prospectively to analyse their outcomes.

the prognosis of epilepsy study, and therefore, 20 children with a recurrence out of these 31 were not included in the 5-year cohort. Of the remaining 139 children, 70 had a recurrence, and were followed for five years like all children with epilepsy. Of the 54 children who were considered to have had an unclear event, 14 had a recurrence. Five of these were diagnosed as epilepsy and added to the 5-year cohort, but one was again removed at two years because the diagnosis was still not clear (the child probably had event-related vagal spells).

After multiple events, 536 were referred; 412 were considered to have epilepsy. Three children received another diagnosis during follow-up, and in 16, doubts on the diagnosis after two years were such that they were not included in the 5-year cohort. In 124, the diagnosis at intake was unclear; 72 had at least one recurrence within one year. Seven of the latter were diagnosed as epilepsy.

Diagnosis

Reliability

This part of the study was undertaken to assess the inter-observer agreement on the diagnosis of a single paroxysmal event in childhood. The description of the events of 100 children out of 233 (170 deemed to have had an epileptic seizure, 54 an unclear event and 9 an event of definitely other nature) were submitted to six paediatric neurologists, grouped in two panels, one consisting of three observers experienced in this interactive approach, and the other of three observers not used to working in this way. They were asked to answer the question whether the event had been a seizure, first on the basis of their clinical insight, and secondly on the basis of the predefined descriptive criteria for the diagnosis of a seizure mentioned above. Next, the observers classified the type of seizure and its mode of onset. The results were then discussed within each panel. Finally, data on the EEG and imaging studies were provided and the panels were asked to score the aetiology and make a syndrome diagnosis, if at all possible. Intra- and inter-panel agreement was calculated with the help of kappa statistics.

The agreement on the epileptic nature of the event was only moderate (median kappa 0.44, range 0.19-0.52). The use of the criteria improved the agreement slightly but not significantly (median 0.48, range 0.23-0.56). The inter-panel agreement after intra-panel discussion was 0.60. Without and with use of predefined criteria, the median kappa for partial or generalised seizure onset was 0.47 (range 0.32-0.60) and 0.54 (range 0.37-0.66), respectively, and for seizure classification 0.45 (range 0.29-0.60) and 0.60 (range 0.34-0.69). Inter-panel agreement after intra-panel discussion reached 0.68 without and 0.69 with criteria. In all analyses, the experienced panel scored slightly but not significantly better than the inexperienced panel. The agreement on aetiology between the panels after intra-panel discussion was 0.75, but for syndrome diagnosis only 0.40. The latter figure was due to a discrepancy in the way of classifying seizures with unclear onset. The experienced panel used the classification "isolated seizure or isolated status" or "epilepsy without obvious generalised or partial features"; the other panel tried to classify each of these as either "cryptogenic localisation-related" or "idiopathic generalised not otherwise defined" [11].

We conclude that these results are disappointing both from a clinical and from a scientific point of view. Insufficient description or unstructured history taking may have caused the disagreement, and the use of predefined criteria does not appear to improve it. Only discussion between (groups of) specialists in the field may improve the agreement, but it is far from the level necessary to call the result a "gold standard" for the diagnosis of a seizure. Moreover, under daily-life clinical circumstances, larger error margins between observers may be present.

Whatever their cause, the apparent mistakes in the diagnosis of a single seizure (both false positive and false negative) may have important consequences for the life of that particular child. Studies on single seizures, in which one or more single observers have made the diagnosis, may contain children with a false-positive diagnosis and may have missed children with a false-negative diagnosis. Perhaps this is one of the explanations for the widely discrepant recurrence ratios reported in the literature [12]. Moreover, clinically relevant syndrome classification is after one seizure possible in only a small minority of the children [11].

Accuracy

Since there is no gold standard for the diagnosis of one or more epileptic seizures, we tried to confirm or disprove the original diagnoses made by the panel by checking them after follow-up. Of 170 children with a diagnosis of a single seizure, none proved to have another diagnosis after two years of follow-up. Of the 54 children recruited after a single unclear event, 14 had a recurrence within one year. Of these, five were considered to have epilepsy after one year, but in one of these five, the correctness of this diagnosis was again doubted after two years of follow-up (false positive rate 0%, 95% confidence interval [CI] 0-2.8%; false-negative rate 7.4%; 95% CI 2.4-18.7%; sensitivity 97.7%, specificity 100%).

A diagnosis of epilepsy was made in 412 children seen after multiple events. After two years of follow-up, this diagnosis appeared to be incorrect in 3, and was doubted in 16. In contrast, seven out of 124 children with multiple unclear events at intake received a diagnosis of epilepsy after one year of follow-up (false-positive rate 4.6%, 95% CI 2.9-7.2%; false-negative rate 5.6%, 95% CI 2.5-11.7%; sensitivity 98.3%, specificity 86.0%) [13].

In conclusion, even with the use of the rigid diagnostic procedures of the DSEC, we made a fair amount of false-positive and false-negative diagnoses. We suppose that our findings are a minimum estimate, since these figures will probably be higher in more usual clinical and research situations. Therefore, we recommend that studies on the prognosis of epilepsy always check the initial diagnosis after follow-up, and remove cases with an incorrect diagnosis from the analysis. On the basis of the findings in our reliability and accuracy studies, a reasonable error margin for the diagnosis of epilepsy should be kept in mind when judging studies on single seizures or newly diagnosed epilepsy [13].

Value of the EEG

A standard EEG was obtained in almost all children after referral. In children with single or multiple seizures according to the panel, 56% of the standard EEGs showed epileptiform abnormalities (59% in children with epilepsy, 46% in children after a single seizure; p = 0.005). Of the 243 children without epileptiform discharges, 73% had a second EEG, performed after partial sleep deprivation (PSD) according to a protocol that defined the amount of sleep deprivation for three age groups. The yield of epileptiform discharges in the PSD EEG was 35%, bringing the yield in the entire group to 67%, and in the group who had had two EEGs to 76% [14].

In the 412 children with epilepsy according to the panel, the diagnosis was based on the clinical history alone in 367 and the EEG results had to be invoked in 45. In three of these 45, the diagnosis was doubted after follow-up. As mentioned above, the number of incorrect or at least doubtful diagnoses of epilepsy amounted to 20 (six with epileptiform EEG abnormalities, 14 without), of whom one had first been labelled as unclear, later as epilepsy, and finally again as unclear, probably vasovagal syncope.

The true positive rate of epileptiform EEG abnormalities in either EEG for the diagnosis of a single epileptic seizure or epilepsy was 89.8% for children after a single paroxysmal event, and 90.1% in children with multiple events. The true negative rate of the absence of epileptiform discharges for any diagnosis other than epilepsy was 33.6% after a single event and 46.9% after multiple events (sensitivity in case of a single event 55.7%, specificity 78%; sensitivity in case of multiple events 70.3%, specificity 77.2%) [14].

Syndrome (re-)classification

Of 494 children with epilepsy, 466 could be followed for at least two years. In these children, the initial classification of the epilepsy type and syndrome was compared with the classification after follow-up. *Table I* details the distribution of the epilepsy types according to the diagnosis at intake and after two years of follow-up. After two years, the classification had to be revised in 32 children (6.9%).

Table I. Distribution of epilepsy types and syndromes at intake and after two years

	Intake (%)	After two years of follow-up (%)
Idiopathic partial epilepsy	28 (6.0)	28 (6.0)
All non-idiopathic partial	143 (30.7)	155 (33.3)
Symptomatic partial epilepsy		69 (14.8)
Cryptogenic partial epilepsy		86 (18.5)
Idiopathic generalised epilepsy	215 (46.1)	194 (41.6)
Absence epilepsy	59 (12.7)	55 (11.8)
Infantile myoclonic epilepsy	8 (1.7)	10 (2.1)
Juvenile myoclonic epilepsy	11 (2.4)	8 (1.7)
Other idiopathic generalised	137 (29.4)	121 (26.0)
All non-idiopathic generalised	51 (10.9)	71 (15.2)
Symptomatic generalised epilepsy		37 (7.9)
Cryptogenic generalised epilepsy		34 (7.3)
Unclear	29 (6.2)	18 (3.9)

We paid special attention to the group of children with non-symptomatic generalised epilepsy who were less than six years of age at intake. In this age group, children in whom syndrome classification at intake is ambiguous or even impossible are seen repeatedly. Some syndromes may overlap, and the literature is not always clear about their delineation. Some children do not comply with the criteria for any syndrome. Moreover, the definition of at least some syndromes seems to depend also on the evolution of the clinical picture, making it necessary to dispose of follow-up data for a correct classification. Examples could be the various types of epilepsy with myoclonic seizures, atonic seizures or atypical absences seen especially in this age group.

Intake and follow-up data of 111 children with a diagnosis of idiopathic or cryptogenic generalised epilepsy (IGE or CGE) either at intake and/or after follow-up were compared. 96 children were classified as IGE both at intake and after two years; however, the majority of them (64) could only be classified as idiopathic generalised epilepsy not otherwise defined, a category that almost certainly contains a number of different syndromes that at present cannot be differentiated. In addition, nine children who received this classification at intake were reclassified: two within the IGE group, but seven to a syndrome with far worse prognostic consequences. Only three children were classified at intake as cryptogenic generalised epilepsy other than West or Lennox-Gastaut syndrome; twice, this diagnosis was maintained and once, the diagnosis changed to benign myoclonic epilepsy of infancy. It should be noted that in this cohort we did not encounter children with severe myoclonic epilepsy (Dravet syndrome), but we did see 10 children with benign myoclonic epilepsy. Reasons for reclassification after follow-up were the occurrence of an additional seizure type, incorrect initial seizure classification (better information or video registrations became available later), or new information about the causal diagnosis [15].

Prognosis

Single seizure

Of 170 children considered by the panel to have presented with a single epileptic seizure (not status epilepticus), 90 (53%) had a recurrence. After exclusion of 14 children (ten because it was deemed possible that fever had elicited the seizure, one because he was accidentally treated with AED, and three because the no-treatment policy was left after multiple recurrences associated with fever), 156 children remained in the analysis of whom 85 suffered a recurrence (54%, 95% CI 46-62%) [8]. Significant variables predictive of a recurrence were aetiology (remote symptomatic) and EEG (epileptiform discharges).

The outcome after two years of the children, who had presented with a single seizure and suffered one or more recurrences, was generally good. The terminal remission (TR) was more than 12 months in 50 children (59%) – 20 of these never had a second recurrence –, 6-12 months in 11 children (12.9%), less than six months in 22 children (25.9%), while two children (2.4%) were lost. 66 Children out of the 85 children with a recurrence were followed for five years with the following results: 41 (62.1%) TR more than two years, eight TR more than one year (12.1%), 17 children TR less than one year (25.8%). Nine out of these 17 had a TR of less than six months at two years after intake (52.9%, i.e. 5.8% of the 156 children in the inception cohort).

We conclude that not starting AED treatment after a single seizure does not worsen the long-term outcome, and therefore, continue to prefer a no-treatment policy in children who present with a single unprovoked seizure.

Do seizures beget seizures?

582 children entered the study with one (170) or multiple (412) epileptic seizures. Twelve children changing from an uncertain diagnosis to epilepsy were added after one-year follow-up. Of these 594 patients, 31 with a single seizure entered the study before August 1, 1988, the official starting date of the prognosis part of the DSEC. To avoid bias, these 31 were excluded from the follow-up studies. Of the remaining 563, 261 had generalised tonic-clonic seizures only. The numbers of seizures and the intervals between them were exactly known in 204 [16]. These children were followed until the start of drug treatment (78), the occurrence of the fourth untreated seizure (41) or the end of the two-year follow-up period (85 untreated children). The length of the successive intervals between the seizures was analysed on a per-patient basis. We distinguished an accelerating pattern (intervals decreased), a decelerating pattern (intervals increased or child became seizure-free without treatment), an erratic pattern (intervals varied) and an uncertain pattern (follow-up after last seizure was too short, or the pattern was impossible to assess because treatment was instituted too early). Ten children were treated after their first seizure (because it had been a status epilepticus), 46 after their second seizure and 22 after their third. Of these 22, the first interval was longer than the second in 14 children, and the reverse was true in eight. These 22 were nevertheless classified as uncertain because a pattern could not be distinguished after only two inter-seizure intervals. After four or more untreated seizures, the pattern was decelerating in three, accelerating in eight and erratic in 30 children. Of the 85 children, who remained without treatment until the end of the two-year follow-up, 83 had a decelerating pattern (having become seizure-free after one (60 children), two (15) or three (8) seizures). In two, the pattern was uncertain, because the last seizure occurred too close to the end of the follow-up to assess the seizure pattern. In summary, the pattern

was decelerating in 86 children (42%, 95% CI 35-49%), uncertain in 110 (54%) and accelerating in eight (4%).

Our conclusion was that the fear that seizures commonly evolve into a progressive disorder with a self-perpetuating mechanism (Gowers' dictum: "Seizures beget seizures") should not be considered as an argument in favour of early treatment of children who present with one or a few generalised tonic-clonic seizures.

Status epilepticus

Presentation by status epilepticus (SE) occurred in 41 children out of the cohort of 494 children with epilepsy. In nine children, the SE was not the child's first seizure, but it was the reason to come to the hospital. Four children had had two or more episodes of SE before presentation; one of these had simple partial SE and one had complex partial SE. After intake, 18 children had at least one SE. In six of these, this was the only SE, the others had also had a SE before presentation. Altogether, 47 children had at least one SE.

When comparing these 47 with all patients without any SE (n = 447), there was a tendency towards a worse outcome two years after intake for the patients with at least one SE, although not significant (TR2 less than 6 months: 40.4% versus 28.6%). Five years after intake, this difference became significant (TR5 less than 1 year: 34.0% versus 21.3%; $p < 0.05$). Remarkably, this difference seemed to be due to the six children who only had a SE after intake. These six children all had a TR of less than six months two years after intake (TR2). Five years after intake, three of these patients still had a poor outcome (TR5 less than one year), one a TR5 of more than one year and for two patients the TR5 could not be assessed. There was no significant difference between all patients without SE and the children who had had a SE before intake: 32% of the latter had a TR2 of less than six months and 32% a TR5 of less than one year. This suggests that a status epilepticus before intake at least in this cohort was not associated with a worse outcome as compared with children who had not had a status epilepticus.

Mortality

For the determination of the mortality, 472 out of the 494 children with a diagnosis of epilepsy could be followed for five years or until death [17]. Nine children died during the follow-up (five boys, four girls), amounting to a mortality rate of 3.8/1 000 person-years. This gives a Standardised Mortality Ratio (SMR) of 7.0 (95% CI 2.4-11.5). For boys, this was 6.6 and for girls 7.4. All deceased children had symptomatic epilepsy and no child conformed to the criteria of Sudden Unexplained Death in Epilepsy (SUDEP). Death in idiopathic epilepsy of childhood may be extremely rare, as is SUDEP in children [17].

Audit of treatment policies

During the course of the study, the treating paediatric neurologists were within certain limits (see Methods paragraph) free to choose the treatment options they preferred. After two to five years of follow-up (endpoint August 1994), we performed an audit of treatment strategies and their results [18].

Within the first three months after intake, the treating paediatric neurologists decided not to treat 29% of the children. Two years after intake, 82 children (17%) had not yet received AED treatment. For this group, the outcome after two years was significantly better than for those who used AED (TR > 1 year 79% vs. 52%). Most of the untreated children had sporadic generalised tonic-clonic seizures; rolandic seizures were only a small minority.

Carbamazepine and sodium valproate were the first-choice AEDs used in almost 90% of the children treated. After two years, 80% were still on monotherapy. The initial AED failed in 40% of the children mainly because of recurrent seizures (28%) and/or intolerable side effects (11%). After the first monotherapy trial, children were treated alternatively with one or more additional monotherapy regimens or with a polytherapy regimen. The number of regimens tried was inversely related to the outcome: after three different regimens, the chance of a TR > 1 year after two years of follow-up was only 10%, and after four regimens, the odds were zero.

Fifty children were after two years of follow-up considered as really intractable. Eighteen of them had not had any change in AED treatment during the last six months of follow-up. In a structured interview, the treating neurologists stated about these 18 children that seizure control had been acceptable in 15 (based on their seizure frequency and/or seizure severity), and that there had been no further treatment options in three of them.

We concluded that experienced paediatric neurologists are able to distinguish at intake a number of children who will not need AED treatment at all. Next, the chances of successful treatment become less after every unsuccessful AED trial and perhaps even negligible after four or more trials. Finally, a child may have acceptable seizure control if the frequency and severity of the seizures has been sufficiently reduced (be it as a consequence of the treatment or not) and need not necessarily become completely seizure-free. Usually, this concerned children who were also seriously handicapped otherwise.

Early withdrawal of medication

One hundred sixty-one children were eligible for withdrawal of AEDs after a short seizure-free period. They were selected because they had become seizure-free within two months after starting treatment and had remained seizure-free for six months after their last seizure. At that point, they were, after informed consent, randomised for either immediate AED withdrawal or continuation of AED therapy for another six months and, if possible, withdrawal at that time. Kaplan-Meier estimates of remission after 24 months were practically equal in both groups (51 vs. 52%). In the group treated for one year, 12% of the recurrences occurred while the child was still treated. In the multivariate analysis, type of epilepsy and age at intake were the only significant risk factors for a relapse. Older age was associated with a higher risk of recurrence after withdrawal, as were symptomatic and cryptogenic partial epilepsy as compared with idiopathic generalised epilepsy. Epileptiform EEG abnormalities before withdrawal were significant in the univariate analysis, but did not remain so in the multivariate analysis.

The overall outcome of this subgroup of the DSEC was favourable. After a median follow-up of 42 months (range 6 to 61 months), a terminal remission of at least one year was attained by 81%. In children with a recurrence, no significant difference between the groups with 6-month and 12-month treatment was found; terminal remission of at least one year occurred in 60 and 66%, respectively [19].

We concluded that early withdrawal of AEDs in a subgroup of children with newly diagnosed epilepsy, selected on the basis of a fast response to AED treatment, is not harmful for the overall prognosis. In more than 50% of the children, recurrences did not occur, justifying the early AED withdrawal. In the other children, the occurrence of a relapse did not influence the overall outcome as compared to the children who had been treated continuously.

Follow-up of newly diagnosed epilepsy during two and five years

Out of the entire cohort, 466 children with epilepsy could be followed for two years and 453 for five years. Eight patients died and five were lost. The outcome of the 453 children could be determined reliably, and was expressed in terms of terminal remission (TR) [9].

Two years after intake, 31% had a TR of less than six months, and 57% of more than one year. Seizure type, type of epilepsy, aetiology, pre-existing neurological signs, CT-scan, number of seizures and 3-month remission during the first six months after intake, and the EEG made after six months were significant univariate predictors of a poor outcome. With stepwise backward multivariate analysis, the intake variables seizure type and number of seizures before intake remained significant. When the variables collected after six months of follow-up were also considered, the most significant variables were a 3-month remission and the number of seizures during these six months.

After five years, 76% attained a TR of one year or more, and 64% a TR of more than two years. Of the 108 children with a TR of less than one year, 24 (22%, 5% of 453) had seizures every month of that last year of follow-up. There was an excellent correlation between the "good" outcome after two and five years. Of the patients with a terminal remission of more than one year after two years of follow-up, 89% had a similar outcome after five years. Of the patients with a TR less than 1 year two years after intake, however, only 41% still had this outcome at the end of the 5-year follow-up, suggesting the possibility of improvement later in the course of the epilepsy for a substantial number of patients. In the univariate analysis, type of epilepsy, aetiology and postictal signs were significant intake variables for a TR of less than one year after five years. The number of seizures and the occurrence of a 3-month remission during the first six months of follow-up, as well as the length of the TR and the EEG results after six months were even more significant. In the multivariate regression model with intake variables only, we found a number of variables to be predictive for the outcome, but only under well-defined conditions (interaction terms; see *table II*). These variables were: aetiology (non-idiopathic versus idiopathic, but only if the number of seizures before intake had been less than 25, and if the child had not had any febrile seizures); age (below versus above four, but only if the EEG was abnormal); EEG (abnormal versus normal, but only if the age at intake was below four); number of seizures before intake (more than 25 seizures versus less than 25) and a history of febrile convulsions (yes versus no), but the latter two variables only if the aetiology was idiopathic. With the intake and 6-month variables combined, we found the following variables to be significant: age (if the EEG did not show abnormalities, age below four was associated with a reduced risk); EEG (if the age at intake was below four); postictal signs; and a TR of less than two months during the first six months of follow-up. It was possible to calculate a prognostic model for a TR of less than 12 months after five years of follow-up *(table II)*.

We concluded that epilepsy in childhood generally has a good prognosis. More than 75% of our cohort remained free of seizures during the last year of follow-up and only about 5% could be considered to be really intractable. Aetiology, type of epilepsy, and – most importantly – the course of the epilepsy during the first half year after the intake were common predictive variables for the outcome both after two years (TR < 6 months) and after five years (TR < 1 year) in the univariate analyses [9]. The early course of the epilepsy was also highly important in the multivariate analyses. This is in accordance with other prospective studies, e.g. the NGPSE [20]. It remains to be seen whether this is due to a pre-existing epileptic disposition of the patient, or really to the influence of the early course on the later outcome. This dilemma can only be solved in a randomised trial.

Table II. Odds ratios (OR) and 95% confidence intervals of the intake, and the intake and 6-month variables, respectively, for a terminal remission (TR) of less than 1 year after 5 years of follow-up. Logistic regression model with interaction

	Odds ratios (95% C.I.)	
	intake variables	intake and 6-month variables
Number of observations	453	453
Number of covariate patterns	88	128
Pearson chi2 (74)	76.44	113.3
Prob > chi2	0.46	0.55
Area under ROC curve	0.72	0.75
INTAKE		
sex (male/female)	1.41 (0.88, 2.27)	1.38 (0.86, 2.23)
pre-existing neurological signs (absent/present)	1.26 (0.65, 2.43)	1.05 (0.49, 2.27)
age at intake (> 4/< = 4 years)		
if age x EEG = 0	0.52 (0.189, 1.43)	0.33 (0.12, 0.91)*
if age x EEG = 1	2.19 (1.24, 3.87)*	1.59 (0.91, 2.78)&
EEG at intake (normal/abnormal)		
if EEG x age = 0	0.55 (0.24, 1.22)	0.56 (0.26, 1.21)
if EEG x age = 1	2.30 (0.98, 5.41)*	2.72 (1.15, 6.43)*
no. of seizures before intake (< = 25/> 25)		
if no. of seizures x aetiology = 0	2.82 (1.25, 6.34)*	
if no. of seizures x aetiology = 1	0.64 (0.34, 1.20)	
aetiology (idiopathic/not idiopathic)		
if aetiol x no. of seiz = 0 and aetiol febrile seiz = 0	6.15 (2.97, 12.75)***	
if aetiol x no. of seiz = 1 and aetiol febrile seiz = 0	1.39 (0.62, 3.13)	
if aetiol x no. of seiz = 0 and aetiol febrile seiz = 1	1.15 (0.29, 4.63)	
if aetiol x no. of seiz = 1 and aetiol febrile seiz = 1	0.26 (0.06, 1.13)	
if aetiology x febrile seizures = 0		1.57 (0.86, 2.87)
if aetiology x febrile seizures = 1		0.75 (0.14, 3.89)
febrile seizures (no/yes)		
if febrile seizures x aetiology = 0	4.41 (1.65, 11.79)**	
if febrile seizures x aetiology = 1	0.83 (0.30, 2.31)	
postictal signs (no/yes)	1.92 (0.95, 3.90)	2.72 (1.34, 5.51)**
6 MONTHS AFTER INTAKE		
3-month remission (no/yes)		0.56 (0.30, 1.04)
terminal remission		
6 months (no/yes)		1.00
2 to 6 months (no/yes)		1.33 (0.68, 2.59)
0 to 2 months (no/yes)		3.44 (1.61, 7.36)**

& 0.05 < p < 0.10; * p < 0.05; ** p < 0.01; *** p < 0.001.

If the highest category (female, present, < = 4 years of age at intake, etc.) for a particular variable is present in a patient, the value of that variable is set at 1, otherwise at 0. The value of the interaction terms can only be 1, if the conditional variable is 1.

The Odds Ratio's of each variable in a model can be transformed into coefficients. The constant of the model with "intake and 6-month variables" is – 1.33. When each coefficient is multiplied by 10 and rounded, the following Score can be derived: 3 x (sex) + 0.5 x (pre-existing neurological abnormalities) – 11 x (age at intake) – 6 x (intake EEG) + 16 x (interaction term of age and EEG) + 4.5 x (aetiology) – 7.5 x (interaction term of aetiology and febrile convulsions) + 10 x (postictal signs) – 6 x (3-month remission) + 3 x (terminal remission of 2-6 months) + 12 x (terminal remission of 0-2 months) – 13.

The odds for a TR < 1 year after 5-year follow-up are calculated using the formula P = 1/(1+ e^{-z}), in which Z = Score/10. In the model, the value of P ranged from 0.046 to 0.796.

References

1. Van Donselaar CA, Geerts AT, Meulstee J, Habbema JDF, Staal A. Reliability of the diagnosis of a first seizure. *Neurology* 1989; 39: 267-71.
2. Commission on Classification and Terminology of the International League Against Epilepsy. Proposal for revised clinical and electroencephalographic classification of epileptic seizures. *Epilepsia* 1981; 22: 489-501.

3. Aicardi J. Epileptic syndromes in childhood. *Epilepsia* 1988; 29: S1-S5.
4. Commission on Classification and Terminology of the International League Against Epilepsy. Proposal for revised classification of epilepsies and epileptic syndromes. *Epilepsia* 1989; 30: 89-99.
5. Hauser WA, Kurland LT. The epidemiology of epilepsy in Rochester, Minnesota, 1935 through 1967. *Epilepsia* 1975; 16: 1-66.
6. Commission on Epidemiology and Prognosis of the International League Against Epilepsy. Guidelines for epidemiologic studies on epilepsy. *Epilepsia* 1993; 34: 592-6.
7. Harrell FE Jr, Lee KL, Mark DB. Multivariable prognostic models: issues indeveloping models, evaluating assumptions and adequacy, and measuring and reducing errors. *Stat Med* 1996; 15: 361-87.
8. Stroink H, Brouwer OF, Arts WF, Geerts AT, Peters ACB, Van Donselaar CA. The first unprovoked, untreated seizure in childhood: a hospital based study of the accuracy of the diagnosis, rate of recurrence, and long-term outcome after recurrence. Dutch study of epilepsy in childhood. *J Neurol Neurosurg Psych* 1998; 64: 595-600.
9. Arts WFM, Geerts AT, Brouwer OF, Peters ACB, Stroink H, Van Donselaar CA. The early prognosis of epilepsy in childhood: the prediction of a poor outcome. The Dutch study of epilepsy in childhood. *Epilepsia* 1999; 40: 726-34.
10. Arts WFM, Geerts AT, Brouwer OF, Peters ACB, Stroink H, Van Donselaar CA, Schmitz PM. Five-year follow-up of a cohort of children with newly diagnosed epilepsy. The Dutch study of epilepsy in childhood. In preparation.
11. Stroink H, Van Donselaar CA, Geerts AT, Peters ACB, Brouwer OF, Van Nieuwenhuizen O, De Coo IFM, Geesink H, Arts WFM. Reliability of the diagnosis and classification of a first seizure in childhood. Dutch Study of epilepsy in childhood. Submitted.
12. Berg AT, Shinnar S. The risk of seizure recurrence following a first unprovoked seizure: a quantitative review. *Neurology* 1991; 41: 965-72.
13. Stroink H, Van Donselaar CA, Geerts AT, Peters ACB, Brouwer OF, Arts WFM. The accuracy of the diagnosis of paroxysmal event(s) in children. Dutch study of epilepsy in childhood. Submitted.
14. Carpay JA, De Weerd AW, Schimsheimer RJ, Stroink H, Brouwer OF, Peters ACB, Van Donselaar CA, Geerts AT, Arts WFM. The diagnostic yield of a second EEG after partial sleep deprivation: a prospective study in children with newly diagnosed seizures. *Epilepsia* 1997; 38: 595-9.
15. Middeldorp CM, Geerts AT, Brouwer OF, Peters ACB, Stroink H, Van Donselaar CA, Arts WFM. Non-symptomatic generalized epilepsy in children under six: axcellent prognosis, but classification should be reconsidered after follow-up. The Dutch study of epilepsy in childhood. *Epilepsia* 2001.
16. Van Donselaar CA, Brouwer OF, Geerts AT, Arts WFM, Stroink H, Peters ACB. Clinical course of untreated tonic-clonic seizures in childhood: prospective, hospital-based study. *Brit Med J* 1997; 314: 401-4.
17. Callenbach PMC, Westendorp RGJ, Geerts AT, Arts WFM, Peters EAJ, Van Donselaar CA, Peters ACB, Stroink H, Brouwer OF. Mortality risk in children with epilepsy: the Dutch Study of Epilepsy in Childhood. *Pediatrics* 2001; 107: 1259-63.
18. Carpay HA, Arts WFM, Geerts AT, Stroink H, Brouwer OF, Peters ACB, Van Donselaar CA. Epilepsy in childhood. An audit of clinical practice. *Arch Neurol* 1998; 55: 668-73.
19. Peters ACB, Brouwer OF, Geerts AT, Arts WFM, Stroink H, Van Donselaar CA. Randomized prospective study of early discontinuation of antiepileptic drugs in children with epilepsy. *Neurology* 1998; 50: 724-30.
20. MacDonald BK, Johnson AL, Goodridge DM, Cockerell OC, Sander JWAS, Shorvon SD. Factors predicting prognosis of epilepsy after presentation with seizures. *Ann Neurol* 2000; 48: 833-41.

Nova Scotia pediatric epilepsy study

Peter and Carol Camfield

The epilepsies of infancy and childhood have many different etiologies, seizure manifestations, remission rates and social outcomes. The Nova Scotia cohort includes all children identified in the Province of Nova Scotia who developed epilepsy between 1977 and 1985 with follow up to assess seizure and social outcomes. These children represent a complete population-based cohort.

Although the sample size is substantial (total n = 693), if all the ILAE epilepsy syndrome categories are considered separately, there are many categories too small for statistical analysis. Therefore, we have created three groups of patients. *Group 1* (n = 511) (Partial and Generalized Tonic-Clonic Epilepsies) is composed of syndromes characterized by generalized tonic-clonic seizures, partial seizures with secondary generalization and partial seizures. *Group 2* (n = 97) (Absence Epilepsies) is composed of syndromes characterized, at least at onset, by absence seizures. *Group 3* (n = 85) (Secondary Generalized Epilepsies) includes syndromes characterized by akinetic/atonic seizures, infantile spasms, myoclonus, atypical absence and tonic seizures.

Many of our studies have focused on one of the three groups at a time. The methods for the individual studies are noted in each of the sections below. This chapter explains the method for identification of the cohort and the basic epilepsy features of the children. We then discuss the incidence of epilepsy and mortality. Next, we focus on seizure outcome (rates of remission) and finally social outcome.

Cohort assembly

Investigational area and population [1]

The Province of Nova Scotia has a population of approximately 850 000, and 50% of people live in rural areas. Comprehensive, universally accessible and portable medical insurance has been available to all residents since 1969. The IWK Health Centre in Halifax is the only tertiary pediatric centre for the province. All pediatric neurologists are located

Case finding and study design

One of our earliest studies found that virtually all children presenting to a physician with a first afebrile, unprovoked seizure would have an EEG requested [2]. Therefore, we were confident that all children with two or more unprovoked seizures who were seen by a physician would have an EEG available. We continue to interpret all pediatric EEG records for the Province and provide all pediatric neurologic services. Hence, EEG records were a comprehensive source to identify children with newly developed epilepsy.

By reviewing approximately 15 000 pediatric EEG reports from 1997 to 1985, 4 000 children were identified with a possible history of one or more afebrile seizures. After careful review of the hospital and pediatric neurology charts, and phone calls to the family doctor and family to limit cases to those with two or more definite afebrile, unprovoked seizures, 693 children were confirmed to have newly diagnosed epilepsy. A variety of other information about each child and their seizure disorder was then coded.

More than 95% of these children were followed during the course of their epilepsy by the four Halifax-based pediatric neurologists. Children were included and followed if they had moved out of the province after diagnosis. In all cases, the last contact was directly with us, either in person or by telephone.

Inclusion and exclusion criteria

Inclusion criteria were residence in Nova Scotia at the time of the first 2 unprovoked seizures between 1977 and 1985, and age at first seizure between 1 month and 16 years. Children with neonatal seizures were included only if seizures had stopped by the time of neonatal discharge and later recurred without provocation.

Children were excluded if there were acute provoking factors for their seizures (e.g. febrile seizures only, seizures within 7 days of head injury) or if they had evidence of progressive neurologic disease (e.g. brain tumor or progressive metabolic disorder). Those with seizures only during the neonatal period were excluded.

Cohort description [3]

Overall, there were 347 boys and 346 girls with new onset epilepsy. The initial seizure type is shown in *figure 1* and included: *Group 1*, Partial and Generalized Tonic-Clonic Epilepsies n = 511 (generalized tonic clonic seizures n = 130, partial seizures with or without secondary generalization n = 369, and unclassified n = 12); *Group 2*, Absence Epilepsies n = 97; *Group 3* Secondary Generalized Epilepsies n = 85.

The clinical features of the Nova Scotia Epilepsy Study cohort are shown in *table I*.

Incidence of childhood epilepsy [3]

Additional Methodology: The entire cohort of 693 children was used for analysis.

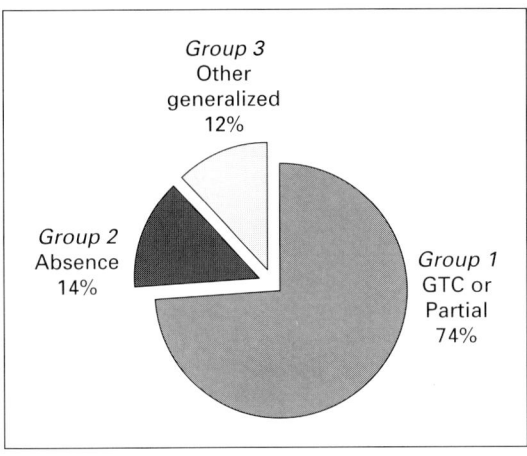

Figure 1. Initial seizure type in 693 children.

Table I. Clinical features of the Nova Scotia epilepsy study

	Group 1 GTC or partial N = 511	Group 2 Absence N = 97	Group 3 Secondary generalized N = 85	Total 693
Males	266 (52%)	38 (40%)	41 (48%)	347
Age onset 1st seizure (months)	81.5	67 ± 32	24.6	
Time 1st to 2nd seizure (months)	4.9 70% in 1st mos	n/a		
1st degree relative with epilepsy	27 (5%)	18 (19%)		
Preceding febrile seizure	88 (17%)	12 (10%)		

Etiology
  Cryptogenic
  Genetic including chromosomal
  Prenatal
  Perinatal
  Neurocutaneous
  Other
	287 (57%)
	97 (19%)
	49 (10%)
	24 (5%)
	9 (2%)
	38 (7%)			

Neurologic findings at time of diagnosis
  Normal
  Mild abnormality
  Major abnormality
	394 (78%)
	55 (11%)
	55 (11%)			

Intelligence estimation at time of diagnosis
  Normal
  Mental handicap
  Learning disorder
	347 (68%)
	50 (12%)
	38 (7%)
		83 (85%)
		
		14 (15%)		

Learning disorder + Behavioral	20 (4%)			

Table II. Age-specific incidence of epilepsy in Nova Scotia between 1977-1985

Age	Group 1 Partia + GTC	Group 2 Absence	Group 3 Sec. Gen.	# Cases	Population at risk	Incidence/ 100 000	CI*
< 13 mos	64	0	48	112	94 800	118	98-143
1 year	27	2	11	40	96 400	42	30-57
2	33	5	7	45	97 600	46	34-62
3	46	6	5	57	98 000	58	44-76
4	38	5	4	47	96 000	49	36-66
5	30	12	3	45	96 800	47	34-63
6	34	18	1	53	100 800	53	40-69
7	34	10	2	46	100 400	46	34-62
8	27	7	–	34	102 800	33	23-47
9	32	7	2	41	105 600	39	28-53
10	49	2	–	51	110 800	46	35-61
11	15	6	1	22	115 600	19	12-29
12	27	6	–	33	116 400	28	20-40
13	24	4	1	29	113 200	26	18-37
14	17	2	–	19	113 600	17	10-26
15	14	5	–	19	117 200	16	10-26
Total	511	97	85	693	1 676 000	41	38-45

* CI = confidence interval.

Documentation of population size of Nova Scotian children

Census data available from family allowance cheques payable monthly to the mother of each child and from Revenue Canada taxation information indicated that there were 226 700 children aged 0-16 years in Nova Scotia in 1981. The number of children, by age groupings, was documented during the census years of 1981 and 1983.

Definitions

Incidence was defined as the ratio of new epilepsy cases compared to the population at risk, expressed as cases/100 000 persons/year. The numerator for the incidence rate was the number of children < 16 years whose diagnosis occurred between Jan 1, 1977 and Dec 31, 1985. The denominator was the total number of children <16 years identified from the census data of the Province (an average of 1981 and 1983 census data).

Multiple seizures in a 24-hour period with complete recovery of consciousness between seizures were counted as separate events. However, an episode of status epilepticus was considered as a single event.

Results

The incidence of epilepsy for each year of age is given in *table II*.

The overall incidence from 1 month – 16 years was 41 cases/100 000 and by age groups was: 118/100 000 for children < 13 months; 48/100 000 for ages 1-5 years, 43/100 000 for ages 6-10 years; and 21/100 000 for ages 11-16 years. The incidence for each year of age between one and ten years was remarkably constant, averaging 46/100 000 ± 7 STD with a range of 33-58/100 000. Comparison of the incidence rates showed significant differences between < 1 year of age as compared with all other ages (p < 0.00001, chi-squared).

Mortality of childhood epilepsy [4]

Additional Methodology: The entire cohort of 692 children was used for analysis.

Follow-up of cohort

In 1999, names and birth dates of the cohort were linked to the Nova Scotia Provincial Death and Marriage Registries (Division of Vital Statistics). For children who were known to have died, the death certificates, autopsy reports, and physician records were reviewed and primary care physicians contacted. For those few likely to have experienced SUDEP, the child's neurologist directly phoned the family for information concerning the death. If a child was known to have died outside of the Province, the death was documented in similar fashion.

For survivors, length of follow up was determined by the last date they were known to be alive. For patients still under our care, the date was the most recent contact. For others who we no longer follow, we had personal contact by telephone or mail from a variety of follow up studies. For some, we had not had contact since the resolution of their epilepsy. We were able to confirm that they were alive at the last date they were seen by a physician in Nova Scotia by linking their name, date of birth and Health Care Number with both the Nova Scotia Admissions-Separations-Day Treatment database and Medical Services Insurance Physician's Services database. These databases document all physician contacts for all persons in Nova Scotia. Patients who moved out of the Province were censored at the last date they were known to be alive.

Statistical methods and analysis

Increased mortality within the cohort was quantified in terms of age and gender standardized mortality ratios (SMR) for the calendar period 1980-1989 and 1990-1999. The SMR was calculated as the observed number of deaths in the study cohort divided by the expected number of deaths based on the control population. Survival of the cohort was compared with the Nova Scotia population standardized with respect to age, gender, and follow up characteristics by Kaplan-Meier survival analysis.

Results

Six patients had no follow up beyond the initial diagnosis, which left 686 patients for long-term outcome studies. For survivors, length of follow up from diagnosis to last date known alive averaged 13 years (median 13.9 years, range 0-22.5) with follow up > 5 years in 91.8%, > 10 years in 71.6%, > 15 years in 41.1% and > 20 years in 5.5%.

Frequency and cause of death and associated epilepsy group

Twenty-six patients died – 25 within Nova Scotia and one in another Province. Death occurred in 12 of 511 (2.4%) children in *Group 1* (Partial and Generalized Tonic-Clonic

Epilepsies). Among the 97 absence patients in *Group 2*, only 1 died – a suicide at 18 years of age. Death was most common in children in *Group 3* with secondary generalized epilepsies - 13 of 85 died (15%).

The deaths of 22 children were not a surprise, because of their severe, associated neurologic disabilities. The average age of death in this handicapped group was 7 years (range 1.5-16 years) and the cause of death was: aspiration with pneumonia (14), infection or sepsis (3), shunt malfunction (1), pulmonary embolism (1), congestive heart failure (1), gastroesophageal reflux and failure to thrive (1), and status epilepticus (1).

In 4 patients, death was unexpected. These were all young adults without severe neurologic deficits (ages 18-30 years). Each had an autopsy and the cause of death was documented as suicide in 2, homicide 1, and probable SUDEP 1. The one case of probable SUDEP occurred in a 21-year old woman with tuberous sclerosis and mild mental handicap. She had partial seizures with secondary generalization beginning at age 11 years that were never well controlled. Medication compliance was poor. Her partner noted several seizures during sleep on the day she died. She was found in dead in bed several hours later. An autopsy failed to reveal a cause of death.

Mortality of children with epilepsy as compared to Nova Scotia children and youth: standardized mortality ratios

Relative to Nova Scotia children and youth, the standard mortality ratio (SMR) of the childhood epilepsy cohort relative to the total Nova Scotia population as a reference standard was 5.30 (2.29-8.32, 95% confidence interval) for January 1980 to December 1989 and 8.80 (4.16-13.43) for January 1990 to December 1999. Twenty years after onset of seizures, 6.1% (3.0%-9.2%) of the cohort had died (*figure 2*, top left panel). This was 5.2% higher than the 0.88% expected in the population reference sample. This difference in survival between the childhood epilepsy cohort and the population reference norms increased with time since onset of seizures (*figure 2*, top left panel). Survival differences with respect to gender were small and not statistically significant. Secondary generalized epilepsies *(Group 3)* were associated with a statistically significant increased mortality relative to absence epilepsies *(Group 2)* and partial and generalized tonic-clonic epilepsies *(Group 1)* (*figure 2*, bottom left panel).

Disparities in mortality between children with and without neurologic handicap were the most apparent finding (*figure 2*, bottom right panel). Children with neurologic handicap were 22.2 times more likely to die than those without handicap. This association remained the same after adjusting for gender, age and epilepsy type.

Seizure prognosis – Partial and generalized tonic-clonic epilepsies – Group 1 (N = 511)

At the time of epilepsy diagnosis, accurate prediction of seizure control and remission has been challenging [1]. We have learned that epilepsy treatment is rarely simple. When a child in our epilepsy cohort *(Group 1)* was started on medication, only 21% had "smooth sailing epilepsy" meaning that they would never have another seizure, either during AED treatment or after AEDs were stopped. While the AEDs used were "traditional" (phenobarbital, carbamazepine, phenytoin and valproic acid), there is no evidence that the newer AEDs are any more effective [5].

An excellent response to the first AED augured well for the future but failure of the first

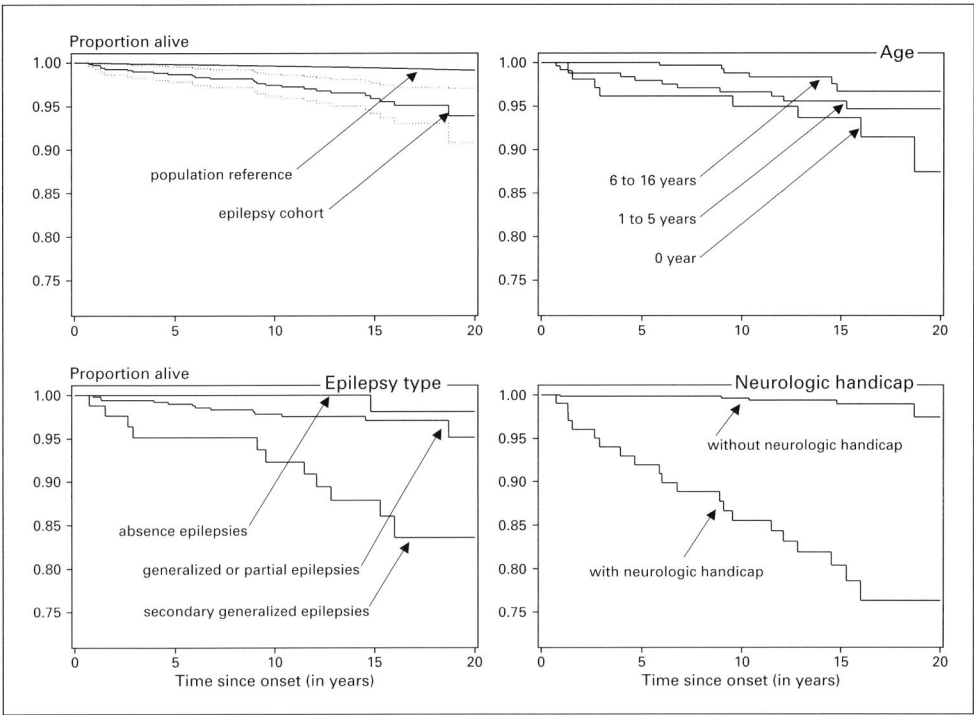

Figure 2. Mortality rates of NS cohort.
Upper left: Overall mortality compared to reference population. Lower left: Mortality within epilepsy types. Upper right: Mortality by age of onset of epilepsy. Lower right: Mortality with and without neurologic handicap

AED to provide seizure control was not as disastrous as previously thought [6]. Among the 17% of children who failed seizure control with a first AED during the first year of treatment, 42% eventually achieved long-term remission. It is interesting that nearly identical results were found in *Group 2* with absence epilepsies [7].

For most of our studies, terminal remission was defined as seizure freedom without daily AED treatment. Only 2% of the overall cohort (n = 693) stopped taking medication even though they continued to have seizures. Overall, the chance of achieving remission for those in *Group 1* (Partial and Generalized Tonic-Clonic Epilepsies) was 54% in the first 7-8 years after diagnosis. Two thirds became seizure free with AED treatment for a long enough time to attempt to discontinue AED treatment and 48% of the entire *Group 1* achieved remission (seizure free without further AED treatment) after a single period of time taking medication, although more than half required more than one AED before achieving complete seizure control. Eighteen percent of *Group 1* discontinued AEDs, had seizures recur and restarted medication. After 2 or 3 attempts to stop AEDs, 5.5% of *Group 1* eventually achieved remission. Overall, about 30% of Group 1 never became seizure free long enough to attempt to discontinue medication.

Based on the evolution of *Group 1*, our general impression is that epilepsy lasts about 1-2 years in about 25% of newly diagnosed patients, 2-4 years in 25% and for many years in 50%.

We developed a scoring system to predict long-term remission on the day of initial diagnosis [1]. Multivariate analysis indicated that the following variables were independent predictors of good outcome – age of onset < 12 years, normal intelligence, lack of preceding neonatal seizures and < 21 seizures before diagnosis. If all of these factors were present, the chance of remission was about 80% by 10 years after beginning AED treatment. If any one factor was absent, remission was anticipated in only 40%. The factors were then weighted as noted below to allow a more graded approach *(table III)*. If the total score was > 495, then remission was predicted. The sensitivity of this scoring system was 74%, specificity 64%, positive predictive value 71%, and negative predictive value 67%. It is important to point out that despite the statistical beauty of this model, remission or no remission was predicted correctly for 68% of patients - 20% of those predicted to be in remission were not and about 40% of those predicted not to be in remission were in fact off medication and seizure free by 10 years after diagnosis.

Table III. Predictive Scoring System

Predictor	Add

1. Age of onset
   < 12 months
   12-144 months
   > 144 months
	
	99
	142
	0

2. Intelligence
   Normal
   Abnormal
	
	111
	0

3. Neonatal seizures
   No
   Yes
	
	218
	0

4. Number of seizures before AEDs
   1 or 2
   3-20
   > 20
	
	72
	123
	0

Total score	If total > 495, predict remission If total < 495, predict no-remission Note if there is a 0 in any predictor variable, predict no-remission

When we attempted to predict long-term remission after 12 months of treatment, we were marginally more successful. The number of seizures after 6 and 12 months of AED treatment entered the statistical model as a powerful predictor, but even including this variable the correct prediction rate only increased to 70%.

We then validated this scoring system using a different cohort with longer follow up – the cohort of Matti Sillanpaa from Turku, Finland [8]. The two cohorts are somewhat different. The Nova Scotia study is an incidence cohort. The Turku study is a prevalence cohort, and therefore includes more children with severe epilepsy. Nonetheless the scoring system was reasonably accurate in this different cohort, with a magnificent follow up of 30 years. *Table IV* compares the scoring system in the two cohorts. It is particularly impressive that on the day of diagnosis, if the scoring system predicts remission, then 84% will be in remission 28 years later. Prediction of no remission is less accurate, reflecting the fact that the longer the follow up, the higher the rate of remission, even though most of those who will remit have done so in the first 4-5 years after diagnosis.

Table IV. Comparison of the predictive scoring system in the Turku and Nova Scotia cohorts

	Nova Scotia (N = 423, average follow up 7 years)	Turku (N = 141, average follow up 28 years)
Overall rate of remission	55%	60%
Correct prediction by the scoring system	67%	61%
Sensitivity	73%	43%
Specificity	64%	88%
Positive predictive value	71%	84%
Negative predictive value	67%	51%

It appears that the 4 factors that we have identified are very basic to the evolution of childhood epilepsy. If epilepsy begins in adolescence, it is likely to persist. If the child is mentally handicapped, there is diffuse brain dysfunction and this appears to have a serious negative effect on the chance of remission. Neonatal seizures are a marker of serious brain injury early in life, which again somehow makes epilepsy more severe.

The issue of seizure number before treatment deserves further comment. It is clear from our experience that if the seizure number before treatment is < 10, then there is no effect on the chance of remission [9]. If the number of seizures is higher, then the prognosis is not as good. It is important to emphasize that children with > 10 seizures (even more so with > 20) before treatment are much more likely to have complex partial seizures than other partial or generalized tonic-clonic seizures. So the effect of many seizures before treatment on remission rate is really the effect of having a more resistant seizure type. There does not appear to be much evidence that repeated seizures somehow become self-replicating.

Seizure prognosis – absence epilepsies – Group 2

Many neurologists and pediatricians seem to be of the impression that absence epilepsies are easily treated with remission guaranteed. In our cohort, prediction of remission at the time of diagnosis with absence epilepsies *(Group 2)* was difficult (10). Of 81 children with typical Childhood Absence Epilepsy, we were able to follow 89% for an average of 14 years. At the end of follow up, 65% were in remission (seizure free and off medication). Fifteen percent went on to develop Juvenile Myoclonic Epilepsy, a life long disorder [10].

Univariate predictors of remission included: absence status, myoclonus while receiving AEDs, generalized tonic-clonic seizures while receiving AEDs, EEG background slowing, family history of generalized tonic-clonic seizures and cognitive difficulties.

Multivariate predictors of remission included: myoclonic seizures while taking AEDs, episode(s) of absence status prior to treatment, family history of generalized epilepsy in a first degree relative, and slowing of the background on the initial EEG. Note that the variable, myoclonic seizures while taking AEDs, becomes available during the clinical course and is not known at the time of diagnosis. Using the 3 factors available at the time of diagnosis allowed prediction of outcome with positive predictive value of 89% and negative predictive value of 73%.

Prognosis for secondary generalized epilepsy (group 3)

We have not studied the long-term outcome of *Group 3* (n = 85) to the same degree as the other two groups. As noted above, 13 children in this group died (4). For consideration of epilepsy remission rate, we have removed those who died from the calculations. Overall, 24 (33%) patients had a terminal remission. Follow up varied from 5 to 25 years. As noted above, the remission rate for *Group 1* and *Group 2* was 54% [1]. The difference in remission between *Group 3* and the other two groups combined is highly significant (odds ratio 3.0, 95% C.I.-1.8-5.1).

Exact characterization of the epilepsy syndromes in *Group 3* is not currently available except that 24 (3.5% of the total cohort) had infantile spasms (West syndrome). About one-half of *Group 3* (48) had the onset of epilepsy in the first year of life. Their death rate was higher (10/48, 21%) than those whose epilepsy began at an older age (3/37,8%), although this difference did not reach statistical significance (p = 0.1). The remission rate for survivors with onset in the first year was 9/38 (24%) compared with 15/33 (45%) in the older age group. It is worth noting that children in *Group 1* who developed epilepsy in the first year of life had the same remission rate (33/64, 52%) as children whose epilepsy started at an older age. The concept that epilepsy beginning in the first year of life is "bad" is dependent on the fact that a high proportion of secondary generalized epilepsies begin before age one year.

Intractable epilepsy

There is no universally accepted definition of intractable epilepsy. We defined intractability as failure of 3 AEDs to provide complete seizure control and at least 1 seizure each 2 months in the last year of follow up [5]. In the overall cohort, 12.4% had intractable epilepsy [5]. The rate of intractability was 7.9% in *Group 1*, 8% in *Group 2* and 54% in *Group 3*. In fact, *Group 3* contributes nearly half of the intractable patients (39/85, 45%).

Long-term psychosocial outcome

Partial and generalized tonic-clonic epilepsies (Group 1)

Additional methodology [11]: Children from the cohort of 511 generalized tonic-clonic and partial with or without secondarily generalized seizures who were *normally intelligent* were followed up after their initial epilepsy diagnosis (90 ± 30 months). These 337 patients were 7-28 years of age. Because of the wide subject age at follow-up, the outcome measures were age-dependent. Of those old enough to be at risk for an adverse outcome, the unfavorable outcomes were examined by univariate and multivariate modeling with step-wise regression analysis.

Results

Overall, 140 patients had a poor social outcome and 197 had a good outcome (11) *(table V)*. Surprisingly, 35% of these normally intelligent children had repeated a grade in school or were placed in a special education class. They had frequently received psychiatric or psychological counseling (23%) and 5% received psychotropic medications. At the last

Table V. *Psychosocial outcomes of the normally intelligent children with epilepsy characterized by generalized tonic-clonic and partial with or without secondary generalization*

Category	Affected Subjects No.	Eligible Subjects* No.	%	(95% CI)
1. Grades repeated or special class	101	200	35	(29,40)
2. Psychiatric or psychologic referral	72	316	23	(18,28)
3. Psychotropic drugs	17	316	5	(3,8)
4. Criminal offense	4	187	2	(0,4)
5. Inadvertent pregnancy	11	88	13	(5,20)
6. Social isolation	11	71	16	(7,24)
7. Financial dependency	21	71	30	(19,40)
8. Unemployment	21	71	30	(19,40)

CI, Confidence Interval.
* Number sufficiently old where exact information was known. Categories 1 to 3 required age at end of follow-up of > 6.9 years, category 4 age > 13.9 years, Category 5 age > 13.9 years and female, categories 6 to 8 age > 17.9 years.

time of follow-up, 16% of these young adults felt socially isolated, 30% were unemployed, and 30% were financially dependent on their families. Four of 187 subjects had been convicted of a criminal offense, and 11/88 (13%) of the women reported an inadvertent pregnancy.

Overall, 42% experienced a poor social outcome. It is surprising that most biologic factors (i.e. seizure type, recurrent seizures after treatment, terminal remission, age onset, cause, etc.) related to the treatment and control of epilepsy did not predict a variety of undesirable social outcomes. Even complete remission of the patient's epilepsy did not alter social outcome. Of children with good social outcome, 67% were in remission, as compared with 58% of children with bad social outcome (p = ns).

Using multivariate analysis, significant predictors of poor social outcome included: learning disorder at the time of diagnosis ($p < 0.0001$) and > 21 seizures before AED treatment ($p < 0.03$). The strongest predictor of poor social outcome was the presence of a learning disorder. This was also evident using stepwise regression and decision tree modeling techniques. Good outcome was predicted by "simple partial" seizure type ($p < 0.008$) with each of these analyses.

Childhood Absence Epilepsy (Group 2)

Additional Methodology [12]: Newly diagnosed children with typical absence epilepsy (CAE) between 1977-85 and ≥ 18 years of age at follow-up in 1994-95 were enrolled. To provide a non-neurological, chronic disease control group, all children with a discharge diagnosis of juvenile rheumatoid arthritis (JRA) between 1977-85 were identified from the hospital medical records database. JRA was defined as inflammation of one or more joints persisting for at least 6 weeks without another cause being identified. The diagnosis was confirmed by chart review and, if necessary, contact with the patient, their family doctor or pediatrician. Patients with JRA were excluded if they had major physical disabilities at the time of follow up.

Both groups participated in a structured interview assessing psychosocial function. Specific areas surveyed in the interview included: academic achievement, drug and alcohol use, social functioning with family and friends, psychological and emotional difficulties, employment and job satisfaction and perceived impact of the illness on present life. In the analysis, issues related to employment and financial security were considered for only those subjects who were not full time students. The socio-economic status of the family of origin was assessed, including parental level of education and employment both at time of diagnosis and at the time of interview.

Results: Eighty-six percent (56/65) of those with CAE and 80% (61/76) of JRA participated in the interview. Mean age at interview was 23 years. Terminal remission occurred in 57% of CAE but only 28% of JRA patients. *Table VI* reveals the significant differences in psychosocial outcome between the young adults with CAE and those with JRA.

Table VI. Significant differences in psychosocial outcome between absence and JRA groups

	Absence		JRA		Odds Ratio (CI)
	%	N	%	N	
Education					
• No high school graduation	36	55	14	59	3.7 (1.3, 10.4)
• Resource or special class	16	56	3	61	5.7 (1.1, 40.5)
• School function below average	29	56	10	61	3.7 (1.2, 11.7)
• Ever repeated a grade	48	56	23	61	3.1 (1.3, 7.6)
• Repeated grade before diagnosis	20	56	3	61	7.6 (1.4, 52.8)
• If yes, repeated a grade for reasons unrelated to illness	100	27	57	14	Undefined (2.8, ∞)
Higher education					
• Never attended university/college	71	55	39	59	3.8 (1.6, 9.1)
Behavior					
• Ever considered a behavior problem	41	56	10	61	6.4 (2.2, 19.9)
Pregnancy					
• Unplanned pregnancy	34	38	3	38	19.3 (2.3, 426.1)
Substance use					
• Past history of heavy drinking	39	56	16	61	3.3 (1.3, 8.7)
Relationships with family and friends					
• Poor relations with sibs	19	53	5	57	4.1 (1.1, 19.7)
• Outings with friend/partner < weekly	14	56	3	61	4.8 (1.1, 34.8)
• No prior involvement with organized religion	52	56	31	61	2.4 (1.1, 5.5)
Psychiatric or emotional problems					
• Past psychiatric or emotional problems	54	56	31	61	2.6 (1.1, 5.9)
Employment					
• Full time months of work in last year	7.6	43	9.3	40	$p < 0.02$
• Unskilled labor	53	30	16	31	5.9 (1.6, 24.0)
• Upper management or professional	0	30	29	31	Undefined (2.3, ∞)
• Poor job satisfaction	33	30	10	31	4.3 (1.1, 21.7)
• Not employed in area of training	50	14	14	21	5.7 (1.2, 33.9)

OR (CI) = Odds ratio (95% Confidence Intervals)

Factor analysis identified five categories of outcome that accounted for 40% of the variance in our sample: Academic-Personal, Behavior, Employment-Financial, Family Relations, Social-Personal Relations. Patients with CAE had greater difficulties in the Academic-Personal and in the Behavior categories ($p < 0.001$ for both) than those with JRA.

Patients with CAE were then divided into 2 groups based on terminal remission. Patients whose epilepsy did not remit were more likely to report that it continued to impact on their lives (71% vs 28%, p < 0.002). Patients without remission scored significantly higher in the Academic – Personal category of the Factor Analysis (p < 0.05) but not in the other 4 categories. Forty-two percent of those with ongoing seizures reported current psychiatric and emotional difficulties, as compared to only 3% of those who were seizure-free (p < 0.0003). Seizure frequency did not correlate with psychosocial outcome, but seizure type did. Patients with ongoing GTC seizures (N = 6) scored significantly higher in the categories Behavior and Employment – Financial (p < 0.002 and p < 0.05).

Prediction of psychosocial outcome in CAE from seizure-related factors present at time of diagnosis or during course of epilepsy was examined. No measure of socioeconomic status of the family of origin correlated with any of the 5 categories of psychosocial outcome identified by factor analysis, suggesting that socioeconomic status of the family of origin. Most seizure-related variables also showed no association with the five categories. Variables examined included: absence subtype, age at seizure onset, duration of seizures prior to treatment, length of treatment until seizure control was achieved, concomitant seizure types (GTC, myoclonic), absence status, types of AEDs used, sex, cognitive difficulties at seizure onset, history of perinatal complications, family history of seizures in first degree relatives, and EEG findings, including slowing of background or photoconvulsive response.

Those without complete seizure control within the first year of AED treatment also scored higher in the category of Social – Personal Relations (p < 0.04). Patients with cognitive difficulties at seizure onset scored higher in the categories Academic – Personal and Family Relations (p < 0.01 for both).

Conclusions

The Nova Scotia Epilepsy Cohort has allowed us to understand some very important basic features of childhood onset epilepsy. The number of seizures before treatment does not effect the clinical course. Long-term remission occurs in only about one-half of children with newly diagnosed epilepsy. Remission can be predicted on the day of diagnosis, albeit not completely accurately. AED treatment is complex and usually not immediately effective. Intractability is unusual but mainly a feature of secondary generalized epilepsy. Death is related to severe neurologic impairment, not seizure control. The social outcome is often unsatisfactory, even in those who are normally intelligent. Biologic features of the epilepsy do not predict social outcome.

Acknowledgements: We thank our pediatric neurology colleagues (Drs. E. Wirrell, J. Dooley and K. Gordon), statistical consultants (B. Smith and P. Veugelers), E. Smith, RN and the patients and families for their help and continued interest in the NS Pediatric Epilepsy Study.

References

1. Camfield CS, Camfield PR, Gordon KE, Dooley JM, Smith BS. Predicting the outcome of childhood epilepsy – a population based study yielding a simple scoring system. *J Pediatr* 1993; 122: 861-8.
2. Camfield PR, Camfield CS, Dooley JM, Tibbles JAR, Fung T, Garner B. Epilepsy after a first unprovoked seizure in childhood. *Neurology* 1985; 35: 1657-60.
3. Camfield CS, Camfield PR, Wirrell E, Gordon KG, Dooley JM. Incidence of epilepsy in childhood and adolescents: a population based study in Nova Scotia from 1977-1985. *Epilepsia* 1996; 37: 19-23.
4. Camfield CS, Camfield PR, Veugelers P. Death in children with childhood onset epilepsy: A population-based study. *Lancet* 2002; 359; 1892-95.
5. Camfield PR, Camfield CS. Antiepileptic drug therapy: When is epilepsy truly intractable? *Epilepsia* 1996; 37 (Suppl 1): S60-65.

6. Camfield PR, Camfield CS, Gordon K, Dooley J. If a first antiepileptic drug fails to control a child's epilepsy, what are the chances of success with the next drug? *J Pediatr* 1997; 131: 821-4.
7. Wirrell E, Camfield CS, Camfield PR, Dooley J, Gordon K. Prognostic significance of failure of the initial anti-epileptic drug in children with absence epilepsy. *Epilepsia* 2001; 42: 760-3.
8. Sillanpaa M, Camfield PR, Camfield CS. Predicting long-term outcome of childhood epilepsy in Nova Scotia, Canada and Turku Finland: Validation of a simple scoring system. *Arch Neurol* 1995; 52: 589-92.
9. Camfield CS, Camfield PR, Gordon KG, Dooley JM. Does the number of seizures before treatment influence ease of control or remission of childhood epilepsy? – Not if the number is less than 10. *Neurology* 1996; 46: 41-4.
10. Wirrell E, Camfield PR, Camfield CS, Dooley JM, Gordon K. Long-term prognosis of typical childhood absence epilepsy: Remission or progression to juvenile myoclonic epilepsy. *Neurology* 1996; 47: 912-8.
11. Camfield CS, Camfield PR, Gordon KE, Dooley JM, Smith BS. Biologic factors as predictors of social outcome in epilepsy in intellectually normal children: A population based study. *J Pediatr* 1993; 122: 869-73.
12. Wirrell E, Camfield CS, Camfield PR, Dooley J, Gordon K, Smith B. Long-term psychosocial outcome in typical absence epilepsy: sometimes a wolf in sheep's clothing. *Arch Pediatr Adol Med* 1997; 151: 152-8.

Long-term prognosis in Finnish childhood-onset epilepsy

Matti Sillanpää

There are few very population-based long-term follow-up studies on epilepsy in terms of medical outcome [1-8], or social consequences [2, 8]. The long-term studies are important to figure out more and more the life-cycle and living circumstances of people with epilepsy who have long been more or less misunderstood and marginalized in the society.

In 1961, at start of my 40-year work in the Department of Pediatrics, Turku University Hospital, my interest in the epidemiology and prognosis of epilepsy was evoked by clinical needs, good clinical laboratory facilities, well-organized collaboration with primary health care and, finally, by the monography of Rodin [9] which showed how great a challenge epilepsy was for the subject, family, and society. Designing of the epidemiological study on childhood epilepsy was started in 1971. Later, the project has been a joint venture in a close collaboration between the Departments of Pediatric Neurology and Epidemiology & Public Health.

Background for the study

Finland is divided into 21 central hospital districts, with 5 districts having a university hospital district status associated with a medical faculty. Every central hospital has the catchment area of its own. However, if needed, the patients may be treated in other hospitals regardless of where they are resident. A unique social security number enables the tracing of the person wherever in the country he is staying or living. From 1961 to 1964, the catchment area of the Turku University Central Hospital (TUCH) district covered the middle total population of approx. 405 000 persons, with the child population < 15 years of approx. 102 000. In the TUCH area, in the 1960s, all children with any seizures were referred to hospital for evaluation.

The primary health care is organized on the basis of health authority areas, the smallest administrative unit of the Finnish public health care system, numbering 20 in the catchment area of the TUCH. A special care for mentally or other developmentally handicapped is also organised districtwise, with a virtually 100% overlapping with central hospital districts.

The National Health Service legislation came into power in 1964 and enabled, by means of personal social security number, identification of every person. A national register of reimbursed medications prescribed by doctor (including 100% reimbursement of licensed antiepileptic drugs), linked to the National Health Service register made it possible to trace all subjects who had been identified as having epileptic seizures whether they were medicated or not.

The identification of the patients was based, not only on the records of the TUCH and other hospitals and special institutions, but also public outpatient clinics, EEG laboratories and private offices and, finally on a review of the National Health Service records. Two or more unprovoked seizures were considered as epilepsy. There were five patients who had two but not three unprovoked seizures. Three patients met the inclusion criteria but could not be traced. Three further patients, were revealed by an ongoing surveillance but too late to be included in the clinical analyses. After the exclusion of non-eligible subjects, 245 remained who constituted the final study group *(table I)*.

Table I. Recruitment of patients for the incidence study

Patients	N
Subjects aged 1 month to 15 years, resident in the Turku University Hospital area, seen by doctor for at least one epileptic seizure in 1961-1964	711
Excluded	
Patients with a progressive brain disease	- 16
Patients with occasional seizures only	- 260
Patients with less than two unprovoked seizures	- 79
Patients referred prior to and seizure-free 1961-64	- 100
Patients with prevalence cases	- 99
Included	157

Incidence

Altogether, 157 patients with incidence cases were identified, which yield the annual incidence rate of 38/100 000. In recent studies, the incidence rates of epilepsy vary from 41 to 89/100 000 [3, 10-14], and those of a first unprovoked seizure from 11 to 375/100 000 [13-15].

The annual incidence for idiopathic epilepsies was 12/100 000, for cryptogenic epilepsies 9/100 000 and for symptomatic epilepsies 16/100 000. The distribution was similar to that of previous reports [10]. The incidence rate was 23/100 000 for partial-onset epilepsies, was 10/100 000 for generalized epilepsies, and 4/100 000 for epilepsies undetermined whether partial-onset, generalized, or unclassifiable.

Mortality

During the follow-up period of 35 years, at the age of 28 to 46 years, 20 (13%) patients had died. The standardized mortality ratio (SMR) was 4.76-fold (4.38-5.25) compared with the general population [8]. In patients with incidence cases, the SMR was 3.48 (2.23-5.15). The figures are comparable with those from similar age groups of other studies [16, 17], who got the SMR of 8.5, for patients with epilepsy as the first diagnosis, at age 0-24 and 7.7 at age 25-44. In our study, the male mortality was higher than the female mortality in line with other studies [18]. The seizure-specific SMR was almost doubled compared with the general population. The mortality was strongly bound to the etiology of seizures. Among patients with an idiopathic or cryptogenic etiology, the mortality was markedly lower than in patients with a remote symptomatic etiology. On the other hand, a symptomatic etiology strongly increased the risk for death. Similar differences have been found in several previous studies [17, 19].

A vast majority (75%) of the patients who died were not in remission. An epileptic seizure was definitely or probably associated with death in 45%. In the 55% whose death was seizure-unrelated had pneumonia as the most common cause of death. Among all who died, the most common cause of death was pneumonia, which most usually occurred in the mentally retarded boys. Most of them had also a cerebral palsy syndrome. A sudden unexpected death (SUDEP), defined in accordance with Annegers [16], mostly occurred in mentally normal girls. One of the five patients with SUDEP was less than 16 and two less than 19 at death. Our figures show that SUDEP is an apparently common cause of death but its underlying mechanisms are still largely unknown [20, 21].

The risk of death was higher in patients with epilepsy and mental retardation and the risk was in relation to the degree of intelligence level (unpublished data). On the other hand, in population studies, the mentally retarded with epilepsy tend to die younger than those without epilepsy [22, 23].

Medical outcome

Remission

After the first five-year remission of seizures, the 5-year terminal remission was maintained by the patients with incident epilepsy in 57%, 58% and 68% on 10, 20, and 30 years from the diagnosis, respectively *(table II)*. Our figures are lower than those of Oka *et al.* [4], whose remission rates included 98% for primary generalized epilepsy, 87% for partial epilepsy and 69% for complex partial epilepsy. Their remission rates are very high; rates less than 40% for complex partial epilepsy, for example, are usually reported in long-term studies [1, 24]. The marked differences may depend on either the different study design or genetic factors, or both.

Table II. Five-year terminal remission (5YTR) of epilepsy after 5-year seizure-freedom in long-term studies of patients with incident cases

Author(s) and year	Duration Yrs	5YTR %
Oka *et al.* (1989)	≥ 10	79
Annegers *et al.* (1979)	≥ 10	65
	≥ 20	76
Sillanpää (1973, 1983, 1990, Sillanpää *et al.* 1998, 2000)	≥ 5	45
	≥ 10	57
	≥ 15	59
	≥ 20	58
	≥ 25	61
	≥ 30	68

The study design of Annegers *et al.* [1] was somewhat different but the figures were largely comparable with our ones. Their patient cohort of 618 patients of all ages who had a diagnosis of epilepsy between the years 1935 and 1974 was retrospectively collected from the state of Minnesota. Of them, 457 fulfilled the inclusion criteria and could be examined. The study was based on medical records data. On follow-up of at least 10 years, the terminal remission of five years or more was achieved by 61% of 328 patients. Of 141 who could be followed for 20 years or more 70% were in terminal remission.

In a Japanese retrospective multi-institutional study [2], which was based on the medical records of patients of all ages, 56% were seizure free for the last five years but, unfortunately, the results from the 10-year follow-up period were not reported separately. The remission rate was significantly higher in the idiopathic group (62%) than in the "recidual" (52%) or symptomatic (50%) epilepsy.

Predictors of remission

A good early effect of drug therapy was the best predictor of a favorable seizure outcome, followed by absence of complex partial or atonic seizure, and idiopathic or cryptogenic etiology of seizures [8]. A good drug effect within early months or one year after onset of therapy has been reported as a determinant of a favorable long-term outcome [1, 25-30]. An idiopathic epilepsy without neurological deficit predicts a virtually good seizure outcome [1, 3, 8, 24].

Predictors of seizure persistence

Factors reported to contribute to an unfavorable outcome mostly belong to three groups: brain structural pathology, intensive seizure occurrence, and poor therapeutic drug effect.

Factors arguing for a brain structural pathology and associated seizure persistence include definite mental retardation [3, 21, 24, 27], symptomatic etiology [8, 31, 32], partial seizures [8, 21, 32], and diffuse slowing [32] or focal spike and wave activity in EEG [31, 32]. A high intensity of seizure occurrence is manifested by early childhood-onset seizures, prior neonatal seizures, and high number of seizures prior to or during early drug therapy [25, 27, 32, 33]. An unsuccessful response to an adequate drug schedule during the first few months or two years of therapy is the third ominous feature [1, 8, 25]. In the long-term follow-up study by Sillanpää *et al.* [8], poor early response to drug therapy, presence of complex partial seizures, and symptomatic etiology of epilepsy predicted an unfavourable outcome of seizures *(table III)*.

Table III. Predictors of seizure persistence on long-term follow-up of childhood-onset epilepsy (Sillanpää et al. 1998) (OR = odds ratio; 95%CI = 95% confidence interval)

Predictor	OR	95% CI	p
Poor early response to therapy	4.50	2.53-8.06	0.004
Complex partial seizures	3.57	1.69-7.69	0.001
Cause of epilepsy			0.002
– Remote symptomatic	1.0		
– Cryptogenic	2.95	1.37-6.37	
– Idiopathic	3.82	1.77-8.26	

Recurrence of seizures

On 35-year follow-up, one fifth of our patients never achieved terminal or temporary 5-year remission of seizures. At the end of follow-up, up to last contact or death, 50% were in their first and still continuing remission of five years or more. Twenty-nine per cent of patients wityh incidence cases and 38% of those who had been in at least 5-year remission experienced one or more relapses after five years of seizure freedom. The mean annual relapse rate was 1.2% in our 116 patients (followed for 3720 person-years) compared with 1.6% in the study of Annegers *et al.* [1]. In the vast majority (83%), there was only one recurrence of seizures.

Risk factors for recurrence

One or more relapses had been significantly more exprienced by patients who had a poor early response to an adequate drug therapy, or who were mentally retarded. Patients with a symptomatic etiology tended to have relapses more often than those with an idiopathic or cryptogenic etiology. The risk was higher in case of the occurrence of status epilepticus, in temporal lobe seizures compared with extratemporal, primarily generalized or other seizures, in males compared with females, and high frequency of seizures, but these variables did not reach statistical significance. Annegers *et al.* [1], too, reported a higher risk of relapse in patients with complex partial epilepsy.

Comorbidity

Mental retardation (IQ < 70) occurred in 33% of our patients with incident cases. It was mild in 12% and severe in 21%. In the literature, mental retardation is associated with epilepsy in 21 to 41% [2, 34-36]. Cerebral palsy occurred in 17%; in 12% with mental retardation and in 5% without mental retardation. The corresponding total figure in Forsgren's [36] study was 14%. In a comparative study between patients with uncomplicated epilepsy, derived from a long-term follow-up study, and general population controls, matched for age, sex and domicile [37], insomnia, psychiatric and psychosomatic disorders occurred significantly more often in people with epilepsy.

Psychotic disorders have been reported in 3% to 5% of people with epilepsy [2, 37]. Camfield *et al.* [38] found behavior disturbances which needed mental health consultation in 22% of normally intelligent patients with childhood-onset epilepsy. Any somatic comorbidity was more commonly associated with epilepsy (89% *vs* 68%) but did not reach statistical significance.

Social outcome

In our study, patients with childhood-onset incident epilepsy who were in remission without medication differed significantly from the matched controls in terms of single marital status, having no children, no driver's license, and no paid work. The marriage status appears to be more associated with emotional adjustment than to mental abilities [39]. Fertility was lower in people with uncomplicated epilepsy than in matched controls. Spontaneous abortions occurred in 36% of patients still on medication, in 19% in patients off medication and in 13% of controls. The average number of children was significantly lower in the patients' families compared with controls [40].

Basicly, three factors may affect social outcome in epilepsy: cognitive function, antiepileptic drug therapy, and psychosocial factors. Short-term medication (< 6 months) of epileptic seizures causes no significant differences in cognitive functions or behavioural patterns [41]. However, a long-term drug therapy, and polypharmacotherapy in particular, has an effect on neuropsychological performance [42, 43].

Psychosocial factors test the patient's self-confidence in terms of the environmental attitudes of overprotection, prejudices and negligence. The overprotection and underestimation of the child's learning potential often starts at home. Academic underachievement of schoolchildren with epilepsy was related to underestimating parental attitudes and intellectual disability in the study of Hartlage and Green [44]. An underachievement is followed by poor self-esteem, decreased motivation to make efforts at school and subsequent depression and "learned helplessness" [45, 46].

Estimates for various learning problems vary from 5% to 50% [47]. In a Finnish study [48], 20% of young adults with childhood-onset epilepsy living in the community had not passed the primary educational level in a compulsory school system compared with 2% of general population controls.

Sixty per cent of patients with childhood-onset epilepsy were well-adjusted and completely independent in the activities of daily living, while 15% required little assistance [7]. In terms of employment and life arrangements, 60% were completely independent and self-sufficient, 21% were completely independent on other persons' continuous assistance and support, and 18% were living in the community but outside the labour market, in most cases on disability pensions. A self-reported life management was reported by patients with uncomplicated epilepsy as "poor" or "absent" four times as often as matched controls, but life satisfaction was as good in the two groups [49]. A subgroup of patients with persistent seizures and polypharmacotherapy were less satisfied. This is in line with other studies on life satisfaction and quality of life [50-52].

Our study shows that people with epilepsy have good chances to be in remission of seizures. Drug therapy can be discontinued without a great risk of relapse. About 20%, however, cannot so far be treated. Our results can still be considered valid today. This is because data on clinical examinations, neuroimaging studies and other laboratory investigations were cumulatively collected and applied, for example, in the reclassification of epileptic seizures and syndromes in accordance with the most recent ILAE classifications. Similarly, effects of drug therapy, with the newest drugs included, could be observed and included in the analyses.

Social outcome is determined in part by medical factors and in part by social and environmental factors. Our study showed that, in addition to intractable seizures, negative or reserved attitudes toward people with epilepsy at home, school, workplace and society still limit their everyday life, education, work career and social integration. Understanding of the most internal essence of epilepsy in the future may make it easier for both the patients and other people to accept epilepsy as one among many other health disorders.

References

1. Annegers JF, Hauser WA, Elveback LR. Remission of seizures and relapse in patients with epilepsy. *Epilepsia* 1979; 20: 729-37.
2. Okuma T, Kumashiro H, and the Group for the study of epilepsy in Japan. Natural history and prognosis of epilepsy: report of a multi-institutional study in Japan. *Epilepsia* 1981; 22: 35-53.
3. Brorson LO, Wranne L. Long-term prognosis in childhood epilepsy: survival and seizure prognosis. *Epilepsia* 1987; 28: 324-30.

4. Oka E, Yamatogi Y, Ohtsuka Y, Ohtahara S. Clinical course and prognosis of childhood epilepsy. *Acta Paediatr Jpn* 1989; 31: 259-66.
5. Sillanpää M. Medico-social prognosis of children with epilepsy. Epidemiological study and analysis of 245 patients. *Acta Paediatr Scand* 1973; 68 (Suppl 237): 104 p.
6. Sillanpää M. Social functioning and seizure status in young adults with onset of epilepsy in childhood. *Acta Neurol Scand* 1983; 68 (Suppl 96): 81 p.
7. Sillanpää M. Children with epilepsy as adults. Outcome after 30 years of follow-up. *Acta Paediatr Scand* 1990; 95 (Suppl 368): 78 p.
8. Sillanpää M, Jalava M, Kaleva O, Shinnar S. Long-term prognosis of seizures with onset in childhood. *New Engl J Med* 1998; 338: 1715-22.
9. Rodin E. *The prognosis of patients with epilepsy.* Springfield, Ill: Charles C. Thomas 1968, 455 p.
10. Beilmann A, Napa A, Hamarik M, Soot A, Talvik I, Talvik T. Incidence of childhood epilepsy in Estonia. *Brain Dev* 1999; 21: 166-74.
11. Camfield CS, Camfield PR, Gordon K, Wirrel E, Dooley JM. Incidence of epilepsy in childhood and adolescence: a population-bases study in Nova Scotia from 1977 to 1985. *Epilepsia* 1996; 37: 19-23.
12. Doerfer J, Wasser S. An epidemiologic study of febrile seizures and epilepsy in children. *Epilepsy Res* 1987; 1: 149-51.
13. Freitag CM, May TW, Pfäfflin M, König S, Rating D. Indicence of epilepsies and epileptic syndromes in children and adolescents: a prospective population-based study in Germany. *Epilepsia* 2001; 42: 979-85.
14. Olafsson E, Hauser A, Ludvigsson P, Gudmundsson G. Incidence of epilepsy in rural Iceland: a population-based study. *Epilepsia* 1996; 37: 951-5.
15. Palencia R. Prevalence and incidence of epilepsy in childhood. *Rev Neurol* 2000; 30 (Suppl 1): 1-4.
16. Annegers JF. United States perspective on definitions and classifications. *Epilepsia* 1997; 38 (Suppl 11): 9-12.
17. Hauser WA, Annegers JF, Elveback LR. Mortality in patients with epilepsy. *Epilepsia* 1980; 21: 399-412.
18. Massey EW, Schoenberg BS. Mortality in epilepsy. International patterns and changes over time. *Neuroepidemiology* 1985; 4: 65-70.
19. Harvey AS, Nolan T, Carlin JB. Community-based study of mortality in children with epilepsy. *Epilepsia* 1993; 34: 597-603.
20. Shorvon S. Risk factors of sudden unexpected death in epilepsy. *Epilepsia* 1997; 38 (Suppl 11): 20-2.
21. Annegers JF, Coan SP. SUDEP: overview of definitions and review of incidence data. *Seizure* 1999; 8: 347-52.
22. Patja K, Iivanainen M, Vesala H, Oksanen H, Ruoppila I. Life expectancy of people with intellectual disability: a 35-year follow-up study. *J Intellect Disabil Res* 2000a; 44: 591-9.
23. Patja K, Mölsä P, Iivanainen M. Cause-specific mortality of people with intellectual disability in a population-based, 35-year follow-up study. *J Intellect Disabil Res* 2000b; 44: 1-11.
24. Sofijanov NG. Clinical evolution and prognosis of childhood epilepsies. *Epilepsia* 1982; 23: 61-9.
25. Arts WFM, Geerts AT, Brouwer OF, Boydewyn Peters AC, Stroink H, van Donselaar CA. The early prognosis of epilepsy in childhood: the prediction of a poor outcome. The Dutch study of epilepsy in childhood. *Epilepsia* 1999; 40: 726-34.
26. Beghi E, Tognoni G. Prognosis of epilepsy in early referred patients: a multicenter prospective study. *Epilepsia* 1988; 29: 236-43.
27. Camfield C, Camfield P, Gordon K, Smith B, Dooley J. Outcome of childhood epilepsy: a population-based study with a simple scoring system for those treated with medication. *J Pediatr* 1993a; 122: 861-8.
28. Covanis A, Skiadas K, Loli N, Lada C, Theodorou V. Absence epilepsy: early prognostic signs. *Seizure* 1992; 1: 289-91.
29. Keränen T. Epilepsy in adults. *An epidemiological study in Eastern Finland.* Doctoral Thesis. Kuopio: University Printing Office 1988, 77 p.
30. Kwan P, Brodie MJ. Early identification of refractory epilepsy. *N Engl J Med* 2000; 342: 314-9.
31. Äikiä M, Kälviäinen R, Mervaala E, Riekkinen Sr PJ. Predictors of seizure outcome in newly diagnosed partial epilepsy: memory performance as a prognostic factor. *Epilepsy Res* 1999; 37: 159-67.
32. Ko TS, Holmes GL. EEG and clinical predictors of medically intractable childhood epilepsy. *Clin Neurophysiol* 1999; 110: 1245-51.

33. Sillanpää M, Camfield P, Camfield C. Predicting long term outcome of childhood epilepsy in Nova Scotia, Canada and Turku, Finland. Validation of a simple scoring system. *Arch Neurol* 1995; 52: 589-92.
34. Beilmann A. Epidemiology of childhood epilepsy in Kaunas. Doctoral Thesis. Kaunas: Kaunas Medical Academy 1997, 26 p.
35. Brorson LO. *Epilepsi hos barn och ungdom. En klinisk, psykometrisk och social undersökning inom Uppsala län.* I. *Socialstyrelsen förevisar.* Stockholm: Epileptikervården 1970, 84 p. (In Swedish, with English summary).
36. Forsgren L. Prevalence of epilepsy in adults in northern Sweden. *Epilepsia* 1992; 33: 450-8.
37. Jalava M, Sillanpää M. Concurrent illnesses in adults with childhood-onset epilepsy: a population-based 35-year follow-up study. *Epilepsia* 1996; 37: 1155-63.
38. Camfield C, Camfield P, Smith B, Gordon K, Dooley J. Biologic factors as predictors of social outcome of epilepsy in intellectually normal children: a population-based study. *J Pediatr* 1993b; 122: 869-73.
39. Dansky LV, Andermann E, Andermann F. Marriage and fertility in epileptic patients. *Epilepsia* 1980; 21: 261-71.
40. Jalava M, Sillanpää M. Reproductive activity and offspring health of yound adults with childhood-onset epilepsy: a controlled study. *Epilepsia* 1997; 38: 532-40.
41. Williams J, Bates S, Griebel ML, Lange B, Mancias P, Pihoker CM, Dykman R. Does short-term antiepileptic drug treatment in children result in cognitive or behavioral changes? *Epilepsia* 1998; 39: 1064-9.
42. Trimple M, Thompson PJ. Anticonvulsant drugs, cognitive function, and behaviour. *Epilepsia* 1983; 24: 55-63.
43. Trimple M. Anticonvulsant drugs: mood and cognitive function. In: Trimple MR, Reynolds EH, eds. *Epilepsy, behaviour and cognitive function.* Chichester: John Wiley & Sons, 1988: 135-45.
44. Hartlage LC, Green JB. The relation of parental attitudes to academic and social achievement in epileptic children. *Epilepsia* 1972; 13: 21-6.
45. Hermann BP, Trenerry MR, Colligan RC. Learned helplessness, attributional style, and depression in epilepsy. Bozeman Epilepsy. Surgery Consortium. *Epilepsia* 1996; 37: 680-6.
46. Dunn DW, Austin JK, Huster GA. Symptoms of depression in adolescents with epilepsy. *J Am Acad Child Adolesc Psychiatry* 1999; 38: 1132-8.
47. Thompson PJ. Educational attainment in children and young people with epilepsy. In Oxley J, Stores G, eds. *Epilepsy and Ecucation 1987.* London: The Medical Tribune Group, 1987: 15-24.
48. Kokkonen J, Kokkonen ER, Saukkonen AL, Pennanen P. Psychosocial outcome of young adults with epilepsy in childhood. *J Neurol Neurosurg Psychiatry* 1997; 62: 265-8.
49. Jalava M, Sillanpää M, Camfield C, Camfield P. Social adjustment and competence 35 years after onset of childhood epilepsy: a prospective controlled study. *Epilepsia* 1997; 38: 708-15.
50. Hanai T. Quality of life in children with epilepsy. *Epilepsia* 1992; 33 (Suppl 1): 28-32.
51. Baker G, Jacoby A, Buck D, Stalgis C, Monnet D. Quality of life of people with epilepsy: a European study. *Epilepsia* 1997; 38: 353-62.
52. Ribeiro JL, Mendonca D, Martins da Silva A. Impact of epilepsy on QOL in a Portugiese population: exploratory study. *Acta Neurol Scand* 1998; 97: 287-94.

Prognosis of epilepsy in Africa

Amadou Gallo Diop, Fatou Sene-Diouf, Léopold Boissy, Pierre-Marie Preux, Ibrahima Pierre Ndiaye

One of the leading brain disorders in developing countries is represented by epilepsy. It is estimated that 85% of people suffering from epilepsy around the world, reside in developing countries, particularly in Africa. The leading factors are represented by: long delay before modern treatment, reduced number of AEDs or (financial) inaccessibility, and limited human and technical resources for epilepsy. Cultural interpretation of the seizures also contribute to exclude epileptic patients from the educational and productive fields, aggravating the burden they face and favoring a treatment gap estimated to 80 to 85%. These factors lead to alter the prognosis of people with epilepsy in the large majority of African countries. Seizure frequency, evolution, complications related to seizures and/or many secondary etiologies characterize the prognosis factors and epidemiology of epilepsy in Africa.

The general context of people with epilepsy in Africa

The existing healthcare structures in Africa are located in a very specific environment dominated by very different quality levels of education, health and wealth, described below.

Demography

750 millions people live in 29 367 km^2 of the African continent. This population has a mean annual percentage growth of 2.6%. The prevision of the African population in the year 2050 is estimated to 1.5 billion. Females represent 50.3% of the African population. The age distribution (which is interesting to emphasize, because of its relation with epilepsy incidence among the extreme ages of life), reveals that people from ages 0 to 14 represent 43.4% of the population. Those who are more than 65 represent 3.1%. Another fact to consider is the migration phenomenon from rural to urban areas which leads to an actual mean of 36% of African inhabitants living in cities. One may note that these types of inhabitants have the strongest background of sub urban bad conditions characterized by promiscuity, bad sanitation and problems of safe water. Rural habits and behavior are

maintained in a vague urban environment. This sort of *"rurban"* situation leads to a concentration of several brain stress factors, field of future epilepsy and their bad prognosis. The mean general under-five mortality rate in 1997 was 133.6 deaths per 1 000 live births, versus 169.7 in 1980 (World Bank, 1999).

Education and communication means

The mean youth illiteracy rate in both male and female in Africa is near 28.4%, but more important among females (World Bank, 1999). In 1997, for the known rates, 22.8% of male and 33.7% of females ages 15-24 did not attend schools in Africa. The general expected years of schooling is 7.6 for males and 6.7 for females. The rate of illiteracy is an important factor to consider and explains why it is important to utilize and be efficient, radio (available for 158 per 1 000 in 1996), and/or television (56 sets per 1000 people in 1997) [1]. These two means should use local languages to better reach the people.

Health

The information concerning the general health environment in Africa reveals that total expenditure *per capita* (including public and private) is 63.9 $. The ratio of health professionals in the '90s on population demonstrate that in Africa there are 30 physicians for 100 000 (excluding dentists). But there is a big difference from a country to another as shown in *table I* [1]. The MD/population in cities is much better than in rural areas. The perinatal period is a leading factor of disability including epilepsy and other neuropsychiatric and developmental disorders. In 14% of births, it is remarked a low birth weight baby. This phenomenon is correlated with the prevalence of anemia in pregnant African women which was 40% in years 1985 to 1995. The mean rate of child immunization has dramatically improved since 1980: 63.9% of African children under 12 months are vaccinated against diphtheria, polio and tetanus. 54.5% of African inhabitants have access to safe water and 46.7% to sanitation [1]. These factors are very important to notice because of the importance of the disease transmission via water and feces (*i.e.* brain cysticercocis), and several bacterial and parasitical diseases involving the brain with an epileptogenic potency and bad prognosis if untreated.

Epidemiological considerations and their impact on prognosis

Prevalence

Many epilepsy epidemiological researches using various protocols have been performed in the African continent. They have demonstrated a wide range of prevalence rates from 5.2 to 74 per 1 000, even by the door-to-door survey methodology, which is considered as the gold standard *(table II)*. High prevalence rates have been reported in Liberia (28‰) and Nigeria (37‰). The lowest rates were shown in Northern African countries (Morocco, Tunisia, Egypt, Algeria, Libya) and in South Africa where the mean prevalence is close to Eastern European countries (2 to 5‰). Low rates have also been reported in Nigeria (6.2 and 5.3‰), in Ethiopia (5‰). In a recent study in Senegal, it has been demonstrated that when the population benefits from a good concentration of health structure, health personnel and pharmacy, the epilepsy prevalence rate can decrease (to 1.9‰ in Saint-Louis

Table I. Health – General situation

Country	Safe water (% of access)	Sanitation (% of access)	Health expenditure per capita 1990-97 ($)	% of < 12 months old child immunization against diphteria, polio, tetanus
Algeria	–	–	85	76
Angola	32	15	–	60
Benin	72	24	–	80
Botswana	70	55	–	78
Burkina Faso	–	–	17	70
Burundi	58	48	–	57
Cameroon	41	40	7	44
Cape Verde	–	–	–	–
Central African Rep	23	45	–	50
Chad	24	21	6	27
Comorros	–	–	–	–
Congo Dem. Répub.	–	–	–	–
Congo Republic	–	9	77	20
Côte d'Ivoire	72	51	25	69
Dijbouti	–	–	–	–
Egypt	84	70	38	93
Equatorial Guinea	–	–	–	–
Eritrea	7	–	–	56
Ethiopia	–	–	3	57
Gabon	67	76	–	49
Gambia	50	37	–	93
Ghana	65	32	6	59
Guinea	55	14	–	54
Guinea-Bissau	53	21	–	57
Kenya	45	45	8	34
Lesotho	62	–	–	55
Liberia	–	–	–	–
Libya	95	86	–	94
Madagascar	16	34	–	70
Malawi	60	64	–	91
Mali	48	37	8	54
Mauritania	64	32	28	24
Mauritius	100	100	116	87
Morocco	57	68	49	93
Mozambique	24	23	–	89
Namibia	60	42	127	60
Niger	48	17	–	35
Nigeria	50	57	5	57
Rwanda	–	94	–	71
Sao Tome Principe	–	–	–	–
Senegal	51	50	23	92
Seychelles	–	–	–	–
Sierra Leone	34	–	–	65
Somalia	–	–	–	–
South Africa	59	53	258	74
Sudan	60	22	4	85
Swaziland	–	–	–	–
Tanzania	49	86	–	71
Togo	55	41	15	35
Tunisia	90	80	99	94
Uganda	42	67	9	59
Zambia	53	51	17	69
Zimbabwe	77	66	41	43

Table II. Prevalence of epilepsy in subsaharan Africa (door-to-door surveys) (adapted from [24])

Country	Authors	Year	N[1]	P[1] ‰	CI 95%[2]	U ou R[3]
Ivory Coast	Kouadjo	1990	309	74.0	43.0-105.0	R
Cameroon	Nkwi et Ndonko	1989	500	70.0	46.3-93.7	R
Ivory Coast (M'Brou)	Kaudjhis	1995	920	59.0	43.0-75.0	R
Cameroon (Bilomo)	Dongmo et al.	1998	1 900	58.0	46.9-69.1	R
Nigeria (Aiyété)	Osuntokun et al.	1982	903	37.0	24.2-49.8	R
Liberia	Goudsmit et al.	1983	4 436	28.0	23.0-33.0	R
Benin (Agbogbomé)	Gbenou	1995	530	24.5	10.9-38.1	R
Senegal	Diop et al.	1996	2 803	21.0	15.5-26.5	R
Togo (Tone)	Balogou et al.	2000	9 143	18.6	15.7-21.5	R
Kenya	Kaamugisha et Feksi	1988	2 960	18.2	13.2-23.2	R
Togo (Kozah)	Dumas et al.	1989	5 264	16.7	13.1-20.3	R
Mali	Farnarier et al.	2000	5 243	15.6	12.2-19.0	R
Benin (Savalou)	Avodé et al.	1996	1 443	15.2	8.7-21.7	R
Togo (Akebou)	Grunitzky et al.	1996	4 182	13.1	9.6-16.6	R
Uganda	Kaiser et al.	1996	4 743	13.0	9.7-16.3	R
Togo (Kloto)	Grunitzky et al.	1991	19 241	12.3	10.7-13.9	R
Mali (Bamako)	Traoré et al.	2000	4 074	11.3	8.0-14.6	U
Burkina Faso	Debouverie et al.	1993	16 627	10.6	9.0-12.2	R
Tanzania	Rwiza et al.	1992	18 183	10.2	8.7-11.7	R
Senegal	Ndiaye et al.	1986	7 682	8.3	6.2-10.4	R
Ivory Coast	Kouassi et al.	1988	1 176	7.6	2.5-12.7	R
Nigeria	Longe et Osuntokun	1989	2 925	6.2	3.3-9.1	R
Nigeria (Igbo-Ora)	Osuntokun et al.	1987	18 954	5.3	4.2-6.4	U
Ethiopia (Butajira)	Tekle-Haimanot et al.	1990	60 820	5.2	4.6-5.8	R

Note: [1]: N = number of subjects; P = prevalence; [2] = 95% Confidence interval; [3]: U = urban; R = rural

survey) [2] with a better prognosis. Between the extremes, various average rates (ranging from 10 to 20 per 1 000) were shown in different places, using different methodology, including WHO or other protocols: Senegal (8 to 12‰), Burkina Faso (10 to 15‰), Benin (10 to 15‰; with high incidence and prevalence rates in cysticercosis endemic zones), Togo (12 to 18‰), Ivory Coast (7.6%), in Tanzania (20‰). In Libya, an epidemiological and clinical study of epilepsy in Benghazi showed a prevalence rate of 2.3‰ in the population above the age of 15 years. For 70.8% of the patients the onset of epilepsy occurred in the first 2 decades of life, and for 7.6% it started after the age of 40. The duration of epilepsy when first seen in the study period was less than 1 year in 14.6%, and greater than 10 years in 25.7% [3]. This last result is the most common reality in Africa where the majority of patients are first seen in modern medical centers between 1 to 20 years after the first symptoms of their epilepsy. The duration is longer in rural than in urban areas (Diop, unpublished data) and consequently the evolution is worsening.

Etiology

This is the leading point which must be considered for analyzing the prognosis of epilepsy in Africa. Many etiologic factors make epilepsy to be considered as a great public health problem in Africa. Such as in low-income developing countries, many epileptogenic factors exist. Perinatal and post-natal causes are brain-stresser in many people, especially those suffering from malnutrition and difficult economical conditions. These causes determine a large part of the evolution of the disease treated or not. Studies have been conducted in known high risk factor areas such as "meningitis belt", cysticercosis in Christian pork consumers, malaria endemic zones, maternity and pediatric structures. In a study performed in South Africa, the survey of 43% of epileptic patients demonstrated historic, clinical, and radiological evidence suggesting epilepsy symptomatic of underlying brain damage or defect [4].

In Nigeria, there were 60 patients representing 4% of admissions into the Newborn Unit during the period. Birth asphyxia, infections and hypoglycaemia were the important identifiable etiological factors which operated either singly (48% of cases) or in concert (in another 48%) of the infants. Detectable infections included meningitis and septicemia caused predominantly by coliforms and *Staphylococcus aureus* [5]. Febrile convulsions were reported in Tanzania and Nigeria. The Benin City experience, in Nigeria revealed that about 20% of children admitted during the study period had febrile convulsions, of which 5% were aged under 5 months or over 5 years. This study confirmed the view that there is a strong familial predisposition in febrile seizures. Major causes of the rise in temperature in those studied included malaria, which accounted for 32.7%, followed by bronchopneumonia (16.8%), measles (15.4%), otitis media (13.4%) and tonsillitis (10.5%). Furthermore, the morbidity and mortality have been attributable to the socio-cultural background of the community which practices modes of therapy that are often detrimental to the health of patients [6]. Other associated factors included unspecified encephalitis (4.7%), cerebral malaria (1.9%), birth injury (1.4%), and other (3%). In 38% of the cases, there was a positive family history of epilepsy [7]; Obi *et al.*, 1994 [8]. In over 50% of children with recurrent seizures in a South African hospital population the onset of attacks was before the age of 2 years. In 32% of patients there was a history of perinatal complications and 11% had a history of meningitis; 38% of the children had abnormalities on physical examination and 55% were intellectually handicapped [4]. In the Kenyan series, etiologies of secondary epilepsy were represented by: head injury (31.2%), congenital CNS abnormality and birth trauma (27.3%), febrile convulsions (8.7%), tumors (5.6%), vascular (2.8%), mesial temporal sclerosis (2.1%) and metabolic (0.7%) [9, 10]. Prevalence of cysticercosis in epileptics and members of their families have been conducted in various countries, including Benin and Togo [11, 12]. Parental consanguinity was found in 65% of the total sample, which emphasizes the role played by that factor in the etiology of mental subnormality [13].

Outcome and prognosis

There is very few data on prognosis in Africa, in particular no true incidence cohort study. Outcome of the same clinical – epileptic or not – feature can differ from an epileptic patient to another, depending on the general situation (between different areas of an African country or from Africa to the developed world). This situation is reflected by the general mortality rate in Africa *(table III)*. The mean duration at first attendance was of 6.5 years in Malawi [14], 13.4 ± 4.1 (ranging from 3 months to 26 years) in Dakar, capital of Senegal. Another one-year follow-up conducted in the second city of Senegal (Thies) [15] revealed that among 73 newly diagnosed epileptic patients treated for the very first time with phenobarbital or carbamazepine, 60% became seizure-free at the end of the one-year follow-up; 30% experienced dramatic reduction of seizures; and 10% did not have any improvement. It was found that as the duration of active epilepsy increased, the number of patients having epilepsy of a given duration decreased. With local assistance and overseas donations of phenobarbital, a clinic founded in a rural community in Tanzania [16], treated approximately 200 patients for less than or equal to 10 years. The area was revisited 30 years later to trace these patients. Of the 164 patients who had started treatment, 52.4% achieved complete seizure suppression, 36.0% experienced reduction in seizure frequency, 7.9% experienced no change, and in 1 (0.6%) seizures were worse. The effect of treatment could not be assessed in 5 (3.0%) patients. After 30 years, only 36 (21.9%) of the 164 pa-

Table III. Mortality and births conditions

Country	Adult male Mortality rate (per 1 000)	Adult female Mortality rate (per 1 000)	Maternal Mortality (/100 000 births)	Under-5 Mortality rate (per 1 000)	% of births Attended by health personnel	Low-birth weight babies (% of births)
Algeria	160	125	140	39	77	9
Angola	412	355	1 500	209	17	–
Benin	362	304	500	149	60	–
Botswana	600	552	250	88	77	8
Burkina faso	540	520	930	169	41	21
Burundi	550	491	1 300	200	24	16
Cameroon	390	352	550	78	58	13
Cape Verde						
Central African Rep	567	476	700	160	46	–
Chad	448	383	840	182	15	–
Comorros	–	–	–	–	–	–
Congo Dem. Répub.	–	–	870	148	–	–
Congo Republic	464	402	890	145	50	16
Côte d'Ivoire	510	490	810	140	45	14
Dijbouti	–	–	–	–	–	–
Egypt	198	174	170	66	46	12
Equatorial Guinea	–	–	–	–	–	–
Eritrea	450	403	1 000	95	21	–
Ethiopia	550	510	1 400	175	8	16
Gabon	380	340	500	136	80	10
Gambia	404	339	1 050	–	44	–
Ghana	278	226	740	102	44	17
Guinea	399	400	880	182	31	13
Guinea-Bissau	469	416	910	220	25	20
Kenya	425	397	650	112	45	16
Lesotho	320	382	610	137	50	–
Liberia	–	–	–	–	–	–
Libya	187	135	220	30	94	5
Madagascar	332	295	500	158	57	15
Malawi	454	471	620	224	55	–
Mali	416	334	580	235	24	17
Mauritania	344	294	800	149	40	9
Mauritius	205	97	110	23	97	–
Morocco	207	150	370	67	40	4
Mozambique	400	354	1 100	201	44	20
Namibia	366	341	220	101	68	–
Niger	450	342	590	–	15	15
Nigeria	398	335	1 000	122	31	16
Rwanda	585	534	1 300	209	26	17
Sao Tome Principe	–	–	–	–	–	–
Senegal	453	381	510	110	47	12
Seychelles						
Sierra Leone	544	483	–	286	25	–
Somalia	–	–	–	–	–	–
South Africa	261	160	230	65	82	–
Sudan	373	328	370	115	86	15
Swaziland	–	–	–	–	–	–
Tanzania	502	460	530	136	38	14
Togo	477	432	640	138	32	20
Tunisia	171	153	170	33	–	16
Uganda	580	590	550	162	38	–
Zambia	512	524	650	189	47	13
Zimbabwe	449	388	280	108	69	14

tients were known to be alive. Of the patients, 110 (67.1%) had died, and the whereabouts of 18 (11%) could not be traced. The causes of death were epilepsy related (status epilepticus, drowning, burns, dying in or after a seizure) in greater than 50% of the patients. Epilepsy-related deaths were proportionately higher after drug supply was stopped and among patients who were receiving drugs irregularly or who had only partial seizure control. Studies about death among people with epilepsy are very scarce in Africa. In Kenya, during a two year community-based investigation of mortality 3.5% of the deaths to individuals over the age of 5 years were reported by bereaved relatives to have occurred to epileptics and 77% of these deaths were thought to have occurred whilst the patient was in status epilepticus [17]. In Ethiopia, during a period of 2 years, 8 persons died of status epilepticus and 1 from severe burns as a result of falling into a domestic fire during a seizure [18]. In this study, the SMR was estimated to be around 3 (Forsgren, personal communication). Patients with epilepsy showed an increased mortality rate, which was twice that of the general rural population of similar age. In Malawi, the number of patients of a given duration of active epilepsy decreased as this duration increased. Possible explanations for this result, such as an increasing incidence of epilepsy or a high mortality rate, are considered, but thought to be unlikely; spontaneous remission seems to be the better explanation of this finding [14]. In a rural zone of Cameroon, 128 pairs of untreated patients and matched controls were followed-up during 10 years. The mortality was 28.9% among patients from which 57% from status epilepticus and only 4.7% among controls (Boussinesq, personal communication). In Kenya Feksi [19] found 53% of seizure-free patients among 302 treated patients in 1 year. Duration of epilepsy and number of fits were not prognostic factors. In Nigeria in an urban zone Ogunniyi [20] found in 1998 only 30% seizure free patients after a 2 years follow-up among 345 treated patients. The factors associated with the absence of remission were the low compliance and a number of fits higher than 6 prior treatment. On the contrary, in rural Mali Nimaga [21] have treated 96 patients and found 80% seizure free patients within 1 year.

Therapeutical itinerary of patient with epilepsy in Africa

Specialized personnel and means of diagnosis

The majority of people suffering from seizure do not consult MD as first intention. Either they have no opportunity to do it or they cultural background does not prepare them for such an initiative. In a study recently conducted in Dakar, Senegal, we found that 63% of patients coming for an EEG to unique service of Neurology of the country, have been seen in the traditional system 1 to 14 years before reaching the modern structures. In "Central" Africa, the mean ratio is 1 Neurologist for 4,1 Million *(table IV)*. The "best" ratio are found in Ivory Coast, Kenya and Senegal (1 Neurologist for 1 Million people). As for the other health data the exceptions are represented by North Africa and South Africa with a ratio of 1 Neurologist for 300 000 to 400 000 people. In the central part of Africa, the diagnosis means necessary for a good and minimal practice are represented by 75 EEG, less than 25 CT-Scans, and 5 MRI. For South Africa and Maghreb countries the conditions are comparable to Eastern Europe condition *(table V)*.

Modern treatment management

The main circulating molecules in the Africa continent are: Phenobarbital (prescribed in 65 to 90%); Carbamazepine (5 to 25%); Phenytoine (2 to 25%); Valproate (2 to 8%)

Table IV. Health personnel: general and neuroscience

Country	Physicians (number)	Physicians (per 100 000)	Nurses and Midwives (number)	Nurses and Midwives (per 100 000)	Neurologist (number)	Neurosurg. (number)	Psychiatry (number)
Algeria	22 202	141	–	–	260	210	–
Angola	–	–	–	–	–	–	–
Benin	318	6	1 226	33	2	0	–
Botswana	–	–	55	–	–	–	–
Burkina faso	–	–	–	–	2	1	2
Burundi	333	6	986	17	2	0	–
Cameroon	1 250	7	–	–	6	4	4
Cape Verde	103	29	205	57	0	0	–
Central African Rep	174	6	1 374	45	0	0	–
Chad	144	2	365	6	0	0	1
Comorros	–	–	–	–	1	0	0
Congo Dem. Répub.	–	–	–	–	33	2	–
Congo Republic	688	27	1 158	49	2	1	–
Côte d'Ivoire	–	–	–	–	9	–	–
Djibouti	115	20	–	–	0	0	–
Egypt	127 121	202	139 707	222	310	160	–
Equatorial Guinea	83	21	129	34	0	–	–
Eritrea	64	2	–	–	–	–	–
Ethiopia	2 214	4	4 209	8	10	0	–
Gabon	248	19	722	56	4	1	–
Gambia	17	2	250	25	0	–	–
Ghana	747	4	–	–	3	5	–
Guinea	920	15	202	3	3	0	–
Guinea-Bissau	187	18	476	45	0	–	–
Kenya	3 554	15	5 879	23	18	20	10
Lesotho	93	5	650	33	–	–	–
Liberia	–	–	–	–	–	–	–
Libya	6 916	137	18 476	366	2	1	–
Madagascar	3 614	24	7 398	55	18	3	3
Malawi	257	2	638	6	1	2	–
Mali	413	4	918	9	2	0	–
Mauritania	233	11	574	27	2	0	3
Mauritius	916	85	2 598	241	–	–	–
Morocco	9 006	34	24 899	94	35	60	–
Mozambique	–	–	–	–	–	–	–
Namibia	330	23	1 153	81	–	–	–
Niger	225	3	1 379	17	0	0	1
Nigeria	21 325	21	144 952	142	11	5	–
Rwanda	–	–	–	–	0	0	–
Sao Tome Principe	40	32	–	–	0	–	–
Senegal	649	7	2 663	35	9	6	12
Seychelles	75	104	–	–	–	–	–
Sierra leone	–	–	–	–	0	0	–
Somalia	358	4	269	3	–	2	–
South Africa	22 208	59	67 843	175	98	118	474
Sudan	2 736	10	19 153	70	–	–	–
Swaziland	–	–	–	–	–	–	–
Tanzania	1 205	4	12 509	46	–	5	–
Togo	225	6	1 259	31	6	1	3
Tunisia	5 960	67	25 176	283	54	30	100
Uganda	722	4	5 351	28	–	3	–
Zambia	–	–	–	–	–	–	–
Zimbabwe	1 632	14	17 654	164	3	6	10

Table V. Means of neuro-diagnostic

Country	EEG	CT-SCAN	MRI
Algeria	50	30	3
Angola	–	–	–
Benin	2	0	0
Botswana	–	–	–
Burkina Faso	1	0	0
Burundi	2	0	0
Cameroon	9	2	–
Cape Verde	–	0	0
Central African Rep	0	0	0
Chad	0	0	0
Comorros	0	0	0
Congo Dem. Répub.	14	1	–
Congo Republic	–	0	0
Côte d'Ivoire	7	3	0
Djibouti	1	–	–
Egypt	–	40	15
Equatorial Guinea	0	0	0
Eritrea	–	–	0
Ethiopia	3	0	0
Gabon	4	0	–
Gambia	0	0	0
Ghana	–	–	–
Guinea	1	0	0
Guinea-Bissau	–	–	0
Kenya	8	6	2
Lesotho	–	–	–
Liberia	0	0	0
Libya	–	–	–
Madagascar	4	1	0
Malawi	–	–	–
Mali	1	0	0
Mauritania	1	1	0
Mauritius	–	–	–
Morocco	25	30	6
Mozambique	–	1	0
Namibia	–	–	–
Niger	1	0	0
Nigeria	10	9	1
Rwanda	0	0	0
Sao Tome Principe	–	–	0
Senegal	5	4	0
Seychelles	–	–	–
Sierra leone	–	0	0
Somalia	–	0	0
South Africa	–	130	46
Sudan	–	–	–
Swaziland	–	–	–
Tanzania	–	–	–
Togo	4	2	0
Tunisia	50	15	3
Uganda	–	–	0
Zambia	–	–	–
Zimbabwe	5	8	3

and diazepam for emergency. Only Morroco, Tunisia, Egypt, Zimbabwe and South Africa have some of the brand new drugs such as Oxcarbazepine, Lamotrigine and Vigabatrin. The prices of drugs are comprised in the annual range of 25 to 50 $ for Phenobarbital and Phenytoine; 200 to 300 $ for Carbamazepine; 300 to 500 $ for Valproate. This price range must be commented by the basis of the financial status of the continent described bellow.

The drugs available in Senegal and the price of a box in US $ are indicated in the following table:

Drug	Strength	Public Price	Generic Price
Phenobarbitone	10 mg	1	0.4
Phenobarbitone	50 mg	1.02	0.4
Phenobarbitone	100 mg	1.24	0.6
Carbamazepine	200 mg	8.7	–
Phenytoin	100 mg	2.18	–
Valproate	200 mg	8.3	–
Valproate	500 mg	9.45	–
Clonazepam	2 mg	8.5	–
Diazepam	10 mg/l	6.9	–
Diazepam	5 mg/ml	6.7	1.24

Bad prognosis of epilepsy in Africa is mainly determined by factors of management gap and treatment gap

The vast majority of patients with epilepsy in developing countries do not receive adequate medical treatment and an estimated percentage of 80-90% are without any treatment. Poor infrastructure, insufficient availability of drugs and scarcity of trained medical personnel are relevant factors for this situation. The impact of infrastructures on prognosis has been demonstrated in a University Hospital of Dakar, Senegal [22] with a overall mortality rate of 24.8% in period of 11-year follow-up. Epilepsy is well known in African societies. Several denominations express epilepsy and specify, in some cultures, different presentations of general or partial simple or complex seizures. Terms such as *morbus sacer*, denoting both a sacred and demoniac condition, or folk names indicating divine punishment, have expressed these feelings in European societies from antiquity to the Middle Ages and beyond. An atmosphere of fear, shame and mysticism surrounds epilepsy even in our days in many non-Western and also in Western cultures. Epilepsy is conceived of as an "African" affliction, a manifestation of supernatural forces that makes it difficult to reach epilepsy sufferers with modern medical treatment. Epilepsy is traditionally looked on as caused by ancestral spirits or attributed to possession by evil spirits. It is also thought to be due to witchcraft, and "poisoning", and often taken to be contagious. One of the prognosis factor, the distance from health care facilities is a problem of the know-how available at the community health care level. It has been shown that a reasonable level of seizure treatment can be achieved by primary healthcare workers, however, given the objection to vertical programs (i.e. primary healthcare workers only involved in epilepsy care), sufficient back-up for the primary healthcare workers should be available in order to give epilepsy care its proper place among their many other duties. A interesting experience has been reported from Zimbabwe [23]. This team evaluated the effectiveness of primary health care nurses in the diagnosis and management of epilepsy, as well as the impact of patient-information pamphlets on drug compliance and clinic attendance of patients with epilepsy in 24 clinics of a district in Zimbabwe. The personnel attended a workshop to improving their knowledge in the diagnosis and management of generalized tonic-clonic seizures. Half of these clinics (experimental group) subsequently received patient-information pamphlets for distribution to patients and relatives, whereas the other half (control group) did not. Frequency of clinic attendance, mean seizure frequencies, and mean serum levels of phenobarbitone were compared at baseline and at 6 months after intervention in patients within each group, and at 6 months after intervention between both groups. They found that Community health worker education led to a 74% increase in patient recruitment as well as a marked improvement in patient drug compliance and outcome over the 6-month study period. The use of patient-information pamphlets led to a marked reduction in patient default from clinic follow-up, but did not appear to influence drug compliance or seizure frequency.

Conclusion

In summary, the effort which must be conducted to reduce treatment gap in Africa have to be a multidisciplinary and multidimensional approach conducted by trained health and social workers, educated patients and families, communicators, community and opinion leaders, with the support of bilateral and multilateral cooperation, international Institutions and NGOs and pharmaceutical companies. The improvement of predictable causes of epilepsy, including a better and convincing management of seizures, pregnancy, and child health must be considered as priorities.

References

1. World bank. World development indicators, 1999.
2. Ndiaye M. Enquête épidémiologique sur l'épilepsie à Saint-Louis (milieu scolaire). Thèse Med., Dakar, 1997, n° 52.
3. Sridharan R, Radhakrishnan K, Ashok PP, Mousa ME. Epidemiological and clinical study of epilepsy in Benghazi, Libya. *Epilepsia* 1986; 27: 60-5.
4. Leary PM, Morris S. Recurrent seizures in childhood. Western Cape profile. *S Afr Med J* 1988; 3: 579-81.
5. Asindi AA, Antia-Obong OE, Ibia EO, Udo JJ. Neonatal seizures in Nigerian infants. *Far J Med Sci* 1995; 24: 243-8.
6. Obi JO, Ejeheri NA, Alakija W. Childhood febrile seizures (Benin City experience). *Ann Trop Paediatr* 1994; 14: 211-4.
7. Rwiza HT, Kilonzo GP, Haule J, Matuja WB, Mteza I, Mbena P, Kilima PM, Mwaluko G, Mwang'Ombola R, Mwaijande F. Prevalence and incidence of epilepsy in Ulanga, a rural Tanzanian district: a community-based study. *Epilepsia* 1992; 33: 1051-6.
8. Iloeje SO. Febrile convulsions in a rural and an urban population. *East Afr Med J* 1991; 68: 43-51.
9. Ruberti RF, Mwinzi SMG, Dekker N, Stewart JD. Epilepsy in the Kenyan. *Afr J Neurol Sci* 1985; 41: 36-40.
10. Ruberti RF. Post-traumatic epilepsy. *Afr J Neurol Sci* 1986; 5: 9-17.
11. Grunitzky E, Dumas M, M'Bella M. Les épilepsies au Togo. *Epilepsies* 1991; 3: 295-303.
12. Avode DG, Bouteille B, Houngbe F, Adjien C, Adjide C, Houinato D, Hountondjl A, Dumas M. Epilepsy, cysticercosis and neurocysticercosis in Benin. *Eur Neurol* 1998; 39: 60-1.

13. Temtamy SA, Kandil MR, Demerdash AM, Hassan WA, Meguid NA, Afifi HH. An epidemiological/genetic study of mental subnormality in Assiut Governorate, Egypt. *Clin Genet* 1994; 46: 347-51.
14. Watts AE. The natural history of untreated epilepsy in a rural community in Africa. *Epilepsia* 1992; 33: 464-8.
15. Boissy LG. Prise en charge de patients épileptiques dans un programme décentralisé de santé mentale: le centre Dalal Xël de Thiés. Thèse Med., Dakar, 2001, n° 38.
16. Jilek-Aall L, Rwiza HT. Prognosis of epilepsy in a rural African community: a 30-year follow-up of 164 patients in an outpatient clinic in rural Tanzania. *Epilepsia* 1992; 33: 645-50.
17. Snow RW, Williams RE, Rogers JE, Mung'Ala VO, Peshu N. The prevalence of epilepsy among a rural Kenyan population. Its association with premature mortality. *Trop Geogr Med* 1994; 46: 175-9.
18. Tekle-Haimanot R, Forsgren L, Ekstedt J. Incidence of epilepsy in rural central Ethiopia. *Epilepsia* 1997; 38: 541-6.
19. Feksi AT, Kaamugisha J, Gatiti S, Sander JW, Shorvon SD. A comprehensive community epilepsy programme: the Nakuru project. *Epilepsy Res* 1991; 8: 252-9.
20. Ogunniyi A, Oluwole OSA, Osuntokun BO. Two-year remission in nigerian epileptics. *East Afr Med J* 1998; 75: 392-5.
21. Nimaga K, Desplats D, Doumbo O, Farnarier G. Treatment with phenobarbital and monitoring of epileptic patients in rural Mali. *Bull World Health Organ* 2002; 80: 532-7.
22. Mbodj I, Ndiaye M, Sene F, Sow PS, Sow HD, Diagana M, Ndiaye IP, Diop AG. Prise en charge de l'état de mal épileptique dans les conditions de pays en développement. *Neurophysiol Clin* 2000; 30: 165-9.
23. Adamolekun B, Mielke JK, Ball DE. An evaluation of the impact of health worker and patient education on the care and compliance of patients with epilepsy in Zimbabwe. *Epilepsia* 1999; 40: 507-11.
24. Preux PM. Contribution à la connaissance épidémiologique de l'épilepsie en Afrique sub-saharienne. Ph D Thesis, University of Limoges, 2000, 385 p.

Prognosis of temporal lobe epilepsy after surgery

H. Gregor Wieser

Introduction

Problems

The postoperative long-term prognosis of patients after temporal lobe surgery remains a difficult topic, although there exist a large number of studies dealing with postoperative outcome [1-8]. One major difficulty is that results from older series do no longer reflect the present state of art. Many of the older series refer to temporal lobectomy and included a high proportion of patients operated on prior to MRI and microsurgical techniques [9-12]. Clearly, the techniques employed in these pioneering centers have since improved. In addition, problems arise because of inconsistent use of seizure outcome classifications, short post-operative follow-ups, relatively small numbers of patients, and limited data with regard to complications, and functional and psychosocial outcome. Underlying etiologies are often not sufficiently taken into account. Furthermore, group results are usually reported what prevents in most instances to trace the individual patient with respect to both, seizure recurrence and the "running down phenomenon" of auras and seizures over time. In addition, antiepileptic treatment management, quality of life and the degree of disability, as well as mortality, are often not adequately addressed although they represent central outcome measures of epilepsy surgery.

Several attempts have been made to obtain comprehensive surveys on the prognosis of temporal lobe epilepsy after surgery. Jensen had collected 2 282 published patients who had undergone anterior temporal lobectomy (ATL) between 1928 and 1973 [1]. The 1985 Palm Desert survey included 2 336 ATLs. In the 1985 survey only ATLs were specified. At this time a few amygdalohippocampectomies (AHEs) had been performed (mainly from Zurich) and were included in the ATL resection category. In the 1992 Second Palm Desert survey ATL and AHE were segregated and the following numbers were given (*table I* [10]). However, ATL were both standard and tailored, and the data in this category did not take into account that some of these resections included only neocortex.

As can be seen from *table II*, in the 1992 Second Palm Desert Survey neocortical resections were not specified further, but opposed to lesionectomies. The results in the temporal lobe surgery category clearly show that there was considerable increase in the percentage of patients who were seizure-free after surgery, and that selective limbic resection were at least no worse than those obtained from larger ATL, when specific selection criteria are met. The 1985 Palm Desert survey specified only neocortical resections and included surgical procedures that were considered lesionectomies in the 1991 survey. At 1991 centers were asked to list the data for neocortical resections and lesionectomies separately. What is clearly reflected in *tables I and II* is that results of AHE and ATL were similar and that results of neocortical resections remained inferior compared to temporal-limbic resections.

Table I. Outcome for temporal lobe surgery (1992 Second Palm Desert survey; [10])

	Before 1985 (%)		1986-1990			
			ATL (%)		AHE (%)	
Seizure-free	1 296	55.5%	2 429	67.9%	284	68.8%
Improved	648	27.7%	860	24.0%	92	22.3%
Not improved	392	16.8%	290	8.1%	37	9.0%
Total	2 336	100%	3 579	100%	413	100%

ATL, anterior temporal lobectomy; AHE, selective amygdalohippocampectomy.

Table II. Outcome for neocortical resections (1992 Second Palm Desert survey; [10])

	Before 1985 (%)		1986-1990			
			Extratemporal resection (%)		Lesionectomy (%)	
Seizure-free	356	43.2%	363	45.1%	195	66.6%
Improved	229	27.8%	283	35.2%	63	21.5%
Not improved	240	29.1%	159	19.8%	35	11.9%
Total	825	100%	805	100%	293	100%

Classification of temporal lobe epilepsy

The new "diagnostic scheme for people with epileptic seizures and with epilepsy" [13] segregates in the axis epilepsy syndromes and related conditions the "Symptomatic (or probably symptomatic) focal epilepsies" into
– Limbic epilepsies
  • Mesial temporal lobe epilepsy with hippocampal sclerosis
  • Mesial temporal lobe epilepsy defined by specific etiologies
  • Other types defined by location and etiology
– Neocortical epilepsies
– Rasmussen syndrome
– Other types defined by location and etiology

Long-term outcome of patients operated in Zurich with the selective amygdalohippocampectomy as treatment for mesial temporal lobe epilepsy

In a retrospective long-term seizure outcome study we re-assessed 400 patients who underwent selective amygdalohippocampectomy (AHE) as treatment for mesial temporal lobe epilepsy (MTLE) at the Zurich University Hospital between 1975-1999 [14]. We report some data of this study and present a summary of several studies on consecutive samples of this series which dealt with quality of life, memory and disability assessment [15-19].

Methods and definitions

Seizure outcome classification

We report seizure outcome with the widely used classification system of Engel I to IV [9, 10] *(table III) and* the new classification system 1 to 6 proposed by the International League against Epilepsy (ILAE [20] *table IV*). In this new system the ILAE class 1a indicates those patients who remained completely seizure and aura free *since surgery*. Furthermore, the ILAE classes 1-4, for the first time, allow a direct comparison with antiepileptic drug (AED) studies in which a more than 50% seizure reduction against baseline is the most common end point.

Table III. Seizure outcome classification according to Engel [9, 10]

Class I: Free of disabling seizures
  A Completely seizure free since surgery
  B Nondisabling simple partial seizures only since surgery
  C Some disabling seizures after surgery, but free of disabling seizures for at least 2 years
  D Generalized convulsions with AED discontinuation only
Class II: Rare disabling seizures ("almost seizure free")
  A Initially free of disabling seizures but has rare seizures now
  B Rare disabling seizures since surgery
  C More than rare disabling seizures since surgery, but rare seizures for the last 2 years
  D Nocturnal seizures only
Class III: Worthwhile improvement
  A Worthwhile seizure reduction
  B Prolonged seizure-free intervals amounting to greater than half the followed-up period, but not < 2years
Class IV: No worthwhile improvement
  A Significant seizure reduction
  B No appreciable change

Table IV. Proposed new ILAE-classification of outcome with respect to epileptic seizures [20]

Outcome Classification	Definition
1	Completely seizure free; no auras
[1a]	[Completely seizure- and aura-free *since* surgery]
2	Only auras; no other seizures
3	1 to 3 seizure days per year; ± auras
4	4 seizure days per year to 50% reduction of baseline seizure days; ± auras
5	Less than 50% reduction of baseline seizure days to 100% increase of baseline seizure days; ± auras
6	More than 100% increase of baseline seizure days; ± auras

Definitions and subgroups

In order to account for differing etiology of TLE we differentiated between "non-lesional" (including "classical" and "non-classical" hippocampal sclerosis, HS), and "lesional" (gross anatomical lesions) AHEs. Most anatomical lesions were identified preoperatively, but there were 32 patients who had lesions identified intraoperatively and/or by histopathological examination of the surgical specimen, particularly before the use of MRI. The definitive classification "lesional" was according to histopathology. Patients with dual pathology, i.e. a lesion *and* hippocampal sclerosis, are indicated too.

Also, differentiation was made between "curative" and "palliative" surgeries. With the preoperatively assigned attribute "curative" we labeled patients with electrophysiologically documented seizure origin in the resected mesial temporal lobe structures or with a lesion in this structures highly concordant with the seizure semiology and the non-invasive electroencephalographic (EEG) and positron emission tomography (PET) findings. "Palliative" was preoperatively attributed to patients in whom the seizure generating structures were not within, or exceeded the borders of the resection but with the proof that the resected mesial temporal lobe structures were of importance for the maintenance of the seizure in the sense of a secondary epileptogenic "pacemaker" or seizure sustaining substrate.

Surgery related complications

Surgery related complications were defined as unwanted, unexpected and uncommon events. Minor complications were defined as complications that resolve within 3 months without sequel. A major complication affects activities of daily living and lasts longer than 3 months. Surgery related complications were determined for all sAHE patients who had undergone a follow-up of more than 3 months (n = 453).

Quality of life assessment

Neuropsychological assessment

Ninety-three patients of this AHE series underwent the same neuropsychological pre- and postoperative testing and were included. The patient population consisted of consecutively operated patients since 1975 [19]. Inclusion criteria were (1) same pre- and postoperative test procedure, using parallel versions, of the following test battery: Rey Auditory Verbal Learning Test (AVLT), a modified Rey Visual Design Learning Test (VDLT), Rey-Osterrieth Complex Figure Test, Word Fluency Test, Five-Point Test, Stroop Test, Kramer Two-Group Test, Goldenberg Association Learning, and Tachistoscopic Lexical Decision Task. (2) Time of testing was within 3 months before, and 3 to 4 months after surgery. Excluded were patients (1) with "palliative" AHEs, (2) with semi-malignant or malignant tumors and (3) with surgery related complications.

Assessment of psychosocial outcome

Kurmann-Bärlocher [18] examined the psychosocial outcome in non-lesional AHE-patients by sending a questionnaire to all AHE patients of this series. Ninety patients responded in a sufficiently detailed fashion to 32 questions, and were included. Besides on epileptological data, the questions concentrated on the following main categories: *Employment (professional career and income), housing, support by family and/or a partner, social contacts, sexual life, sport and leisure activity (including hobbies), depression, self-confidence, independence*, and judgment of *overall quality of life*.

Results

Characteristics of the Zurich AHE series

Of 400 retrospectively studied consecutive sAHE patients 218 (55%) were operated on for a gross anatomical lesion presumably causing their seizure ("lesional"). In the "lesional" group the pathological findings were grouped into: *Tumors* (n = 162; 74.3%): WHO I (mainly ganglioglioma and DNET): n = 50, 23.0%; WHO II (mainly astrocytoma, oligodendroglioma, and ganglioglioma): n = 64; 29.4%; WHO > II (mainly astrocytoma III): n = 48; 22%; *Vascular malformations and vascular tumors*: n = 41; 18.8%; *Others* (including cortical dysplasia, hamartoma, tuberous sclerosis): n = 15; 6.9%.

In the "non-lesional" group (182 patients) pathological examination revealed 151 (83%) with hippocampal sclerosis and 31 (17%) with no pathological findings. In 16 patients with no histopathological findings only small tissue samples were available, preventing reliable judgement.

Dual pathology, i.e. a gross lesion and hippocampal sclerosis, was present in 47 patients (11.7%).

All surgical procedures in patients with gross lesions were defined as "curative", as compared to 76.4% of the surgeries in the "non-lesional" group. The rest of the surgeries of patients from the "non-lesional" group (n = 43) were considered "palliative" *(table V)*.

Age at first seizure (onset of the disease) and preoperative duration of epilepsy were significantly different ($P < 0.01$) between "lesional" and "non-lesional" groups. Age at first seizure (mean ± SD) was 23.0 ± 16.1 and 11.8 ± 9.8 years for the "lesional" and "non-lesional", respectively. Preoperative duration of epilepsy (mean ± SD) was 7.5 ± 8.7 versus 21.4 ± 10.3 years, respectively. There was no significant difference with respect to age at surgery (30.5 ± 15.0 versus 33.2 ± 10.8 years, for the "lesional" and "non-lesional", respectively), however the percent of patients treated concomitantly by > 3 AEDs prior to surgery differed significantly ($P < 0.001$): 10.6% in the "lesional" versus 36.7% in the "non-lesional" group had concomitantly > 3 AEDs.

The severity of epilepsy prior to operation is indicated in *table VI* giving the baseline seizure days, i.e. days in the year prior to surgery with one or more seizures, including status epilepticus.

Seizure Outcome

Patients seizure outcome was followed up to 24 years following surgery, with a median of 7.1 years. In 125 patients, follow-up period was 10 years or more.

Table VII displays the annual (year by year) seizure outcome over 17 years follow up and the last available outcome (lao) for our entire population, with regard to the widely used Engel classification system (see *table I*).

Table VIII displays the year by year seizure outcome over 17 years follow-up and the last available outcome for our entire population using the new ILAE classification system [20]; see *table II*.

Table IX gives the percent changes of seizure days (preoperative baseline/postoperative last available outcome) for all AHE patients, and the break-down for lesional and non-lesional groups. Neglecting auras, a 100% reduction in the number of seizure days occurred in 242 patients (65.5%), a 50-100% reduction in 92 (25%) patients, and a less than 50% reduction in 35 patients (9.5%).

Table V. Gender, side of AHE, "curative" versus "palliative" indication

	n	Males	Females	Right	Left	Curative	Palliative
Lesional	**218**	**116**	**102**	**108**	**110**	**218**	
	54.5%	29%	25.5%	27%	27.5%	54.5%	
Non-lesional	**182**	**110**	**72**	**98**	**84**	**139**	**43**
	45.5%	27.5%	18%	24.5%	21%	34.75%	10.75%
Total	**400**	**226**	**174**	**206**	**194**	**357**	**43**
	100%	56.5%	43.5%	51.5%	48.5%	89.25%	10.75%

Table VI. Mean preoperative seizure days in the last year before surgery ("baseline") and postoperative follow-up (months)

	Baseline[b] (seizure days[a])		Postoperative follow-up (months)	
	Mean	SD	Mean	SD
Lesional	**176.9**	151.3	**77.2**	68.1
Non-Lesional	**131.7**	120.7	**94.7**	63.4
Total	**152.9**	137.8	**85.2**	66.6

[a] *Seizure day*: 24-h period with one or more seizures; this may include an episode of status epilepticus.
[b] *Baseline seizure days*: seizure-day frequency during the 12 months before surgery, with correction for the effects of AED reduction during diagnostic evaluation.

During follow-up period, in each point in time, more than 49% of the patients were completely seizure- and aura free (ILAE, class 1), more than 59% were free of "non-disabling" seizures (Engel, class I), and more than 87% had a "worthwhile" improvement (Engel classes I-III). *Figures 1 + 2 and 3 + 4* compare the "non-lesional" and "lesional" subgroups.

Table X correlates the last available outcome with the severity of hippocampal sclerosis in the "non-lesional" group, and *table XI* the last available outcome with the type of lesion (vascular and tumors WHO I and WHO II).

Figure 5 compares the year to year follow up and last available outcome of those patients who remained completely seizure- and aura free since operation (ILAE Class 1a) differentiating between "lesional" and "non-lesional" and between "curative" and "palliative" subgroups.

Table XII compares the group results in Class Engel I, Class ILAE 1 and ILAE Class 1a one year, 10 years and 17 years after AHE.

In order to study the individual seizure outcome we undertook an individual regression analyses for each patient's own score in the new ILAE outcome classification. These analyses revealed that 76% of the patients had a tendency to improve or stayed stable during the follow-up period *(table XIII)*. 19% improved (negative slope); 57% remained stable (slope = 0). Patients in the "curative" group did better than in the "palliative" group.

Surgery related complications

There was no surgery-related mortality. In a total of 453 sAHE patients 26 complications occurred in 21 patients (4.64%). In 5 patients 2 concommittant complications occurred. Seventeen patients (3.75%) had minor complications, 4 patients (0.88%) had major complications (underlined).

Table VII. Annual and last seizure outcome – All patients (n = 369), Engel classification

N = 400	1	2	3	4	5	6	7	8	9	10	11	12	13	14	15	16	17	Lao
	369	331	287	261	234	203	188	169	147	125	111	100	80	67	47	38	24	369
Ia	208	188	154	141	129	125	117	104	86	72	64	58	43	33	23	20	14	212
Ib	48	38	27	21	21	16	13	12	10	7	6	5	6	4	4	3	2	29
Id	5	6	10	8	4	1	5	1	2	0	1	0	0	1	1	1	0	6
IIb	26	28	22	18	16	11	8	11	8	10	8	7	6	5	2	0	0	32
IId	8	5	7	5	7	6	7	6	7	5	4	2	2	2	2	2	0	8
IIIa	49	43	43	44	36	29	22	21	21	18	16	16	13	12	10	8	7	54
IVa	3	4	4	3	4	3	3	3	3	3	3	3	2	2	2	2	0	4
IVb	22	19	19	20	17	12	13	11	10	10	9	9	8	8	3	3	1	23
IVc	0	0	1	1	0	0	0	0	0	0	0	0	0	0	0	0	0	1
I	70.7%	70.1%	66.6%	65.1%	65.8%	70.0%	71.8%	69.2%	66.7%	63.2%	64.0%	63.0%	61.2%	56.7%	59.6%	60.5%	66.7%	**66.9%**
II	9.2%	10.0%	10.1%	8.8%	9.8%	8.3%	8.0%	10.1%	10.2%	12.0%	10.8%	9.0%	10.0%	10.5%	8.5%	5.3%	0.0%	**10.9%**
III	13.3%	13.0%	15.0%	16.9%	15.4%	14.3%	11.7%	12.4%	14.3%	14.4%	14.4%	16.0%	16.3%	17.9%	21.3%	21.0%	29.1%	**14.6%**
IV	6.8%	6.9%	8.3%	9.2%	9.0%	7.4%	8.5%	8.3%	8.8%	10.4%	10.8%	12.0%	12.5%	14.9%	10.7%	13.2%	4.2%	**7.6%**

Lao = last available seizure outcome; Columns 1 to 17 are postoperative years.
Please note that follow-up years with n < 20 patients are not plotted.

Table VIII. Annual and last seizure outcome – All patients (n = 369), ILAE classification

N = 400	1	2	3	4	5	6	7	8	9	10	11	12	13	14	15	16	17	Lao
	369	331	287	261	234	203	188	169	147	125	111	100	80	67	47	38	24	369
1	56.4%	56.4%	54%	53.7%	55.5%	61.1%	62.2%	62.1%	59.2%	56.8%	56.8%	57%	53.7%	49.2%	48.9%	52.6%	58.4%	**57.1%**
1a	56.4%	50.1%	42.2%	39.1%	38.0%	38.9%	38.3%	34.9%	32.7%	33.6%	33.4%	33.0%	32.5%	25.3%	23.4%	23.7%	29.2%	**36.8%**
2	13.3%	11.5%	9.4%	8.0%	9.0%	8.4%	6.9%	6.5%	6.8%	5.6%	6.3%	6.0%	7.5%	6.0%	8.5%	7.9%	8.3%	**8.4%**
3	7.3%	9.1%	10.5%	9.6%	9.0%	5.9%	7.5%	6.5%	6.8%	10.4%	9.0%	6.0%	5.0%	6.0%	6.4%	5.3%	0.0%	**9.8%**
4	13.5%	13.3%	15.0%	17.2%	14.5%	11.8%	10.1%	11.9%	13.6%	11.2%	13.5%	15.0%	17.5%	19.4%	19.2%	18.4%	20.8%	**15.2%**
5	9.5%	9.7%	11.1%	11.5%	12.0%	12.8%	13.3%	13.0%	14.3%	16.0%	14.4%	16.0%	16.3%	19.4%	17.0%	15.8%	12.5%	**9.5%**

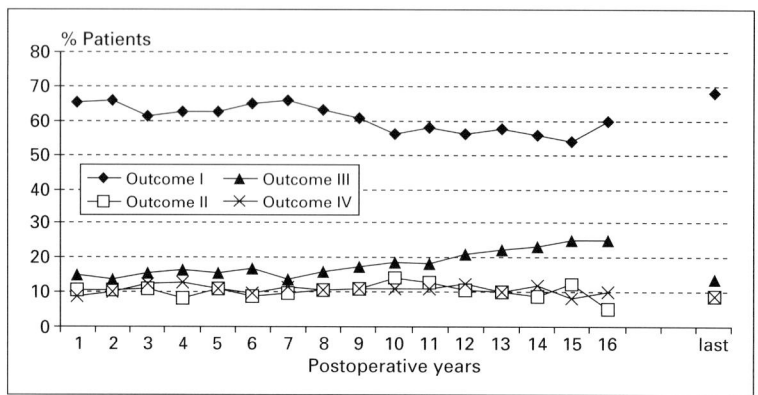

Figure 1. Annual and Last Seizure Outcome – "Non-lesional" AHE (n = 180), Engel.

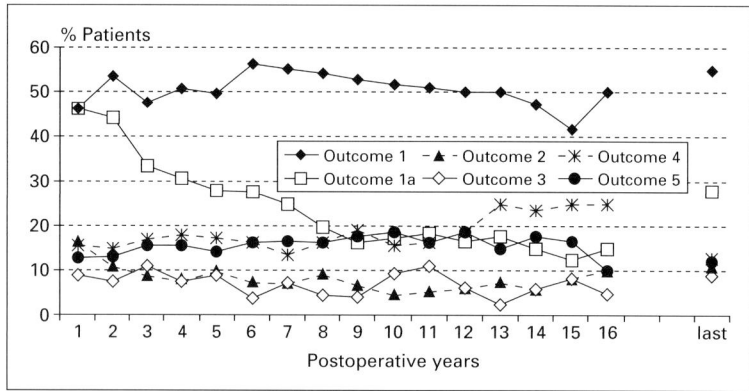

Figure 2. Annual and Last Seizure Outcome – "Non-lesional" AHE (n = 180), ILAE.

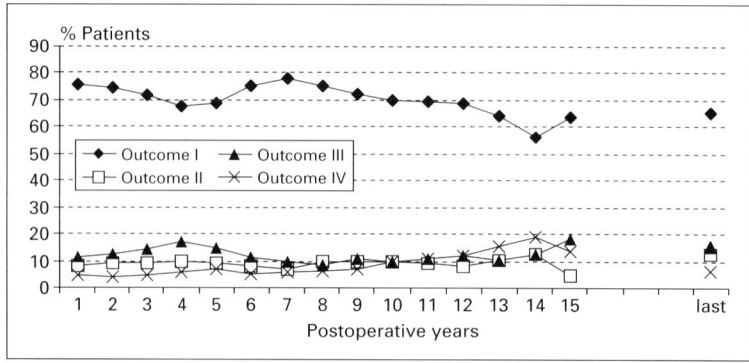

Figure 3. Annual and Last Seizure Outcome – "Lesional" AHE (n = 189), Engel Classification.

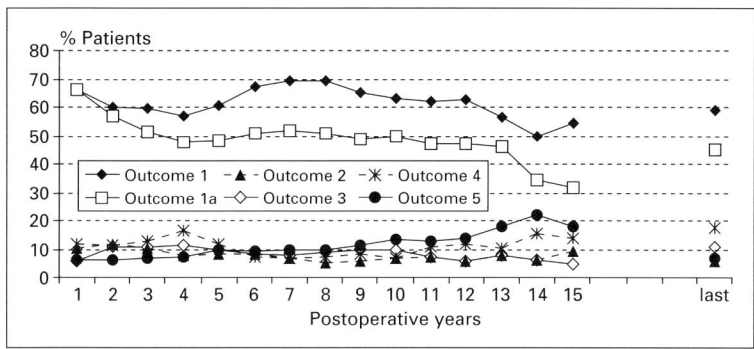

Figure 4. Annual and Last Seizure Outcome – "Lesional" AHE (n = 189), ILAE Classification.

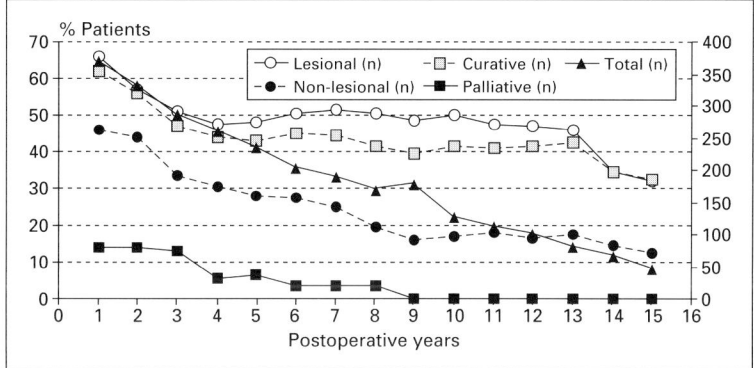

Figure 5. ILAE Class 1a: Annual Seizure Outcome for "Lesional" versus "Non-lesional" and "Curative" versus "Palliative" Subgroups.

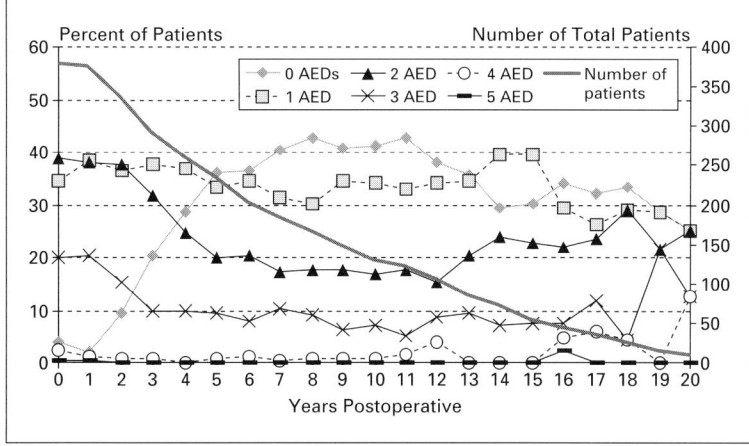

Figure 6. Annual changes (plotted over 20 years after AHE) of the number of antiepileptic drugs taken concomitantly by AHE patients.

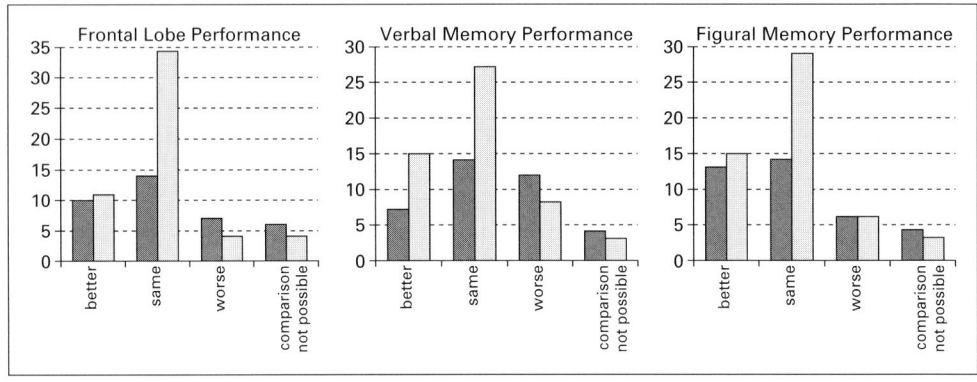

Figure 7. Comparison of pre-/postoperative neuropsychological outcome of 90 patients after AHE (Left AHE: dark; right AHE: white).

The *major* complications were as follows: Persistent hemiparesis (duration > 3 months) was observed in 3 patients. One patient had preoperatively a severe seizure disorder accompanied by a marked "schizophrenia-like" personality disorder. He had a left-sided sAHE with removal of a cavernoma situated in the left posterior parahippocampal gyrus. Surgery itself was uncomplicated, but the patient continued to have seizures, deteriorated in his memory and had a homonymous hemianopia.

Minor complications: Four patients were re-operated for intracranial hematomas. Three patients (2 epidural, 1 sub-dural hematoma) were re-operated on the same day of the first surgery. One patient presented with headache three months after surgery and was re-operated with a chronic subdural hematoma. Another patient with a small intracranial hematoma at the site of operation and no neurological deficit was not operated on.

Cranial nerve injuries (n = 5; oculomotor 4, trochelar 1) resolved within three months following surgery. Wound infection occurred in 2 patients, meningits in 1 patient, and deep leg vein thrombosis in 2 patients. A transient dysphasia occurred in 1 patient.

Antiepileptic drug treatment pre-/postoperative changes

Postoperatively, 70% of the patients had reduced their antiepileptic drugs. At the postoperative year 10, 36 of the 42 (85.7%) patients in the seizure- and aura-free group took no AEDs, 6 (4.6%) took 1 AED, and no patient took two or more AEDs. In contrast, of the 83 patients who suffered seizures, only 13 (15.7%) did not take any medication, 38 (45.85%) took 1 AED, 20 (24.1%) took two different AEDs, and 12 (14.5%) took 3 AEDs.

At the time of the last available outcome 49.4% of patients had reduced the number of AEDs compared to pre-operatively, and 96 patients (27%) of the whole population were without AEDs *(table XIV)*. The annual AED treatment changes (number of AEDs used concomitantly) are shown in *figure 6*.

Table IX. Percent changes of seizure days (preoperative baseline/postoperative last avaliable outcome) for all AHE patients, and the break-down for "lesional" and "non-lesional" groups

Seizure Days Reduction	[ILAE class]	All AHE		Lesional AHE		Non-lesional AHE	
100%	[1, 2]	**65.5%**		**64.9%**		**66.1%**	
90-99%	[3, 4]	13.9%		16.1%		11.9%	
80-89%		3.6%		3.2%		4%	
70-79%		4.7%	**25%**	7.4%	**28.2%**	1.7%	**21.7%**
60-69%		1.4%		1%		1.7%	
50-59%		1.4%		0.5%		2.4%	
40-49%	[5]	1.8%		0%		3.7%	
30-39%		0.7%		1.6%		0%	
20-29%		0.7%	**9.5%**	0.7%	**6.9%**	0.9%	**12.2%**
10-19%		0.3%		0%		0.6%	
0-9%		6%		4.6%		7%	

Table X. "Non-lesional AHE": last available seizure outcome correlated with severity of hippocampal sclerosis (HS; n = 162[a])

	Engel (%)				ILAE class (Wieser et al. [20]) (%)						
	I	II	III	IV	1	1a	2	3	4	5	6[b]
Severe HS (n = 46)	86.9	4.3	4.3	4.3	67.4	39.1	15.2	8.7	4.3	4.3	
Moderate HS (n = 34)	76.5	8.8	11.8	3.0	55.9	29.4	14.7	11.8	11.8	5.9	
Mild HS (n = 51)	58.8	9.8	19.6	11.8	54.9	23.5	3.9	5.9	15.7	19.6	
No pathology[c] (n = 31)	48.4	12.9	19.3	19.3	38.7	12.9	9.8	9.7	19.3	22.6	

[a] 18 patients excluded, because degree of HS not exactly stated.
[b] No entries in ILAE class 6.
[c] Includes patients with insufficient tissue (other studies!).

Table XI. "Lesional" AHE: last available seizure outcome correlated with type of lesion (vascular and tumors[a])

	Engel (%)				ILAE class (Wieser et al. [20]) (%)						
	I	II	III	IV	1	1a	2	3	4	5	6[b]
Vascular (n 41)	73.7	10.5	10.5	5.3	76.7	50.0	0	7.9	15.8	2.6	
Benign tumors WHO I (n 50)	72.7	15.9	9.1	2.3	65.9	47.7	6.8	13.6	11.4	2.3	
Semibenign tumors WHO II (n 64)	60	13.3	18.3	8.3	51.7	43.3	6.7	11.7	18.3	11.7	

[a] Tumors with WHO > II (mainly astrocytoma III) and the category "Others" were excluded. Excluded were also 3 patients from the vascular group, 6 patients from the benign tumors WHO I, and 4 patients from the semibenign tumors WHO II due to short-follow-up.
[b] No entries in ILAE class 6.

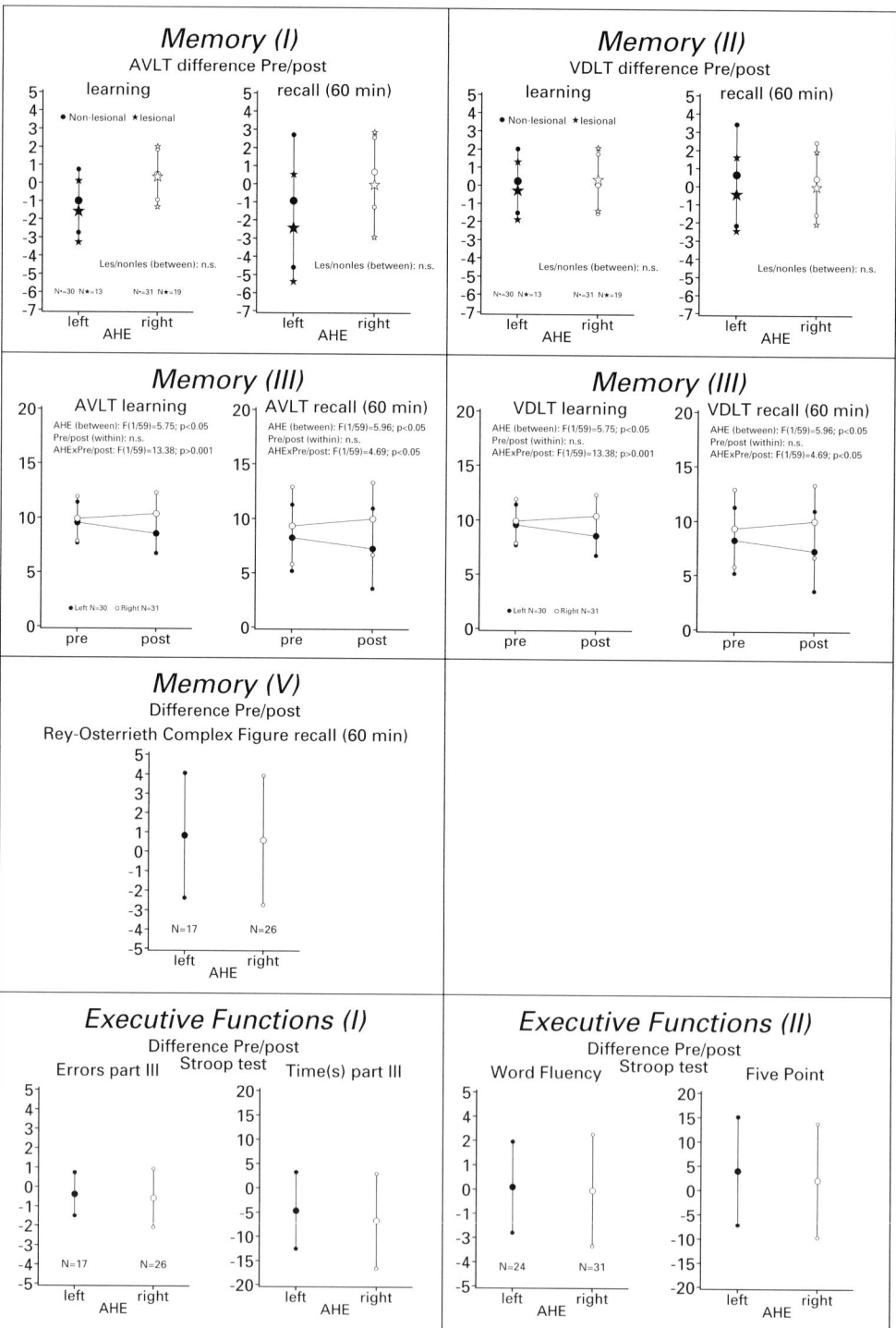

Figure 8. Pre-/postoperative neuropsychological test performances [changes of memory (I to V) and executive functions].

Table XII. Percentage of "seizure-free" patients qualifying for Engel class I, ILAE class 1 and ILAE class 1a one year, 10 years and 17 years after AHE

	1 yr. after AHE (n 369)	10 years after AHE (n 125)	17 years after AHE (n 24)
Free of "disabling seizures" (Engel class I)	**71%**	**63%**	**67%**
Completley seizure-free, no auras (ILAE class 1)	56%	57%	58%
Completley seizure-and aura free since surgery (ILA class 1A)		34%	29%

Table XIII. Regression analyses for each patient using the ILAE scale results in three groups: patient who improved during the follow-up period (negative slope), stable patients (slope = 0) and patients who deteriorated (positive slope). Stable patients were further divided to outcome classes ILAE 1 & 2 and to outcome classes ILAE 3 & 4

	Total n	Improved %	Stable ILAE class 1 & 2 %	Stable ILAE class 3 & 4 %	Deteriorated %
Palliative	43	23	9	56	12
Curative	326	19	43	12	26
Total	369	19	39	18	24

Table XIV. Antiepileptic drug (AED) therapy at last available outcome in comparison with AED therapy before AHE[a]

Same as pre-operatively		
	n	
1 AED	74	20.8%
2 AEDs	66	18.5%
3 AEDs	36	10.1%
4 AEDs	4	1.1%
Total	**180**	**50.6%**
Preoperative AED treatment reduced to		
	n	
0 AED	96	27%
1 AED	57	16%
2 AEDs	22	6.2%
3 AEDs	1	0.3%
Total	**176**	**49.4%**

[a] 13 patients were excluded because of conflicting or missing data at the time of this survey.

Quality of life

Pre-/postoperative changes of neuropsychological test performances

Figure 7 displays the individual neuropsychological data for those 90 "non-lesional" AHE patients of this series (out of 182 "non-lesional" patients) who were included in the psychosocial outcome data. For this subpopulation neuropsychological test criteria were less stringent. We included patients with slightly differing test batteries preoperatively compared to postoperatively, and allowed for a larger time window postoperatively (postoperative testing up to 9 months). Thirty-seven patients of this subpopulation had a left AHE and 53 a right AHE. (In the whole series of "non-lesional" AHEs (n = 182) there were 84 left and 98 right AHEs). Concerning the frontal lobe functions 48 patients (53%) were postoperatively unchanged, 21 patients (23%) improved postoperatively (left AHE n = 10, right AHE n = 11), and 10 patients (11%) deteriorated (left AHE n = 6, right AHE n = 4). Thus, in the latter group left AHE were twice as often compared to right AHE (6/37 = 16% versus 4/53 = 8%). With regard to verbal memory 22 patients (24%) were postoperatively better (left AHE n = 7, right AHE n = 15) and 20 patients (22%) worse (left AHE n = 12, right AHE n = 8). With regard to figural memory 28 patients (31%) were postoperatively better (left AHE n = 13, right AHE n = 15), and 12 patients (13%) worse (left AHE n = 6, right AHE n = 6).

In the AHE sample of Treyer [19] there were 45 females and 48 males. 43 AHEs were left and 50 right. Mean age at surgery for this subgroup was 33.41 years (left *versus* right AHE: n.s.). There were 13 left-handers. Sixty-one patients were "non-lesional – curative" (25 females, 36 males; 30 left, 31 right AHEs; age at surgery was not significantly different between left and right AHEs; 6 patients were left-handers).

Figure 8 displays the main group results for memory (Memory I-V) and for the Stroop Test (Executive Functions I) as well as for the Word Fluency and Five Point Test (Executive Functions II) of this sample. Data are shown comparing the changes pre- to postoperative. Left AHE patients have a slight to moderate decline of memory in the auditory verbal learning test (AVLT), which is more marked for lesional than for non-lesional patients. In all other modalities no significant pre- to postoperative changes were detected in this selected subpopulation. Similar neuropsychological outcome data on AHE patients have been reported earlier by Regard *et al.* [22].

Psychosocial outcome

From the 90 non-lesional AHE-patients, who had responded in a sufficiently detailed fashion to 32 questions, 62 patients (68.9%) reported to be seizure free at the time of responding to the questionnaire, 5 patients (5.6%) indicated that they had less than 3 seizures per year, and 7 patients (7.8%) reported a worthwhile improvement with a seizure reduction of 90% or more compared to pre-operatively, i.e., 82.2% of these subset of patients claimed to experience a postoperative seizure-reduction of 90% or more.

The analysis of the questions within the main categories revealed: (1) **Employment**: Preoperatively 82 patients were employed, postoperatively 84 patients. Pre-/postoperative changes in the percentage of employment: improved 30%, unchanged 48%, and deteriorated 22%. (2) **Housing**: Preoperatively 32 patients were living with their parents, 24 with a partner, 23 with partner and child(ren) and 11 alone. Postoperatively the housing situation changed in 33 patients (37%): Only 18 patients were living with their parents, but 23 patients alone; 49 patients lived either married or with a partner (10 patients found a new partner and lived together, and 10 patients got one or more children since the surgery). (3) **Support by family and/or a partner**: Postoperatively 73 patients were very satisfied with their support, 8 found it sufficient, 4 too less, and 5 had no support at all. According to the scaling of the patients' their support has postoperatively "very improved" in 22%, "improved" in 11%, was "unchanged" in 57%, had slightly diminished in 5%, and markedly diminished in 4%. (4) **Social contacts**: Postoperatively social contacts were good in 67 patients, sufficient in 7 patients; insufficient 6 patients and 10 patients had no social contacts at all. Compared to preoperatively social contacts were improved in 53% (++: 31%, + 22%), unchanged in 41% and less good in 6% (-- 5%, - 1%). (5) **Sexual life**: Postoperatively 49 patients found their sexual life very satisfying, 12 had no problems, 6 some problems and 16 found it unsatisfactorily (no response 7). In comparison to pre-operative 19% found it much better, 11% better, 50% unchanged, 2% less good, and 7% markedly deteriorated (11% no response). (6) **Sport and leisure activity**: Postoperatively 25 patients engaged in regular sportive activity, 17 were moderately active, 12 rarely, 36 did not engage in sportive activities. In comparison to pre-operative 32% had increased their sportive activity (++ 10%, + 22%), 64% were unchanged, and 3% diminished. Concerning **hobbies**: Postoperatively 64 patients engaged regularly in a hobby, 12 randomly, 4 very rarely, 10 never. In comparison to pre-operative 41% improved in their hobbies (++ 23%, + 18%), 52% patients were unchanged, 7% reduced their hobbies (-- 4%, - 2%). Overall 57 patients (63%) stated that the AHE had a beneficial effect on their leisure activities (++ 37%, + 27%); unchanged 28%, decline 9% (-- 6%, - 3%). **Depression**: Postoperatively 17 patients (19%) claimed to have a depressive mood change (D) and 15 (17%) anxiety (A). In comparison to pre-operative 44 patients (49%) improved in D (++ 31%, + 18%), and 51% in A (++ 30%, + 21%); 36 patients (40%) were unchanged in D and A, 10 patients (11%) deteriorated in D (-- 6%, - 6%) and 9% in A (-- 2%, - 7%). **Self-confidence**: Postoperatively 56 patients rated it with good, 16 with moderate, and 18 with poor (-- 11, - 7). In comparison to pre-operative 54% improved (++ 36%, + 19%), 38% were unchanged, 8% diminished (-- 3%, - 4%). **Independence**: Postoperatively 73 patients rated it with good, 6 with moderate, 11 with poor (--- 6, - 5). In comparison to pre-operative 47% improved (++ 26%, + 21%), 48% were unchanged, and 6% less independent (-- 2%, - 3%). **Overall quality of life**: Postoperatively 68 patients rated it with good, 13 with moderate, 9 with poor (--- 5, - 4). In comparison to pre-operative 66% improved (++ 43%, + 22%), 27% were unchanged, and in 8% of the patients the quality of life declined postoperatively (-- 4%, - 3%).

A multivariate logistic regression analysis revealed that the presence of a *postoperative psychiatric diagnosis* had the highest impact on psychosocial outcome (6 times $P > 0.05$ for 11 tested items). The *seizure situation* was for 5 items significant (3 times severe seizures with falls, 2 times complex partial seizures). Next were the *side effects of AEDs* (with 4 significant items). The *duration of active epilepsy* was 3 times significant and *sex* 2 times. The variables *neuropsychological deficits* were 2 times significant (once verbal, once figural). The *side of AHE* had no significant influence on the tested 11 variables.

The following variables had the strongest correlation (listed in the sequence of their importance): *Income* with (a) psychiatric diagnosis; *professional position* with (a) psychiatric diagnosis, and (b) AED side effects; *support by family and/or life partners* with (a) duration of active epilepsy, (b) a psychiatric diagnosis, and (c) sex; *social contacts* with (a) severe seizures with falls, (b) postoperative depression, and (c) sex; *sexual life* with (a) complex partial seizures, and (b) duration of active epilepsy; *sport and leisure activities* with (a) age at operation; *depression* with (a) AED side effects; *anxiety* with (a) postoperative seizures with falls, (b) neuropsychological deficits (mainly figural) and (c) side effects of AEDs; *self-confidence* with (a) postoperative psychiatric diagnosis, and (b) side effects of AEDs; *independence* with (a) postoperative seizure outcome, and (b) side effects of AEDs; and *general quality of life* with (a) seizures with severe falls, and (b) postoperative psychiatric diagnosis.

Discussion

A review of the larger temporal epilepsy surgery series (including surveys) reveals that 37%-71% of patients operated on because of drug-refractory TLE become completely seizure free [10, 23-35]. In the ILAE Global Survey [25], 57% of patients undergoing anterior temporal lobectomy and 60% of patients undergoing selective AHE became post-operatively seizure free, and 82-85% benefited from surgery. Patients with hippocampal sclerosis, a history of complex febrile seizures, and patients with "foreign tissue lesions" have significantly higher success rates with 80-94% of patients becoming seizure free. Prognostic factors for good postoperative outcome are unilateral hippocampal atrophy in qualitative MRI, and small quantitative hippocampal volume on the side of seizure onset. Qualitative MRI reveals lateralizing abnormalities in 74% and hippocamapl atrophy in 52-63% of patients undergoing epilepsy surgery for TLE [36-38].

Concerning more recent temporal lobectomy series most centers report rates of seizure free patients of 70% or more. These numbers are group results, reported either at a given postoperative year or year by year or as the last available seizure outcome. Sperling *et al.* [32] reported on 89 patients consecutively treated by temporal lobectomy between 1986 and 1990. All had noninvasive preoperative evaluation and 31 were evaluated with intracranial electrodes prior to surgery. Five years after surgery 62 patients (70%) were seizure free, 8 (9%) had seizuers on fewer than 3 days per year or exlusively had nocturnal seizures, 10 (11%) had greater than 80% reduction in seizure frequency, and 5 (6%) had less than 80% reduction in seizure frequency. Four (4%) died of causes unrelated to surgery. 55% of seizure recurrence rate happened within the 6 months of surgery and 93% occurred within 2 years after surgery. Outcome at 1 year related only moderately well to outcome at 5 years. No significant cognitive and/or linguistic deficits occurred. Underemployment and unemployment declined significantly after surgery, with improvement noted in seizure-free patients.

In general, our long-term seizure outcome results after selective amygdalohippocampectomy suggest that AHE is associated with at least as good a seizure control as temporal lobe resection, a conclusion supported by the prospective study of Robinson and co-workers on 22 consecutive children and adolescents who underwent trans-parahippocampal sAHE [39]. From our long-term assessment of the Zurich AHE series we conclude, that AHE, carried out by an experienced neurosurgeon, is a safe surgical procedure, with low rates of complications and morbidity. In well-selected patients (medically-intractable seizures, and a preoperative evaluation documenting seizures origin in the mesial temporal lobe), AHE results in a stable, long-term significant reduction in seizure days and in the use of AEDs in most patients. Complete disease-cured state was achieved in one third of these patients for a time period of more than 10 years after sAHE. Seizure outcome results are excellent both in patients with a distinct anatomical lesion (vascular anomaly or benign tumor), especially when the preoperative duration of disease is less then 5 years, and in patients with hippocampal sclerosis. They are, however, better in the "classical" hippocampal sclerosis (with relative sparing of the Cornu Ammonis field CA2) compared to the more diffuse "non-classical" HS with pathological changes also marked in CA2. In terms of severity scores of hippocampal sclerosis seizure outcome is better with marked or severe hippocampal pathology as compared to mild pathology.

The calculation of percentage of decrease in the number of seizure days of last available outcome in relation to the year before surgery revealed a more than 50% reduction in the number of seizure days in 90.5% of patients. These numbers, for the first time, allow a direct comparison with AED studies in which a more than 50% seizure reduction against baseline is the most common end point.

The significant differences between "palliative" and "curative" AHEs in the Zurich AHE outcome study is ample evidence for the importance of a careful presurgical evaluation, since these differences suggest that the pre-operative evaluation is able to predict the existence of epileptogenic tissue outside the resected area. On the other hand, the less than good results with the "palliative" AHE raise the question of AHE in this sub-group. These patients might have been candidates for a tailored larger temporal resection including lateral neocortex.

That surgery in a certain population of patients yields better results than medical treatment has been shown by Wiebe et al. in their recent intention-to-treat randomized, controlled trial of surgery for TLE. Wiebe et al. [35] reported that 64% of 36 patients who actually underwent surgery were *free of disabling seizures* 1 year after temporal lobectomy. The cumulative proportions who were free of seizures impairing awareness at one year were 58% in the surgical (n 40) and 8% in the medical group (n 40) (P < 0.001). Four patients (10%) had adverse effects of surgery: small thalamic infarct (n 1); wound infection (n 1); decline in memory (n 2). Asymptomatic superior subquadrantic visual field defects were present in 22 patients (55%) in the surgery group.

Seizure outcome in our selective AHE series is comparable to that of Wiebe et al. [35] (1 year after sAHE 70.7% of the patients being Engel class I and 56,4% ILAE class 1). Thus, these outcome data corroborate our philosophy that surgical resection in MTLE should be limited to the structures responsible for seizure initiation, sparing as much of the "healthy" neocortical temporal lobe as possible. AHE may be a more time-consuming and technically challenging operation, but with an experienced neurosurgeon morbidity following AHE is similar to other surgical treatments of MTLE [40]. Indeed, the limited resection in AHE may account for the surprisingly low percentage of patients suffering postoperatively from severe global memory deficits or persistent dysphasia (0.22% in our ZH AHE series compared to 1-5% [27, 40-42]). In addition the re-assessment of postoperative neuropsychological performance revealed overall satisfying results. Previous studies in a sub-group of our AHE patients revealed that neuropsychological performance was better in patients with AHE compared to patients with temporal lobectomies [43]. Similar findings were reported by Goldstein and Polkey [44]. However, we have to underline that in Zurich candidates for AHE who are considered to be at risk for postoperative memory loss undergo preoperative selective temporal lobe amytal testing with co-injection of SPECT tracer [45]. This modified selective Wada test with inactivation of the vascular territory of the anterior choroidal artery predicts memory outcome very well [46]. Nevertheless verbal memory loss following left temporal resection remains a problem in patients who have only a slight preoperative verbal memory deficit and do not become seizure-free after surgery, and our data confirm that AHE performed in the language-dominant hemisphere and without marked verbal memory problems preoperatively show a slight decline in verbal memory postoperatively.

Overall quality of life assessment in our AHE series shows satisfactory results. Postoperatively 68 patients rated their quality with good, 13 with moderate, and only 9 with poor. In comparison to pre-operative 66% improved, 27% were unchanged, and in 8% of the patients the quality of life declined postoperatively.

In the study of Khan and Wieser [15], which assessed the psychosocial outcome in 90 patients of this series three variables were studied: (1) psychosocial adjustment, (2) personal career, and (3) family support, and correlated with: (1) postoperative seizure outcome, (2) personal career outcome; and (3) psychosocial outcome. There was a positive correlation between psychosocial outcome and postoperative seizure outcome; and there was a positive trend between personal career outcome and postoperative seizure outcome. Furthermore the functional outcome was the better the shorter the pre-operative duration of epilepsy, and the postoperative psychosocial outcome was better with a more radical removal of the parahippocampal gyrus. From this study it was concluded that complete postoperative seizure control is the most important single variable predicting psychosocial outcome. *Career outcome* was as follows: Pre-operatively 61% [n 55] were employed, 28% were students (regular school), 3% lived in special institutions; and 8% were housewives. Postoperatively 53/55 (96%) continued to be employed (11 patients at markedly higher demand level, 26 patients at a slightly higher demand level, 13 patients at the same level and 3 patients at a slightly inferior level); 2/55 (= 3.6%) lost their job (1 patient with paranoid psychosis; 1 patient due to headache and insomnia); 16 patients became employed and there was no change with regard to the 7 housewives.

With regard to the *psychosocial outcome* (n 90) 72.2% of patients improved after AHE, in 14.4% there was no change, and in 13.3% deterioration was obvious. All of the 12 patients with a deterioration of their psychosocial status had "behavioral disorders" pre- and post-operatively.

Concerning seizure control and mortality, Sperling *et al.* [47] have studied 393 patients who had epilepsy surgery between 1986 and 1996 (347 had focal resection or transection, and 46 had anterior or complete corpus callosotomy). Overall, seizure-free patients had a lower mortality rate than those with persistent seizures. In the subset of patients with localized resection or multiple subpial resection, no patients died among 199 with no seizure recurrence, whereas of 194 patients with seizure recurrence, 11 died. Six of the deaths were sudden and unexplained. Thus the standardized mortality ratio for patients with recurrent seizures was 4.69, and the risk of death in these patients was 1.37 in 100 person-years, whereas among patients who became seizure free, there was no difference in mortality rate compared with an age- and sex-matched US population.

Because surgical intervention early in the course of medically refractory MTLE provides the greatest opportunity for complete psychosocial rehabilitation [48-52], early diagnosis is important. From the review of the literature and of our Zurich AHE series we strongly feel that intractability should be defined as early as possible. Kwan & Brodie [53] suggested that this can be done following treatment with 2 different antiepileptic drugs (AEDs) of first choice successively and with one combination.

References

1. Jensen I. Temporal lobe surgery around the world: results, complications and mortality. *Acta Neurol Scand* 1975; 52: 354-73.
2. Rasmussen T. Cortical resection for medically refractory focal epilepsy: results, lessons and questions. In: Rasmussen T, Marino R, eds. *Functional Neurosurgery*. New York: Raven Press, 1979: 253-69.
3. Lüders H, ed. *Epilepsy Surgery*. New York: Raven Press, 1992.
4. Engel J Jr, ed. *Surgical Treatment of the Epilepsies*. New York: Raven Press, 1993: 609-21.
5. Shorvon S, Dreifuss F, Fish D, Thomas D, eds. *The Treatment of Epilepsy*. Oxford: Blackwell Science, 1996.
6. Tuxhorn I, Holthausen H, Boenigk H, eds. *Paediatric Epilepsy Syndromes and their Surgical Treatment*. London, Sydney: John Libbey & Comp. Ltd, 1997.
7. Oxbury J, Polkey C, Duchowny M, eds. *Intractable Focal Epilepsy*. London: W.B. Saunders, 2000.
8. Wieser HG, Silfvenius H. Overview: epilepsy surgery in developing countries. *Epilepsia* 2000; 41 (Suppl 4): 3-9.
9. Engel J Jr. Outcome with respect to epileptic seizures. In: Engel J Jr, ed. *Surgical Treatment of the Epilepsies*. New York: Raven Press, 1987: 553-71.
10. Engel J Jr, Van Ness P, Rasmussen TB, *et al*. Outcome with respect to epileptic seizures. In: Engel J Jr, ed. *Surgical treatment of the epilepsies*. 2nd ed. New York: Raven Press, 1993: 609-21.

11. Rasmussen T, Branch C. Temporal lobe epilepsy. Indications for and results of surgical therapy. *Postgrad Med* 1962; 31: 9-14.
12. Pilcher WH, Roberts DW, Flanigin HF, Crandall PH, Wieser HG, Ojemann GA, et al. Complications of epilepsy surgery. In: Engel J Jr, ed. *Surgical treatment of the epilepsies*. New York: Raven Press, 1993: 565-81.
13. Engel J Jr. Classification of epileptic disorders. *Epilepsia* 2001; 42: 317-20.
14. Wieser HG, Ortega M, Friedman A, Yonekawa Y. Long-term seizure outcome following amygdalohippocampectomy. Submitted 2002.
15. Khan N, Wieser HG. Psychosocial outcome of patients with amygdalohippocampectomy. *Journal of Epilepsy* 1992; 5: 128-34.
16. Wieser HG. Behavioural consequences of temporal lobe resections. In: Trimble MR, Bolwig TG, eds. *The Temporal Lobes and The Limbic System*. Petersfield: Wrightson Biomed, 1992: 169-88.
17. Hajek M, Wieser HG, Khan N, et al. Preoperative and postoperative glucose consumption in mesiobasal and lateral temporal lobe epilepsy. *Neurology* 1994; 4: 2125-32.
18. Kurmann-Bärlocher A. *Veränderung der psychosozialen Situation von 90 Patienten der Zürcher AHE-Serie nach Amygdalohippokampektomie*. Thesis, Medical Faculty, University Zürich, 2000.
19. Treyer V. *Nuropsychologische Leistungen vor und nach selektiver Amygdalohippokampektomie*. Lizentiatsarbeit, Philosphical Faculty I, University Zürich, 2000.
20. Wieser HG, Blume WT, Fish D, et al. ILAE Commission Report. Proposal for a new classification of outcome with respect to epileptic seizures following epilepsy surgery. *Epilepsia* 2001; 42: 282-6.
21. Häne A. *Langzeitergebnisse der Antepileptika-Therapie nach selektiver Amygdala-Hippokampektomie*. Thesis Medical Faculty University Zürich (submitted 2002).
22. Regard M, Schiess R, Landis T. Höhere Hirnfunktionen und Epilepsie – mit besonderer Berücksichtigung der Leistungen vor und nach Amygdala-Hippokampektomie. *Z EEG-EMG* 1996; 27: 257-62.
23. Penfield W, Flanigin H. Surgical therapy of temporal lobe seizures. *Arch Neurol Psychiatry* 1950; 64: 491-500.
24. Falconer MA, Serafitinides EA. A follow-up study of surgery in temporal lobe epilepsy. *J Neurol Neurosurg Psychiatry* 1963; 26: 154-65.
25. ILAE Commission report. A Global survey on epilepsy surgery, 1980-1990. *Epilepsia* 1997; 38: 249-55.
26. Rasmussen TB. Surgical treatment of complex partial seizures: results, lessons, and problems. *Epilepsia* 1983; 24: 65-76.
27. Walczak TS, Radtke RA, McNamara JO, Lewis DV, Luther JS, Thompson E, Wilson WP, Friedman AH, Nashold BS. Anterior temporal lobectomy for complex partial seizures: Evaluation, results and long-term follow-up in 100 cases. *Neurology* 1990; 40: 413-8.
28. Rasmussen T, Feindel W. Temporal lobectomy: Review of 100 cases with major hippocampectomy. *Can J Neurol Sci* 1991; 18: 601-2.
29. Rougier A, Dartigues J, Commenges D, Claverie B, Loiseau P, Cohadon F. A longitudinal assessment of seizure outcome and overall benefit from 100 cortectomies for epilepsy. *J Neurol Neurosurg Psychiatr* 1992; 55: 762-7.
30. Davies KG, Weeks RD. Temporal lobectomy for intractable epilepsy: experience with 58 cases over 21 years. *Br J Neurosurgery* 1993; 7: 23-34.
31. Salanova V, Markand ON, Worth R. Clinical characteristics and predictive factors in 98 patients with complex partial seizures treated with temporal resection. *Arch Neurol* 1994; 51: 1008-13.
32. Sperling MR, O'Connor MJ, Saykin AJ, Plummer C. Temporal lobectomy for refractory epilepsy. *JAMA* 1996; 276: 470-5.
33. Salanova V, Markand O, Worth R. Longitudinal follow-up in 145 patients with medically refractory temporal lobe epilepsy treated surgically between 1984 and 1995. *Epilepsia* 1999; 40: 1417-23.
34. Foldvary N, Nashold B, Mascha E, Thompson EA, Lee N, McNamara JO, Lewis DV, Luther JS, Friedman AH, Radtke RA. Seizure outcome after temporal lobectomy for temporal lobe epilepsy. A Kaplan-Meier survival analysis. *Neurology* 2000; 54: 630-4.
35. Wiebe S, Blume WT, Girvin JP, Eliasziw M. A randomized, controlled trial of surgery for temporal-lobe epilepsy. *New Engl J Med* 2001; 345: 311-8.
36. Kuzniecky R, Burgard S, Faught E, Morawez R, Bartolucci A. Predictive value of magnetic resonance imaging in temporal lobe epilepsy surgery. *Arch Neurol* 1993; 50: 65-9.

37. Berkovic SF, McIntosh AM, Kalnins RM, Jackson GD, Fabinyi GCA, Brazenor GA, Bladin PF, Hopper JL. Preoperative MRI predicts outcome of temporal lobectomy: An actuarial analysis. *Neurology* 1995; 45: 1358-63.
38. Garcia PA, Laxer KD, Barbaro NM, Dillon WP. Prognostiv value of quantitative magnetic resonance imaging hippocampal abnormalities in patients undergoing temporal lobectomy for medically refractory seizures. *Epilepsia* 1994; 35: 520-4.
39. Robinson S, Park TS, Bourgeois BFD, Blackburn LB, Arnold S. Transparahippocampal selective amygdalohippocampectomy in children and adolescents: Efficacy and cognitive morbidity. *J Neurosurg* 2000; 93: 402-9.
40. Pilcher WH, Rusyniak WG. Complications of epilepsy surgery. *Neurosurg Clin N Am* 1993; 4: 311-25.
41. King D, Flanigan H, Gallagher B, et al. Temporal lobectomy for partial complex seizures: evaluation, results and 1 year follow-up. *Neurology* 1986; 36: 334-9.
42. Wieser HG, Yasargil MG. Selective amygdalohippocampectomy as a surgical treatment of mesiobasal limbic epilepsy. *Surg Neurol* 1982; 17: 445-57.
43. Birri R, Perret E, Wieser HG. Der Einfluss verschiedener Temporallappenoperationen auf das Gedächtnis von Epileptikern. *Nervenarzt* 1982; 53: 144-9.
44. Goldstein LH, Polkey CE. Short-term cognitive changes after unilateral temporal lobectomy or unilateral amygdalo-hippocampectomy for the relief of temporal lobe epilepsy. *J Neurol Neurosurg Psychiatry* 1993; 56: 135-40.
45. Wieser HG, Müller S, Schiess R, et al. The anterior and posterior selective temporal lobe amobarbital tests: angiographical, clinical, electroencephalographical PET and SPECT findings, and memory performance. *Brain and Cognition* 1997; 33: 71-97.
46. Wieser HG. Anterior cerebral artery amobarbital test. In: Lüders HO, ed. *Epilepsy surgery*. New York: Raven Press, 1992: 515-23.
47. Sperling MR, Feldman H, Kinman J, Liporace JD, O'Connor MJ. Seizure control and mortality in epilepsy. *Ann Neurol* 1999; 46: 45-50.
48. Wieser HG, Engel J Jr, Williamson PD, Babb TL, Gloor P. Surgically remediable temporal lobe syndromes. In: Engel J Jr, ed. *Surgical Treatment of the Epilepsies*. New York: Raven Press, 1993; 2: 49-63.
49. Engel J Jr, Williamson PD, Wieser HG. Mesial temporal lobe epilepsy. In: Engel J Jr, Pedley J, eds. *Epilepsy: A Comprehensive Textbook*. New York: Raven Press, 1997: 2417-26.
50. Meyer FB, Marsh WR, Laws ER Jr, Sharbrough FW. Temporal lobectomy in children with epilepsy. *J Neurosurg* 1986; 64: 371-6.
51. Thadani VM, Williamson PD, Berger R, et al. Successful epilepsy surgery without intracranial EEG recording: criteria for patient selection. *Epilepsia* 1995; 36: 7-15.
52. Mihara T, Inoue Y, Matsuda K, et al. Recommendations of early surgery from the viewpoint of daily quality of life. *Epilepsia* 1996; 37 (Suppl 3): 33-8.
53. Kwan P, Brodie MJ. Early identification of refractory epilepsy. *N Engl J Med* 2000; 3: 314-9.

Prognosis of frontal lobe epilepsy after surgery

Suzanne Trottier, Jean-Marie Scarabin

Frontal lobe epilepsy (FLE) today represents a formidable challenge in the field of epilepsy surgery because this chronic disorder has many medical and psychosocial implications. Partial seizures originating in the frontal lobe are the second most common type of seizures that are evaluated for surgery. However, the outcome of the frontal surgery is less favourable as compared to that of the temporal lobe epilepsy surgery [1-5]. Several reasons have been proposed to explain the failures after surgery: the variety of the frontal seizure patterns [6-10] that do not always clearly correlate with anatomical subdivisions of the frontal lobe, the poor localising or lateralizing value of some clinical signs, the difficulty to record frontal seizures with scalp-EEG because complex clinical manifestations (agitated and hyperkinetic automatisms) [6, 11] the high speed propagation of the ictal electrical discharges within the frontal lobe and to the opposite side through the corpus callosum and the large extent of the epileptogenic areas [1, 5, 12, 13].

Many efforts have been made to improve the preoperative assessment of the refractory frontal lobe seizures with the main objective to better define the limits of the frontal tissue volume to be resected and to ameliorate the prognosis of FLE after surgery. During this last decade, the practise of long-lasting EEG-video recordings, the systematic use of magnetic resonance imaging (MRI) by searching for causative structural lesions not identified with computer tomography scanning (CT-Scan) and the stereoelectroencephalography (SEEG) with depth and chronically implanted electrodes for some days necessary to determine the epileptogenic area to be removed have constituted the fundamental approach for FLE surgery.

The present study reports the long-term outcome on seizure control from a selected patient population who underwent FLE surgery performed at the Departments of Neurosurgery of Sainte-Anne (Paris, France) and Pontchaillou (Rennes, France) hospitals between 1990-2000.

Methods

Population and presurgical evaluation

We selected 53 epileptic patients operated on at these two institutions because they were similarly evaluated for FLE surgery. This allowed us to decrease, at least partially, the difficulty in collecting a cohort large enough of patients with FLE to be analysed after surgery. The choice of this relatively short period (1990-2000) was certainly a limiting factor for estimating the long-term surgical outcome over ten years or more, but this last decade corresponded to a "modern period" as compared with that before 1985-1990, because prolonged EEG-video recordings, MRI and (except one) chronic SEEG procedure have been systematically achieved in all patients. For all patients the same presurgical evaluation strategy was used to define the origin of seizures and the limits of the epileptogenic area to be removed [5, 14, 15]. When a lesion existed, it was crucial to determine if the epileptic activity starts within and/or near the lesion before surgery. *Figure 1* shows the morphological (MRI), electrical and surgical data (SEEG) of an illustrative case of a mediodorsal resection around the right F1-F2 sulcus.

Type of frontal resections

The advent of MRI, combined with the three-dimensional reconstructions, has significantly improved the anatomical surgery of the frontal lobe by illustrating the gyral and sulcal anatomy and some individual anatomical variations.

Related to the striking development of the frontal lobe, the various clinical and intracerebral EEG findings, the presence or not of a structural lesion, the FLE surgery warranted several types of frontal resections. We propose to class them in 9 anatomical categories, the extent of the resective zone being more or less large: 1) the *frontopolar* resections included the polar region and more or less the orbital cortex 2) the *mediodorsal* resections were of various extents of the first frontal gyrus (F1) and they involved either the supracallosal extent of the inner surface corresponding to the anterior part of the motor supplementary area (MSA) or the lateral surface reaching the F1-F2 sulcus or the superior part of F2 3) the *frontal intermediate* resection involved the lateral convexity F1-F2 with or without the medial extent of F1 4) the *central* resection involved either the opercular low part of the pre- and post-central gyri or a more extended part of these two gyri 5) the selective resection of the precentral gyrus spared the central gyrus 6) the *large medial* resection included F1, the central gyrus and the cingulate 7) only two *frontopolar* resections similar to type 1 were secondarily extended with the ablation of the *anterior part of the temporal lobe* 8) a "special" anatomical category included the resection of the opercular region with that of the orbital cortex or of the cingulate gyrus 9) the largest resection was "en bloc" *frontal lobectomy*.

Evaluation of seizure outcome after surgery

The follow-up period was from 18 months to 10 years.

The outcome for seizure control was assessed "year-per-year" and according to the widely used classification proposed by Engel with the four main classes I, II, III and IV [16]. We also attempted to determine the seizure outcome by using the new classification system "year-per-year" with the 6 classes proposed by the International League Against Epilepsy (ILAE) [17].

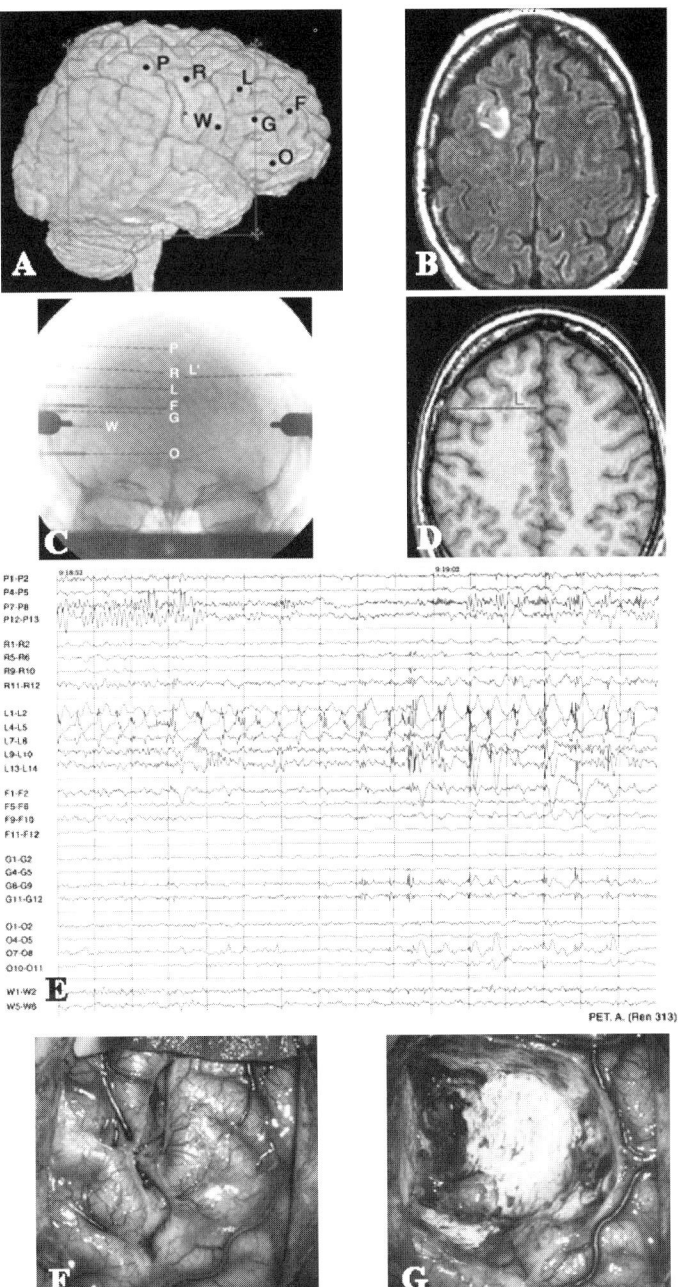

Figure 1. Illustrative case of frontal epilepsy related to a focal cortical dysplasia
A – 3D Preoperative MRI with the localization of the depth electrodes implanted for SEEG
B – MRI (FLAIR sequence) showing on an horizontal section a lesion involving the F1-F2 sulcus
C – Coronal diagram of the implantation of the depth electrodes for SEEG
D – Horizontal section of MRI indicating that the electrode L was placed within the lesion
E – SEEG recordings showing the typical intralesional activity of rhythmic spike discharges on the internal plots of the electrode L
F-G – Operative photographs before (F) and after (G) surgery.

Finally, we also determined the seizure outcome according to the pathological final diagnosis and the types of brain resections.

Results

Description of the cohort

The cohort comprised 53 patients (35 males and 18 females).

The mean age at the first seizure (the epilepsy onset) was 10 years (range: 2 months-33 years) *(figure 2)* and at surgery was 26 years (range: 11-52 years) *(figure 3)*. The mean duration of the disease from the onset of seizures to the age of surgery was 16 years (range: 5-42 years).

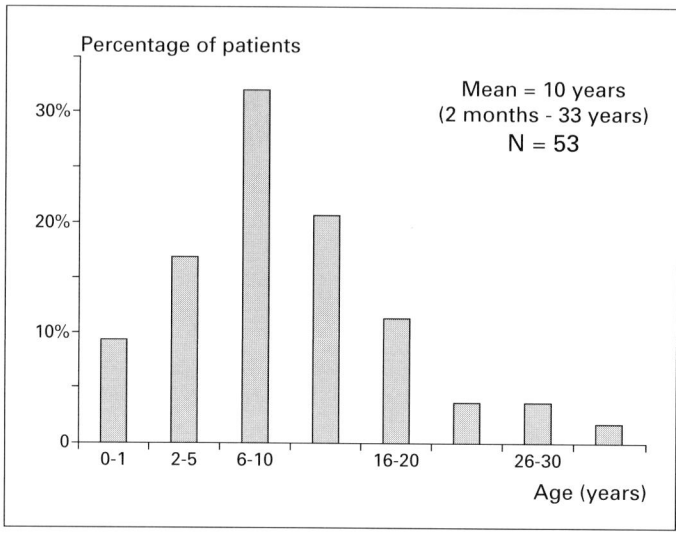

Figure 2. Age of the first seizure

Neurological examination was normal for 41 patients (77.3%). 11 patients (20.7%) had a cerebral infantile hemiplegia and 1 patient had a slight facial paresis. In this series, 45 patients were right-handed patients (84.9%), 6 patients were left-handed (11.3%) and only 1 patient was ambidextrous (1.8%). However all patient except one right-handed patient had a left hemisphere dominant for language *(table I)*.

MRI was performed for each patient and detected frontal lobe structural lesions for 35 patients.

Brain side and type of cortical resections

Table I illustrates the side of resection and the dominant hemisphere for language. The majority of resections was in the right brain (N = 43, 81.1%), only 9 (16.9%) resections were performed in the left brain.

The types of cortical resections are indicated in *table II* which illustrates the variety of the frontal resections.

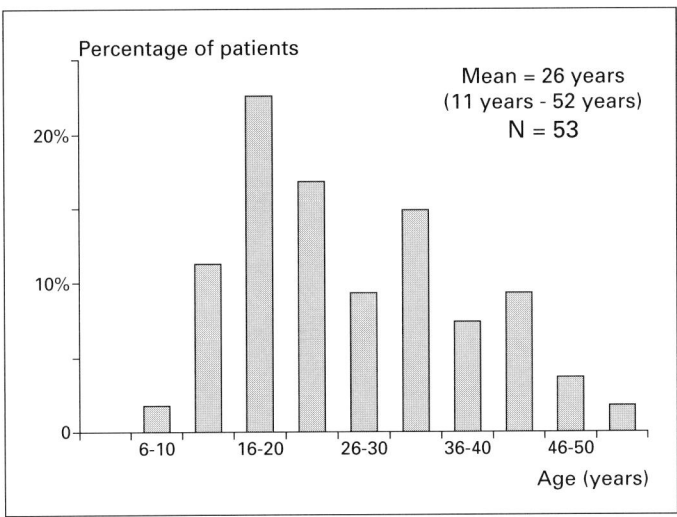

Figure 3. Age at frontal surgery

Table I. Side of surgery and manual and language hemispheric dominance

Side of surgery		Right 43 (81.1%)	Left 9 (16.9%)
Manual lateralization	Right-handed	42 (79.2%)	3 (5.6%)
	Left-handed		6 (11.3%)
	Ambidextrous	1 (1.8%)	
Langage dominant hemisphere		Right	Left
	Right-handed	1 (1.8%)	45 (84.9%)
	Left-handed		6 (11.3%)
	Ambidextrous		1 (1.8%)

Pathological findings

In the majority of cases, structural frontal lesions were preoperatively identified but the pathological diagnosis was only confirmed after examination of all surgical brain samples. Thus 6 cases with focal cortical dysplasia not evidenced by MRI were identified at the pathological examination.

Figure 4 summarizes the incidence and category of the structural brain lesions. Histopathology was negative for 12 patients (25%) and positive in the 40 remaining cases (75%). The neurodevelopmental lesions, the most common pathology found in 24 patients (45%) were either cortical dysplasia (n = 16, 30%) or dysembryoplasic neuroepithelial tumors (DNET) (n = 8, 15%). The other lesions were sequella of birth trauma (neonatal pathology) for 8 patients (15%), head trauma for 4 patients (7.5%), vascular malformations for 2 patients (3.7%), astrocytoma (1.8%) for 1 patient and infectious disease for 1 patient (1.8%).

Table II. Types of frontal resections

Type of frontal resections		Number of patients
Frontopolar	+ partial resection of the orbital cortex	4
	+ total resection of the orbital cortex	12
Mediodorsal	around the F1-F2 sulcus	6
	Selective resection of SMA without lesion	1
	Selective resection of SMA with lesion	1
Intermediate frontal	With lesion	8
	Without lesion	3
Central	Restricted to the opercular area	3
	Extended to the lateral and medial surface	7
Selective of the precentral gyrus	without lesion	1
Large medial surface (F1, central gyrus and cingulate)	with lesion	1
Frontal and temporal	without lesion	2
Special anatomical category		3
Frontal lobectomy		1

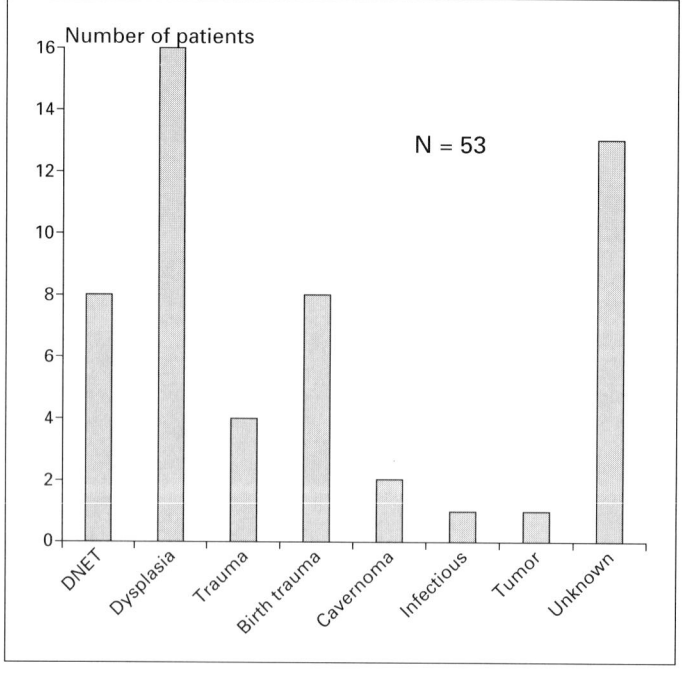

Figure 4. Histopathological findings

Evaluation of surgical outcome

Mortality

In this study no mortality resulted from invasive procedures. Two males patients, apparently seizure-free died during the second post-operative year. One 22-year old patient died after a road accident but he was not the driver. For the second 28-year old patient who had epilepsy without defined aetiology there was a sudden death during sleep.

Few complications were encountered after FLE surgery. There was no major persistent neurologic deficit. An early postoperative motor and speech deficit was the result of a large resection of the precentral gyrus including the supplementary motor area. Although the deficit was immediately profound, it rapidly recovered in the first post-operative weeks after surgery as reported [18, 19]. Some patients (n = 12) with cerebral infantile hemiplegia exhibited a transitory increase of their motor deficit. Only one patient has had a more persistent motor deficit. One patient, although seizure-free, experienced a pulmonary thrombosis rapidly treated but a long-lasting and severe infection of the skull that needed plastic surgery 2 years later.

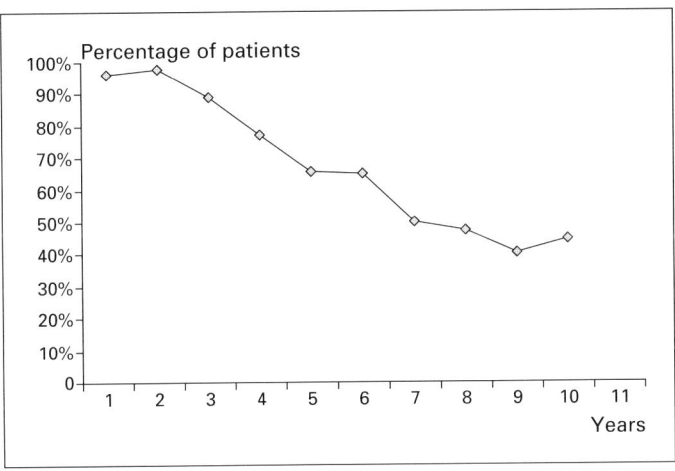

Figure 5. Follow-up of patients after frontal surgery

Seizure control

In spite of efforts to maintain contact after surgery, some patients have been lost for long-term follow-up as illustrated in *figure 5*. Thus, the percentage of patients who were regularly followed-up "year per year" progressively decreased over time *(figure 5)*. Outcome was available for most patients at the first (51/53 patients, 96.2%), second (41/42 patients, 97.6%) and third (34/38 patients, 89.4%) post-operative yea. At year 5, 65.5% of patients (19/29) were yet followed and at year 7, the surgical outcome was available for only 50% (12/24).

The surgical results on seizure control estimated "year-by-year" according to Engel's classification [16] in our population are reported in *table III* and indicate that there were changes according to the duration of the follow-up. The percentage of seizure-free patients (Class IA) decreased from 72.5% at the first year to 50% at the end of the follow-up period. Concomitantly the percentage of failures (class IV) progressively increased from

Table III. Seizure outcome according to Engel classification

Post-op. year	1	2	3	4	5	6	7	8	9	10
Number of patients	51	41	34	24	19	17	12	9	4	4
IA	37 72.5%	25 60.9%	21 65.6%	15 62.5%	10 52.6%	9 52.9%	6 50%	4 50%	2 50%	2 50%
IB										
IC										
ID			1 2.9%							
Classe I	37 72.5%	25 60.9%	22 64.7%	15 62.5%	10 52.6%	9 52.9%	6 50%	4 44.4%	2 50%	2 50%
IIA		3 7.3%	1 2.9%							
IIB						1 8.3%				
IIC										
IID										
Classe II	0	3 7.3%	1 2.9%	0	0	0	1 8.3%	0	0	0
IIIA										
IIIB										
Classe III	0	0	0	0	0	0	0	0	0	0
IVA	6 11.7%	6 14.6%	5 14.7%	3 12.5%	3 15.7%	3 17.6%	1 8.3%	1 11.1%	1 25%	1 25%
IVB	7 13.7%	6 14.6%	5 14.7%	5 20.8%	5 26.3%	4 23.5%	3 25%	3 33.3%	1 25%	1 25%
IVC	1 1.9%	1 2.4%	1 2.9%	1 4.1%	1 5.2%	1 5.8%	1 8.3%	1 11.1%		
Classe IV	15 29.4%	13 31.7%	11 2.3%	9 37.5%	5 7.3%	8 47%	5 41.6%	5 55.5%	2 50%	2 50%

30% to 50%. According to the ILAE classification [17] the surgical results were similar *(table IV)*. The distinction between the seizure-free patients with and without antiepileptic drugs (AED) indicated that only two patients were off medication, the other seizure-free patients continued to use one or more AED.

An alternative presentation of these results in *figure 6A and 6B* clearly illustrates the progressive decrease in the seizure control until the fifth year. After that, the ratio of success and failures remained stable. This profile may be biased by the fact that some patients who were seizure-free are most likely to become lost to follow-up and/or by the decreasing number of available outcomes over a 10 year period (see *figure 5*). To overcome these complicating factors, we selected the 18 patients who were regularly followed up "year by

Table IV. Seizure outcome according to ILAE classification

Post-op. year	1	2	3	4	5	6	7	8	9	10
Number of patients	51	41	34	24	19	17	12	9	4	4
Classe 1	37 72.5%	25 60.9%	22 64.7	15 62.5%	10 52.6%	9 52.9%	6 50%	4 44.4%	2 50%	2 50%
Classe 2		2 4.8%								
Classe 3		1 2.4%	1 2.9%			1 8.3%				
Classe 4	8 15.6%	6 14.6%	5 14.7%	3 12.5%	3 15.7%	3 17.6%	1 8.3%	1 11.1%	1 25%	1 25%
Classe 5	6 11.7%	7 17%	6 17.6%	4 16.6%	6 31.5%	3 29.4%	4 33.3%	2 44%	1 25%	1 25%
Classe 6										

year" during the same 5 year-lasting period and we find that the ratio 50% of success/50% of failures was definitively observed at the third post-operative year and remained stable until the fifth year *(figure 6C)*.

When relating the surgical outcome to the pathological findings *(figure 7)*, the global seizure control was better for symptomatic epilepsies than for cryptogenic epilepsies. Of 12 patients for whom no etiology was determined, only 6 patients (50%) were seizure-free (class I), the 6 others were not cured (class IV). On the contrary, among the 38 patients with a brain structural lesion (whatever the type), 27 patients (71%) were seizure-free (class IA), 9 patients (24%) were not cured (class IV) and 2 patients (5%) were improved (class II and III).

There were some differences in the rates of success and failures when comparing the global surgical outcome and the location and extent of the frontal resections *(table V)*: the central resections (n = 10) carried the best seizure outcome prognosis (class I) for 80% of patients, they were followed by the mediodorsal resections (n = 8) for 75% of patients, the intermediate frontal resections (n = 11) for 63% of patients and then the most common frontopolar resections (n = 16) with only 50% seizure-free patients. Finally the uncommon and selective resections (n = 8) were successful for half of patients.

Finally, comparing the lesional versus non lesional epilepsies with the types of frontal resections and with surgical outcome *(table VI)* we confirmed that the better outcome was obtained for symptomatic epilepsies and was about 70-80% and that whatever the anatomical location of the frontal resections *(table VII)*.

Discussion

Our study was mainly concerned with analysis of the long-term surgical outcome with respect to seizure control. The important problem with assessing whether the surgical treatment had neuropsychological consequences and effect on quality will be not detailed in this study.

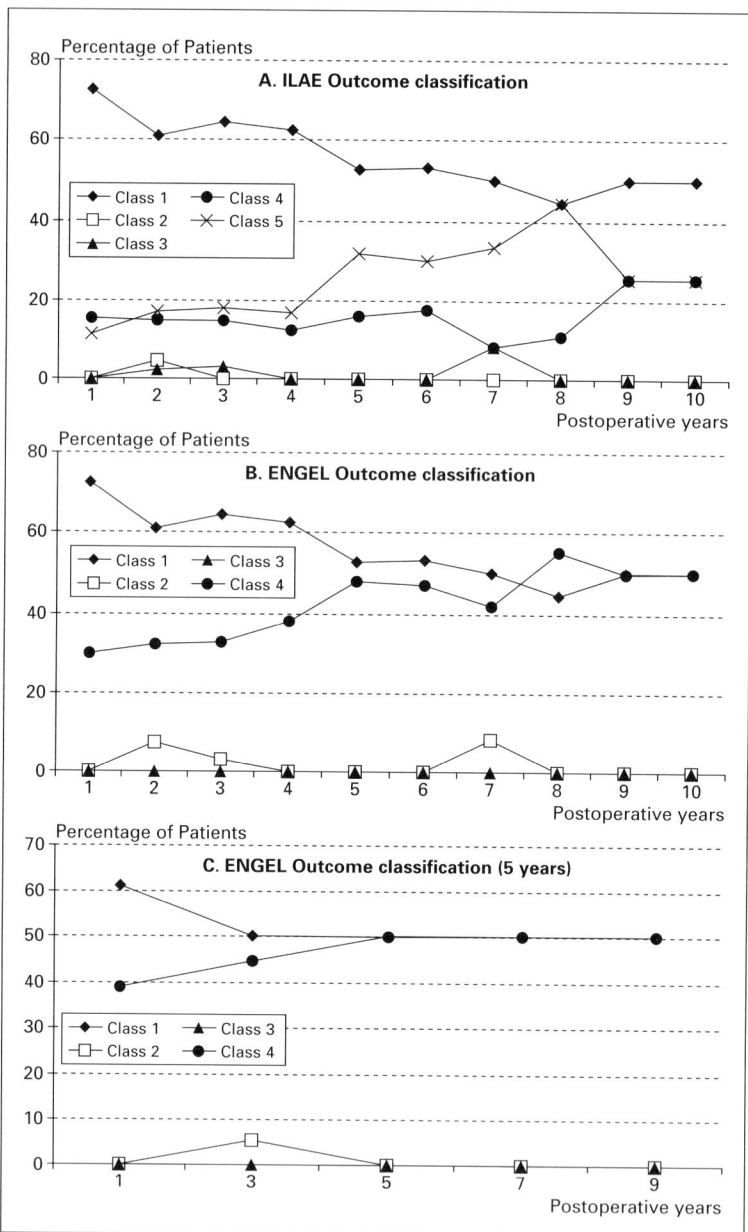

Figure 6 A, B, C. Surgical outcome according to ILAE and Engel classification

Long-term control of seizure reduction and duration of the follow-up

Our results indicate that *FLE surgery was an effective treatment* in this selected cohort: 50% of the patients were seizure-free (class IA or class 1), 25% were really improved (class IVA or class 4) and 25% were not cured at all (class IVC or class 5). *No mortality* (linked to SEEG or surgery) was observed in the immediate postoperative period.

Table V. Results of the various types of frontal resections

Type of frontal resections	Class I	Class II	Class III	Class IV
Frontopolar (N = 16)*	50%			43.7%
Mediodorsal (N = 8)	75%			25%
Intermediate frontal (N = 11)*	63%			27%
Central (N = 10)	80%			20%
Selective of the precentral gyrus (N = 1)	100%			100%
Large medial resection (N = 1)				100%
Frontal and temporal (N = 2)				100%
Special anatomical category (N = 3)	100%			
Frontal lobectomy (N = 1)	100%			

* the percentage of not available outcome is not indicated

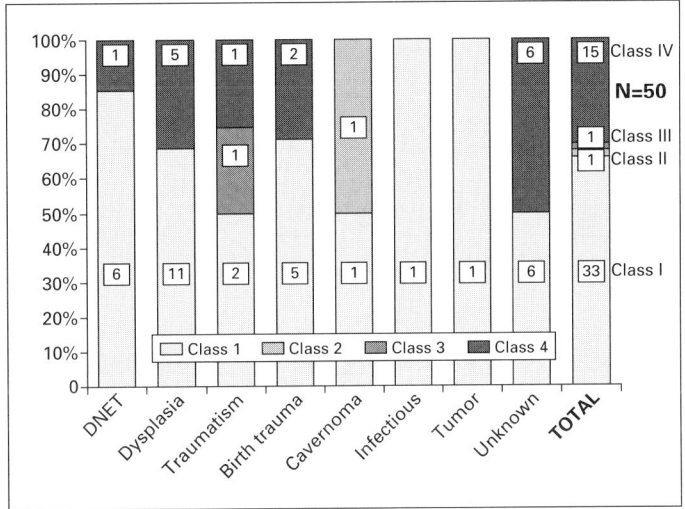

Figure 7. Histopathology and surgical outcome (Engel classification)

The comparison of our results with those previously reported is difficult for several reasons: i) some authors really estimated the percentage of seizure-free patients varying from 11% to 13%, 23%, 34% or 42% [1, 4, 5, 10, 20] others using the Engel class I (which includes seizure-free patients and patients who continue to have rare seizures) or adding class I and class II reported higher but non homogeneous percentage of improvement as 64% [21] or 78% [22] ii) the seizure reduction was sometimes differently estimated from 75 to 90%, the percentage for patients with an important improvement ranging from 21% to 26% and 60% [1, 5, 23] iii) the "rare seizures" term was ambiguous and differently interpreted from center to center and the percentages of patients with "rare seizures" varied from 6% to 26%, 32% or 52 [1, 4, 5, 10] iv) the incidence of failures also greatly varied from 12% to 19% or 44% [1, 3, 5] but the failures mean either patients with no worthwhile reduction, or with seizure reduction from 10 to 50%, or patients in the Class IVB v) finally the last global study on FLE surgery performed between 1980-1990 reported from the Global Survey on Epilepsy Surgery by Silfvenius and Wieser [10] for 330 patients indicates that 41.2% patients were seizure-free, 12.8% had rare seizures, 20% had seizure reduction by less than 90%, 19.1% had no worthwhile improvement and 1.5% had worse seizures.

In our cohort, by using the Engel or ILAE "year-by-year" classifications over a postoperative period from 1 1/2 to 11 years, we observed that the percentage of seizure-free patients

Table VI. Types of frontal resections and surgical outcome

A) Frontopolar resections

Partial resection of orbital cortex	Number of patients	Pathology
Class I	1 1	Unknown DNET
Class II		
Class III		
Class IVA	1 1	Dysplasia Post-trauma
Class IVB		
Class IVC		

Total resection of orbital cortex	Number of patients	Pathology
Class I	4 1 1 1	Dysplasia Birth trauma Post-trauma Unkown
Class II		
Class III		
Class IVA	1 1	Post-trauma Unknown
Class IVB	2	Unkown
Class IVC		

* 1p: outcome not available

B) Mediodorsal resections

Around the F1-F2 sulcus	Number of patients	Pathology
Class I	4	Dysplasia
Class II		
Class III		
Class IVA	1	Dysplasia
Class IVB	1	Dysplasia
Class IVC		

Selective resection of SMA	Number of patients	Pathology
Class I	1 1	Astrocytoma Unknown
Class II		
Class III		
Class IVA		
Class IVB		
Class IVC		

C) Intermediate frontal resections

Intermediate resection	Number of patients	Pathology
Class I	5 1 2	DNET* Post-trauma Unknown
Class II		
Class III		
Class IVA	1	Dysplasia
Class IVB	1	DNET
Class IVC	1	Unknown

* 1 outcome was not available

D) Central resections

Restrited to the opercular region	Number of patients	Pathology
Class I	2	Dysplasia
Class II	1	Cavernoma
Class III		
Class IVA		
Class IVB		
Class IVC		

Extended to the central gyrus**	Number of patients	Pathology
Class I	5	Birth trauma
Class II		
Class III		
Class IVA	2	Birth trauma
Class IVB		
Class IVC		

** All patients had a cerebral infantile hemiplegia

E) Other types of frontal resections

Types of resections	Number of patients and Engel's classes		Pathology
Precentral gyrus	1	Class I	Unknown
Large and medial surface	1	Class IVA	Large dysplasia
Frontopolar + temporal	2	Class IVC	Unknown
Special resections: – Opercular – opercular + orbital cortex – opercular + cingulate gyrus	1 1 1	Class I Class I Class I/II	Cavernoma DNET "* Unknown"
Frontal lobectomy	1	Class I	Large dysplasia

* temporo-insular atrophy and cingulate epileptogenic area

Table VII. Surgical outcome of lesional versus non lesional epilepsies according to the type of frontal resections

	Lesional		Non lesional	
	Class I	Class IV	Class I	Class IV
Frontopolar	70%	30%	25%	75%
Mediodorsal	71%	29%	100%	37%
Intermediate	75%	25%	66%	
Central	80%	20%		

(class IA or class 1) changed with follow-up duration from 72.5% at the first postoperative year to 50% at the end of the follow-up *(table III)*. Accordingly, the percentage of patients in class IV increased from 30% to 50%. The analysis of these data with the ILAE classification *(table IV)* indicated that among this half of not cured patients (Class IV), half of the patients was really improved (class 4) as compared to the preoperative period while the other half patients had definitively no reduction in seizure control (class 5). This classification of patients in class 4 (50% reduction of baseline seizure days) or in class 5 (less than 50% reduction of baseline seizure days) is one of the advantages of the ILAE classification allowing to evaluate with more objectivity the surgical outcome. Thus we can assume that in our cohort 50% of patients were seizure-free, 25% were improved and 25% had no benefit after FLE surgery.

What is the appropriate duration of the follow-up necessary before surgical results can be reported with certainty? A consensus is not yet established probably because the variability of the surgical outcome and the differences in duration of the follow-up in a group of patients consecutively operated over a definite period. A one-year follow-up is undoubtedly too short and a 5-year follow-up appeared too long. A longer period of follow-up than 5 years could be biased by the lost of patients for evaluation.. In our cohort, we had observed that the individual outcome status could change during the first post-operative years. In fact by analysing "year-by-year" the 18 same patients for whom the outcome was available over the 5 years after surgery we found that the effect of surgery on seizure control was stable after the third year *(figure 6C)*. Although this was based upon a small number of patients, we suggest that the third postoperative year might be a good compromise to estimate with certainty the prognosis of FLE surgery. This conclusive point should be confirmed by further studies of larger cohorts by using the "year by year" ILAE classification to avoid conflicting results or misleading data.

Long-term prognosis and predictive value of the presence or the absence of a brain lesion

In this 53 patient cohort, 12 patients (20%) had no radiological nor pathological lesion. Structural lesions were documented in 41 patients (77%) either evident (DNT, cortical dysplasia, porencephalic cysts, vascular malformations, small astrocytoma) or less or more discrete (3%) in the form of post-traumatic or infectious gliosis or atrophy. Only 5 pathological lesions had not been seen by MRI indicating the necessity to perform MRI systematically and possibly before the CT-Scan. Our cohort displayed a high incidence of developmental lesions, DNET (n = 8) and focal cortical dysplasia (n = 16) counting for more the half (58.5%) of the total structural lesions. DNET and focal cortical dysplasia had not been initially reported in the 100 patient series from Sainte-Anne Hospital [5]. In the 180 patient series from the Montreal National Institute (MNI) [24] only nonneoplastic lesions were documented in the form of cortical dysgenesis (15.5%). In fact, in a retrospective analysis of brain histological sections from the whole population of 500 patients operated by Pr. Talairach at Sainte-Anne Hospital, focal cortical dysplasia were found in only 28 patients (less than 6%) and were located within the frontal lobe in 16 patients [25] suggesting that this lesion type would not be related to partial epilepsies. In fact, in the present study, the focal cortical dysplasia were the most frequent lesions (40%) suggesting that in the previous and retrospective studies cortical dysplasia have been diagnosed, probably because they were not seen on the CT-Scan nor found in the surgical samples. Actually when a cortical dysplasia is not seen on the MRI images, the characteristic patterns of ictal and interictal of the EEG and SEEG discharges dictate the pathologist to search carefully for a focal cortical dysplasia in the surgical samples. In the same way, the DNET, initially described by Daumas-Duport [26], had not been identified as such in the different series [27-29]. In fact, since this pioneering study, there has been much debate about whether DNET should be included in the class of lesions having a dysembryoplastic origin or in the class of hamartoma or of low-grade brain tumors (ganglioglioma or oligodendroglioma) [13, 21, 27] and recent reports indicate that DNET must be differenciated from glioma [30, 31]. The most extensive study, reporting the DNET as a specific entity, is that from the National Hospital for Neurology and Neurosurgery (Queen Square, London) with 100 patients and 21 DNET (21%) among the 35 lesions classified as cortical dysgenesis [29]. The following year, at the Montreal National Institute, Clarke *et al.*, reviewed 60 patients with frontal structural lesions and reported 16 lesions mainly named ganglioglioma (9) and hamartoma (1) or oligodendroglioma (6) [32]. It is likely that the some or all microscopical patterns of glioma would be to-day recognized as being DNET. More recently, Errikson *et al.* evaluated the findings of the 103 frontal, temporal and multilobar resections in children and adults performed at the Göteborg Epilepsy Surgery. They distinguished the parenchymal malformations including the cortical dysplasia from the low-grade tumors including the DNET which were rare [33]. Similarly, Jobst *et al.* diagnosed only 1 DNET and 4 low-grade tumors (20%) among the 25 frontal lobe lesions [22]. The true estimation of the DNET in association with partial seizures is difficult because the use of different pathological nomenclatures. However if DNET and some low-grade tumors were intermingled, we could suggest that the percentage of the DNET occurrence might range from 15 to 25% in the whole population of epileptic patients who underwent surgery. In our cohort, 8 DNET but no low-grade ganglioglioma were diagnosed by pathological examination. So, the percentage of 19.5% of DNET in our cohort seems to be in good accordance with that extrapolated above (between 15 to 25%). *Thus the developmental lesions (DNET and focal cortical dysplasia) appear the most frequent and causative lesions to frontal lobe seizures and their presence should be suspected when no aetiology is found leading to repeat MRI.*

As shown in *figure 7*, whatever the brain lesion, 27 patients (71%) were seizure-free (class IA), 2 patients (5%) had a great improvement (class II-III) and 9 patients (24%) had no benefit in seizure control (class IV). Moreover and for the first time, we report that the DNET and focal cortical dysplasia were associated with an excellent prognosis (class IA) for 75% of patients bearing such lesions. The remaining patients (25%) demonstrated a significant reduction of seizure days (ILAE class 4). Among the five cases with dysplasia not identified before surgery, only one was associated with a partial failure indicating that SEEG with depth electrodes had correctly determined the limits of the cortical resection including the epileptogenic area and the lesion histologically found in the surgical samples. This agrees very well with the results showing that in 82% of cases, the dysplatic cortex concides with the epileptogenic area [25]. The failures observed in this series can be related to an incomplete removal of the dysplastic lesion (seen on the MRI performed after surgery) due to the proximity of eloquent cortex.

The other brain lesions (porencephalic cysts related to neonatal trauma, brain head trauma, cavernoma and tumor) were less frequent (n = 15) and the percentages of patients in the four categories were 66% (class I), 13% (class II/III) and only 20% (class IV). The low number of patients with vascular malformations, astrocytoma or sequels of infectious disease did not allow evaluation of the predictive value of such lesions.

Finally, of the 12 patients (24%) classified in the category of cryptogenic epilepsy (no radiological nor pathological abnormality) only 6 patients (50%) were seizure-free (class I) and the 6 others (50%) were not cured (class IV). Moreover, for the two seizure-free patients we retrospectively suspect the presence of a cortical focal dysplasia based upon the characteristic patterns of continuous rhythmic spike discharges during SEEG [25]. If true, the percentage of good surgical outcome would be only 40% in the cryptogenic epilepsies.

Thus, *a frontal lesion (especially neurodevelopmental lesions) is a good predictive value for a good surgical outcome*. This concept already suspected by the pioneering centers of epilepsy surgery [1-3, 5] is actually reinforced by more recent studies [22, 25, 34-36] and our present results.

Long-term prognosis and anatomical location and/or extent of the frontal resections

The different localisations and sizes of the tailored frontal resections *(table II)* were associated with different surgical outcomes *(table VI)*. When considering the 4 main defined categories, the central resections carried the best seizure outcome prognosis (80% seizure free) followed by the mediodorsal resections (75%), the intermediate frontal resections (63%) and then the most common frontopolar resections with 60% seizure-free patients. The other and unusual resection types were associated in the half of cases with a good outcome.

The best outcomes (80% of seizure-free patients) coincided with resections of the central gyrus where structural lesions were present. Seven patients had cerebral infantile hemiplegia with more or less diffuse lesions (porencephalic cyst, brain atrophy), only two patients had a small focal lesion (1 dysplasia and 1 cavernoma) situated in the opercular region. The good outcome was associated for 7 patients with a total excision of the lesion and the epileptogenic area. The 3 failures were probably linked to a too restricted resection of the epileptogenic area as for example, the cavernoma seemed completely excised on the postoperative MRI.

The mediodorsal resections represented 75% of good outcome and were associated with the presence of a cortical dysplasia. We have misgivings about the lack of aetiology for the patient who underwent a limited resection to the SMA with an excellent outcome. Athough the pathological analysis of the broken and small surgical samples failed to detect a lesion, a small but not MRI-identified cortical dysplasia could be suspected. Only two patients with cortical dysplasia were not cured and will be evaluated again with SEEG procedure to explain these failures, possibly incomplete resection of the dysplasia and/or insufficient delineation of the epileptogenic area to be removed.

The intermediate frontal resections lead to a favourable outcome in only 63%. Frequently carried out for DNET (6 of the 8 DNET) they lead to a good outcome as previously reported [26, 30].The failures in one patient (class IVB) with DNET and in an other patient with cortical dysplasia (class IVA) were explained by an incomplete resection of the epileptogenic pathological tissue near the central gyrus to avoid a postoperative motor deficit.

The frontopolar resections, the most frequently done in our cohort, resulted in 60% of seizure-free patients and they represented the largest volumes of excised tissue reaching the third or the half anterior part of the frontal lobe. In this category, the etiology was unknown for 5 patients and was heterogeneous for the other patients such brain head trauma (3), cortical dysplasia (5), DNET (1). All except one patient with developmental lesions were seizure-free. The failure for the only one patient (class IVA) after resection of a focal cortical dysplasia is remained undetermined as the patient has been lost during the second post-operative year. Of 4 patients with head traumatic lesions only two were seizure-free. In this cohort the incidence of head trauma lesions (7.5%) was low as compared to previous series [4, 5] reaching 28% and 15% respectively and leading to 46% of success [5]. Finally the large frontopolar resections carried out when the aetiology was unknown were not associated with a good prognosis *(table VI)*.

The last types of selective frontal resections need some remarks, as half was associated with a favourable outcome. A good prognosis was in fact observed when a structural lesion was present whatever its size leading to a limited resection (opercular or opercular and orbital cortex) or a frontal lobectomy. The selective resection of the premotor area (precentral gyrus) was carried out for only one patient with success but we have been unable to find a causative lesion. The patient with the large cortical dysplasia (megagyrus) on the medial surface was not cured but greatly improved. The lack of complete relief could be due to remaining abnormal tissue suspected on the MRI images at the posterior limit of the resection.

Finally, two patients were not cured nor improved after a large resection involving both the frontal and temporal lobe and no aetiology was diagnosed. This observation based upon only two patients cannot be easily compared to the high rate (80%) of success of frontotemporal resections previously reported [5]. However none of the 26 patients with frontal and temporal resections became seizure free in the MNI series [37]. It is likely that our patients had large epileptogenic area with not well defined boundaries. It is possible that they in fact had bilateral frontal epilepsy.

Thus, *a better long-term prognosis of frontal lobe epilepsy is associated with central and to intermediate and mediodorsal resections providing a structural brain lesion exists and the resections involve both the lesion and the epileptogenic area.*

An other conclusive point *is that a good long-term prognosis is not related to the extent of the frontal resection* as suggested by the bad outcome after large frontopolar and frontotemporal resection. In these cases, the aetiology was unknown and it is probable that the SEEG had not correctly identified the limits of the epileptogenic areas (more extended and even bilateral frontal?).

Finally we have to note that only one complication (wound infection) was directly linked to surgery, the most frequent complication of epilepsy surgery [38].

Conclusions and perspectives

1. Frontal lobe epilepsy surgery is an effective treatment for intractable frontal seizures.

2. No mortality related to the invasive procedures (SEEG and surgery) is observed.

3. Surgical results should be evaluated at the third post-operative year.

4. Magnetic resonance imaging (MRI), an obligatory procedure, will identify the majority of brain lesions related to frontal seizures.

5. Brain lesions, especially developmental lesions, are a positive predictive factor for a better surgical outcome.

6. The resection of the whole lesion seems an important factor for a good outcome.

7. The extent of the epileptogenic area to be removed must be carefully identified and for that the SEEG seems actually the procedure to be done.

8. When no brain lesion is seen in spite of a correct brain neuroimaging, SEEG is absolutely necessary but our feeling is "the more extended are the resections, the worse are the results".

9. The increasing use of chronic monitoring of patients with intractable seizures to document the electrophysiological patterns of frontal seizures (EEG- and SEEG-video) and of sophisticated brain neuroimaging technics associated to a better understanding of the basic epileptogenic mechanisms should result in improvement in frontal lobe surgery to cure the medically refractory frontal lobe seizures.

Aknowledgements

The authors would like to thank the EEG technicians, nurses and physicians who managed the patients: D. Toussaint, J.P. Gagnepain, O. Lebourdais, C. Friquet, P. Tessier, D. Taussig, E. Landré, A. Biraben, F. Chassoux, J.P. Vignal, M. Ghossoub, D. Broglin, P. Chauvel, J.P. Chodkiewicz, E. Seigneuret, B. Devaux, B. Turak, F. Darcel and C. Daumas-Duport.

We dedicate this work to Jean Bancaud, our teacher and to Claudio Munari, our friend, who regrettably departed this life too soon and to Professor Jean Talairach.

References

1. Olivier A. Surgery of frontal lobe epilepsy. *Adv Neurol* 1995; 66: 321-48; discussion 348-52.
2. Rasmussen T. Surgery of frontal lobe epilepsy. *Adv Neurol* 1975; 8: 197-205.
3. Rasmussen T. Characteristics of a pure culture of frontal lobe epilepsy. *Epilepsia* 1983; 24: 482-93.
4. Rasmussen T. Tailoring of cortical excisions for frontal lobe epilepsy. *Can J Neurol Sci* 1991; 18 (Suppl 4): 606-10.
5. Talairach J, Bancaud J, Bonis A, Szikla G, Trottier S, Vignal JP, Chauvel P, Munari C, Chodkiewicz JP. Surgical therapy for frontal epilepsies. *Adv Neurol* 1992; 57: 707-32.
6. Bancaud J, Talairach J. Clinical semiology of frontal lobe seizures. *Adv Neurol* 1992; 57: 3-58.
7. Chauvel P, Trottier S, Vignal JP, Bancaud J. Somatomotor seizures of frontal lobe origin. *Adv Neurol* 1992; 57: 185-232.
8. Munari C, Bancaud J. Electroclinical symptomatology of partial seizures of orbital frontal origin. *Adv Neurol* 1992; 57: 257-65.
9. Salanova V, Morris HH, Van Ness P, Kotagal P, Wyllie E, Luders H. Frontal lobe seizures: electroclinical syndromes. *Epilepsia* 1995; 36: 16-24.
10. Wieser HG, Hajek M. Frontal lobe epilepsy. Compartmentalization, presurgical evaluation, and operative results. *Adv Neurol* 1995; 66: 297-318; discussion 318-9.
11. Bancaud J, Talairach J, Geier S, Bonis A, Trottier S, Manrique M. Behavioral manifestations induced by electric stimulation of the anterior cingulate gyrus in man. *Rev Neurol (Paris)* 1976; 132: 705-24.
12. Quesney LF, Constain M, Rasmussen T, Stefan H, Olivier A. How large are frontal lobe epileptogenic zones? EEG, ECoG, and SEEG evidence. *Adv Neurol* 1992; 57: 311-23.
13. Rasmussen TB. How large are frontal lobe epileptogenic zones? Surgical aspects. *Adv Neurol* 1992; 57: 325-30.
14. Bancaud J, Angelergues R, Bernouilli C, Bonis A, Bordas-Ferrer M, Bresson M, Buser P, Covello L, Morel P, Szikla G, Takeda A, Talairach J. Functional stereotaxic exploration (stereo-electroencephalography) in epilepsies. *Rev Neurol (Paris)* 1969; 120: 448.
15. Talairach J, Tournoux P, Mussolino A, Missir O. Stereotaxic exploration in frontal epilepsy. *Adv Neurol* 1992; 57: 651-88.
16. Engel JJr. Outcome with respect to epileptic seizures. In: Engel J, ed. *Surgical treatment of the epilepsies*. New York: Raven Press, 1987: 553-71.

17. Wieser HG, Blume WT, Fish D, Goldensohn E, Hufnagel A, King D, Sperling MR, Luders H, Pedley TA. ILAE Commission Report. Proposal for a new classification of outcome with respect to epileptic seizures following epilepsy surgery. *Epilepsia* 2001; 42: 282-6.
18. Bleasel A, Comair Y, Luders HO. Surgical ablations of the mesial frontal lobe in humans. *Adv Neurol* 1996; 70: 217-35.
19. Laplane D, Talairach J, Meininger V, Bancaud J, Orgogozo JM. Clinical consequences of corticectomies involving the supplementary motor area in man. *J Neurol Sci* 1977; 34: 301-14.
20. Rougier A, Dartigues JF, Commenges D, Claverie B, Loiseau P, Cohadon F. A longitudinal assessment of seizure outcome and overall benefit from 100 cortectomies for epilepsy. *J Neurol Neurosurg Psychiatry* 1992; 55: 762-7.
21. Schramm J, Kral T, Blumcke I, Elger CE. Surgery for neocortical temporal and frontal epilepsy. *Adv Neurol* 2000; 84: 595-603.
22. Jobst BC, Siegel AM, Thadani VM, Roberts DW, Rhodes HC, Williamson PD. Intractable seizures of frontal lobe origin: clinical characteristics, localizing signs, and results of surgery. *Epilepsia* 2000; 41: 1139-52.
23. Swartz BE, Delgado-Escueta AV, Walsh GO, Rich JR, Dwan PS, DeSalles AA, Kaufman MH. Surgical outcomes in pure frontal lobe epilepsy and foci that mimic them. *Epilepsy Res* 1998; 29: 97-108.
24. Robitaille Y, Rasmussen T, Dubeau F, Tampieri D, Kemball K. Histopathology of nonneoplastic lesions in frontal lobe epilepsy. Review of 180 cases with recent MRI and PET correlations. *Adv Neurol* 1992; 57: 499-513.
25. Chassoux F, Devaux B, Landre E, Turak B, Nataf F, Varlet P, Chodkiewicz JP, Daumas-Duport C. Stereoelectroencephalography in focal cortical dysplasia: a 3D approach to delineating the dysplastic cortex. *Brain* 2000; 123: 1733-51.
26. Daumas-Duport C, Scheithauer BW, Chodkiewicz JP, Laws ER, Jr., Vedrenne C. Dysembryoplastic neuroepithelial tumor: a surgically curable tumor of young patients with intractable partial seizures. Report of thirty-nine cases. *Neurosurgery* 1988; 23: 545-56.
27. Hirose T, Scheithauer BW, Lopes MB, VandenBerg SR. Dysembryoplastic neuroeptihelial tumor (DNT): an immunohistochemical and ultrastructural study. *J Neuropathol Exp Neurol* 1994; 53: 184-95.
28. Prayson RA, Estes ML. Cortical dysplasia: a histopathologic study of 52 cases of partial lobectomy in patients with epilepsy. *Hum Pathol* 1995; 26: 493-500.
29. Raymond AA, Fish DR, Sisodiya SM, Alsanjari N, Stevens JM, Shorvon SD. Abnormalities of gyration, heterotopias, tuberous sclerosis, focal cortical dysplasia, microdysgenesis, dysembryoplastic neuroepithelial tumour and dysgenesis of the archicortex in epilepsy. Clinical, EEG and neuroimaging features in 100 adult patients. *Brain* 1995; 118: 629-60.
30. Daumas-Duport C, Varlet P, Bacha S, Beuvon F, Cervera-Pierot P, Chodkiewicz JP. Dysembryoplastic neuroepithelial tumors: nonspecific histological forms – a study of 40 cases. *J Neurooncol* 1999; 41: 267-80.
31. Stanescu Cosson R, Varlet P, Beuvon F, Daumas Duport C, Devaux B, Chassoux F, Fredy D, Meder JF. Dysembryoplastic neuroepithelial tumors: CT, MR findings and imaging follow-up: a study of 53 cases. *J Neuroradiol* 2001; 28: 230-40.
32. Clarke DB, Olivier A, Andermann F, Fish D. Surgical treatment of epilepsy: the problem of lesion/focus incongruence. *Surg Neurol* 1996; 46: 579-85; discussion 585-6.
33. Eriksson S, Malmgren K, Rydenhag B, Jonsson L, Uvebrant P, Nordborg C. Surgical treatment of epilepsy-clinical, radiological and histopathological findings in 139 children and adults. *Acta Neurol Scand* 1999; 99: 8-15.
34. Kral T, Kuczaty S, Blumcke I, Urbach H, Clusmann H, Wiestler OD, Elger C, Schramm J. Postsurgical outcome of children and adolescents with medically refractory frontal lobe epilepsies. *Childs Nerv Syst* 2001; 17: 595-601.
35. Mosewich RK, So EL, TJ OB, Cascino GD, Sharbrough FW, Marsh WR, Meyer FB, Jack CR, PC OB. Factors predictive of the outcome of frontal lobe epilepsy surgery. *Epilepsia* 2000; 41: 843-9.
36. Lorenzo NY, Parisi JE, Cascino GD, Jack CR, Jr., Marsh WR, Hirschorn KA. Intractable frontal lobe epilepsy: pathological and MRI features. *Epilepsy Res* 1995; 20: 171-8.
37. Salanova V, Quesney LF, Rasmussen T, Andermann F, Olivier A. Reevaluation of surgical failures and the role of reoperation in 39 patients with frontal lobe epilepsy. *Epilepsia* 1994; 35: 70-80.
38. Behrens E, Schramm J, Zentner J, Konig R. Surgical and neurological complications in a series of 708 epilepsy surgery procedures. *Neurosurgery* 1997; 41: 1-9; discussion 9-10.

Identification of epilepsy syndromes at diagnosis and modification with time*

Anne T. Berg

Introduction

The concept of epilepsy syndromes – specific disease entities – is not new. The first widely accepted proposal to classify and organize the epilepsies was published in 1970 [1]. Since then, the classification of the epilepsies has been formalized further and specific syndromes identified and included in the International Classification of the Epilepsies [2]. The classification continues to undergo massive revision and restructuring [3]. The recognition and use of syndromes represents the current mainstream approach to the diagnosis, treatment, management and study of the epilepsies, especially in developed countries.

An epilepsy syndrome is a coherent clinical entity characterized by numerous clinical and other information. Age at onset, seizure type(s), underlying etiology, specific electroencephalographic patterns, and often site of seizure focus are the chief components. Other factors such as acute precipitating provocations and diurnal patterns of seizure occurrence are also key to identifying some specific syndromes.

Prior to and even since the advent of the first officially accepted classification of the epilepsies, the emphasis for clinical and certainly for research purposes was on components of syndromes, age at onset, seizure types, etiology, and selected EEG characteristics. Typical questions were, "is the prognosis associated with generalized tonic clonic seizures different from that associated with complex partial seizures?" or "Does childhood onset epilepsy have a different prognosis compared to adult onset epilepsy?" This approach lumps togethers individuals with vastly varying forms of epilepsy. For example, myoclonic seizures may occur in benign myoclonic epilepsy in infancy as well as in the Lennox-Gastaut syndrome. Both of these syndromes first occur in childhood and would be lumped together in a simple comparison of childhood versus adulthood onset epilepsy. Simple partial seiz-

---

* Supported by Grant RO1 NS 31146 from the National Institutes of Neurological Disorders and Stroke.

ures associated with benign rolandic epilepsy would be lumped together with those associated with various forms of symptomatic partial epilepsy, and so on.

Studying and treating epilepsy in terms of syndromes rather than symptoms could potentially provide a much keener insight into the underlying pathophysiology and prognosis of epilepsy (from all perspectives). Early identification of the syndrome could also be useful in guiding decisions regarding ancillary testing (particularly the use of neuroimaging) and the decision to initiate pharmacologic treatment and which specific medication to use initially and also subsequently if the first medication fails. This is especially important as, in some syndromes, the incorrect choice of a drug can lead to an exacerbation of seizures (e.g. carbamazepine for childhood absence epilepsy). This approach, in theory, should also provide information about the immediate and long-term seizure prognosis.

To achieve these goals, it is essential that syndromes be identifiable very early in the course of the seizure disorder, ideally at the time of initial diagnosis. This a) permits knowledge of the syndrome to aid in evaluation and treatment decisions; b) avoids the problems of selective attrition when studying a prevalent group (because those who have been followed for a period of time and who can still be contacted tend to be different from those who are no longer in contact with the researcher or the site of medical care), c) avoids syndromes being positively identified only after patients have conformed to the expected outcome for that syndrome [4].

Use of the syndromic approach

There are many issues to resolve. At least three will be considered here:
a) Can syndromes be identified at initial diagnosis?
b) Does the initial diagnosis withstand the test of time?
c) Do different investigators utilize the criteria for syndromes in a comparable manner?

Before addressing the evidence that relates to these issues, a few comments are warranted.

1) All disorders associated with the occurrence of seizures are organized within the classification. Thus, syndromes such as febrile seizures, neonatal seizures as well as single unprovoked seizures are included under their own special heading. Although strictly speaking, a single seizure is not yet "epilepsy" [5] it is entirely valid and appropriate to identify specific epilepsy syndromes in patients at the time of a first seizure. This can provide valuable information about the early course of syndromes [6].

2) The classification is hierarchical in nature. At the first level, one distinguishes partial, generalized, and undetermined (whether partial or generalized) syndromes. At the second level, etiology is identified (idiopathic, symptomatic, and cryptogenic) [5]. At subsequent levels, specific syndromes may be identified.

3) Cases can be fit into this classification scheme, but certain groups are more diagnostically specific than others. For example, there is a category for patients who are essentially unclassified (undetermined without unequivocal evidence of either focal or generalized onset seizures). Within the idiopathic generalized grouping, the category for "other idiopathic generalized epilepsy (IGE) not specified above" is a specific designation only in that it identifies IGE. All cases have a generalized spike and wave EEG pattern, but beyond that, the designation is nonspecific and/or heterogeneous [7]. Some categories representing nonidiopathic generalized syndromes and undetermined syndromes with both generalized and focal features are not fully specific. Others are primarily defined by a highly specific etiology the diagnosis of which may not occur immediately.

4) The wording of the classification document for nonidiopathic partial syndromes has created confusion. To avoid misunderstandings, the terms cryptogenic and remote symp-

tomatic will be reserved for etiology [5]. For the fully specified syndrome, evidence sufficient to determine localization or a specific localization-related syndrome will be required. A combination of etiology and localization is needed for complete identification of a nonidiopathic partial syndrome, thus those with unlocalized partial epilepsy would be considered only partially classified. This approach combines methods of several groups of investigators, preserves important distinctions, and permits comparisons across studies. It also underscores the possibility of having an only partially-identified syndrome. Finally, even though, on the surface, this approach to nonidiopathic partial epilepsies appears to provide a high degree of specificity, in fact, there is considerable heterogeneity within these groups that is already recognized, that is being discovered or that we have not yet even imagined.

Identification of syndromes at initial diagnosis

Many studies have examined the distribution of syndromes in selected groups of prevalent or combined prevalent and incident patients. The OREp study in Lombardy examined syndromes in 8 570 patients and is the most remarkable of these studies [8]. Most patients were not newly diagnosed, however, because of the enormous size of the study, it was possible for the investigators to provide information about some of the rarer syndromes. Only a few studies have focused exclusively on the issue of recognition of syndromes at the time of initial diagnosis in representative series of patients. Two of these studies [9, 10] have covered the full gamut by including individuals of all ages, with single seizures as well as newly diagnosed epilepsy. The CAROLE study [10] is particularly noteworthy as it includes nearly 2 000 patients, roughly half children and half adults, half single seizures and half newly diagnosed epilepsy. The other three studies have focused on children and adolescents. One included only individuals with a single seizure and classified the syndromes only in those who went on to have a second seizure [11]. The other two focused on children with newly diagnosed epilepsy [12, 13]. The rest of this discussion will focus largely on the Connecticut study as it was explicitly designed to address early identification of syndromes and their stability over time. By necessity, this discussion will largely be limited to epilepsy of childhood and early adolescent onset.

The methods for the Connecticut study have been published previously [14, 15]. Children and adolescents (1 month-15 years) were identified at the time of initial diagnosis of epilepsy by clinicians in the State of Connecticut between 1993 and 1997. Their syndromes, seizure types, and etiologies were classified according to the published criteria available at that time [2, 5, 16]. Of note, all but five children had an EEG and 80% had a neuroimaging study. An MRI was performed in 63% of participants. Patients are followed intensively by phone and by periodic review of all interim medical records. After two years of follow-up, each child's history was re-evaluated and the syndromes, seizure types and etiology reclassified based upon all information available up through two years after diagnosis. The initial distribution and the distribution after two years of follow-up (which will be discussed in the next section) are presented in *table I*.

From the distribution of syndromes at diagnosis, one can appreciate that fully a third of children were placed in categories that represented completely unclassified epilepsy (~ 11%) or partially classified syndromes (~ 22%). Another 18 (2.9%) were classified as "other idiopathic generalized syndromes", and a few are in the grouping for symptomatic generalized epilepsies or "other undetermined epilepsies not defined above". Both of these last two are not always entirely specific. Although accounting for only a few percent of this cohort, these syndrome groups include perhaps some of the most difficult cases to treat so the accuracy of diagnosis is all the more important for these children.

Table I. Distribution of syndromes in the Connecticut cohort at initial diagnosis and two years later [12]

Syndrome	At Initial Diagnosis N (%)	After 2 years N (%)
1. LOCALIZATION-RELATED	359 (58.6)	366 (59.7)
1.1 **Idiopathic localization related**	61 (10.0)	66 (10.7)
1.1.1 Benign Rolandic epilepsy	59 (9.6)	63 (10.3)
1.1.2 Childhood epilepsy with occipital paroxysms	2 (0.3)	3 (0.5)
1.2. **Symptomatic localization-related**	72 (11.6)	80 (13.1)
1.2.3.a Symptomatic localization-related, unlocalized	21 (3.4)	27 (4.4)
1.2.3.b Symptomatic localization-related, localized	51 (8.2)	53 (8.6)
1.3 **Cryptogenic Localization related**	226 (36.9)	220 (35.9)
1.3.0.a Cryptogenic Localization related, unlocalized	103 (16.8)	91 (14.8)
1.3.0.b Cryptogenic Localization related, localized	123 (20.2)	129 (21.0)
2. GENERALIZED	178 (29.0)	196 (32.0)
2.1 **Idiopathic generalized**	126 (20.6)	135 (22.0)
2.1.0 Idiopathic generalized not further classified	1 (0.2)	1 (0.2)
2.1.3 Benign myoclonic epilepsy in infancy	1 (0.2)	2 (0.3)
2.1.4 Childhood absence epilepsy	74 (12.1)	76 (12.4)
2.1.5 Juvenile absence epilepsy	15 (2.4)	17 (2.8)
2.1.6 Juvenile myoclonic epilepsy	12 (2.0)	15 (2.4)
2.1.7 Epilepsy with GTCS on awakening	2 (0.3)	2 (0.3)
2.1.8 Other idiopathic generalized	18 (2.9)	18 (2.9)
2.1.9 w/ seizures precipitated by specific modes of activation	3 (0.5)	4 (0.7)
2.2 **Cryptogenic/Symptomatic generalized**	43 (7.0)	51 (8.3)
2.2.0 Generalized cryptogenic/symptomatic not further classified	3 (0.5)	3 (0.5)
2.2.1 West syndrome*	24 (3.9)	19 (3.1)
2.2.2 Lennox-Gastaut syndrome	4 (0.7)	19 (2.9)
2.2.3 Epilepsy with myoclonic-astatic seizures (Doose)	10 (1.6)	8 (1.3)
2.2.4 Epilepsy with myoclonic absences	2 (0.3)	2 (0.3)
2.3 **Symptomatic generalized**	9 (1.5)	9 (1.5)
2.3.1 Symptomatic generalized epilepsy (nonspecific etiology)	4 (0.7)	3 (0.5)
2.3.2 Symptomatic generalized epilepsy (specific syndromes)	5 (0.8)	6 (1.0)
3. UNDETERMINED	76 (12.4)	51 (8.3)
3.1 **With partial and generalized features**	5 (0.8)	2 (0.3)
3.1.2 Severe myoclonic epilepsy in infancy	1 (0.2)	1 (0.2)
3.1.3 Epilepsy with continuous spike-wave during slow wave sleep	1 (0.2)	1 (0.2)
3.1.5 Other undetermined epilepsies not defined above	3 (0.5)	0 (0)
3.2 **Epilepsies without unequivocal generalized or focal features (unclassified)**	71 (11.6)	50 (8.2)

In the Bronx, NY study, syndromes were classified only in the 182 patients who experienced a second seizure. As the types of patients included in the two studies differs substantially, one cannot directly compare the distributions of syndromes. For example, West syndrome and childhood absence epilepsy were not represented at all in the Bronx. What is striking, however, is the large proportion of children who do not meet the criteria for a specific syndrome despite most patients having had an EEG; 19% were partially classified and 26% completely unclassified after the second seizure. The French studies [9, 10] and the Dutch study [12] also report a substantial proportion of unclassified or partially classified cases.

Overall, a significant proportion of children with newly diagnosed epilepsy cannot be assigned to a specific epilepsy syndrome even though they have been reasonably well evaluated according to standards in developed countries. The same is true of adults. Currently, and given available technology and standards of care, this seems to be a fair assessment of how well syndromes can be classified in children with newly diagnosed epilepsy. The issues in adults in whom specific syndromes have not been as well defined may, of course, be somewhat different [8-10].

Although these findings leave the interested investigator with a certain sense of dissatisfaction, at the very least, such data help to delimit the areas of weakness in early diagnosis of epilepsy in developed countries and may help in planning future studies into these issues.

How stable is the initial diagnosis over time?

There are at least two reasons for changes in syndromic diagnosis. A change may reflect the evolution of one syndrome to another or it may simply reflect an error in the initial diagnosis.

Evolution of syndromes

In some of the more severe forms of childhood epilepsy, one syndrome can evolve into another. Such a determination is based largely on true changes in seizure type and specific EEG patterns as well as overall impression about the child's clinical status, particularly neurological and development status. These evolutions almost always involve nonidiopthic generalized syndromes either as the initial syndrome, the syndrome to which the epilepsy evolves or both. After two years, 24 cases (4%) in the Connecticut study had clearly evolved to a different syndrome. As might be surmised from the works of others [17], West and Lennox-Gastaut syndrome were implicated the most frequently in such cases *(table II)*.

In the Bronx study, 6 (3%) children experienced an evolution of their syndrome [11]. In all instances, the initial syndrome was non-idiopathic partial which evolved to Lennox-Gastaut. In both studies, Lennox-Gastaut syndrome was relatively rare at initial diagnosis (< 1%) but ultimately accounted for several percent of pediatric onset epilepsy.

Correction of initial errors in diagnosis

After two years of follow-up, 60 (10%) of children in the Connecticut study, had their initial syndromic diagnosis revised. Fully one third (N = 21) of these cases came from the category for unclassified epilepsy and almost another third (N = 18) were only partially classified initially. Thus, the initial diagnosis was in a sense already acknowledged to be in error. These cases were assigned a more specific classification at two years.

In five cases, reclassifications were made between related syndromes, and in only 16 cases (representing < 3% of the entire cohort) apparently major changes were made (e.g. non-idiopathic localization-related epilepsy to idiopathic generalized epilepsy). In all of these cases, there were significant difficulties in the initial classification either because of poor quality of information or contradictory findings. The most salient changes are summarized in *table II*.

A similar pattern of changes was evident In the Bronx study [11], where 28 initial diagnoses were changed. In 18 of these instances, the initial diagnosis was completely (N = 10) or partially (N = 8) unclassified. The Gironde study's results also reflect similar patterns of change after one and five years [9, 18].

The specific changes deserve further comment *(figure 1)*. Once identified, a highly specific syndromic diagnosis rarely is discarded later. None of the cases with idiopathic partial epilepsy (mostly benign Rolandic) was removed from that category after two years and only ~ 2% in the idiopathic generalized syndromes were re-classified, all of whom were initially in the "other" (nonspecific) IGE group. The same observation holds for West syndrome and localized forms of nonidiopathic partial epilepsy (both symptomatic and

Table II. Summary of the more common changes that occurred between initial diagnosis and diagnosis at 2 years*

Connecticut Study		
Initial syndrome (N who changed)	Syndrome at 2 years	N1.
Evolution of Syndrome (N = 24)		
West (N = 9)	Lennox-Gastaut Other	5 4
Non-idiopathic partial (N = 10)	West Lennox-Gastaut Other	3 4 3
Undetermined/unclassified (N = 5)	Lennox-Gastaut Non-idiopathic partial	4 1
Correction to initial diagnosis (N = 60)		
Undetermined/Unclassified (N = 21)	Non-idiopathic partial Idiopathic partial Idiopathic generalized	15 2 4
Cryptogenic partial – unlocalized (N = 15)	Cryptogenic-localized Other	12 3
Cryptogenic partial – localized (N = 5)	Idiopathic generalized Other	3 2
"Other" idiopathic generalized (N = 3)	Juvenile absence Juvenile myoclonic Cryptogenic partial unlocalized	1 1 1
Other undetermined with both focal and generalized features (N = 3)	Nonidiopathic partial Idiopathic generalized	2 1

* Only the most salient changes are represented in the table. For more specific details see [12].

cryptogenic). The groups most susceptible to change are the unclassified and partially classified cryptogenic localization-related categories. Finally, after two years, the categories to which cases were most likely to be added were the nonidiopathic partial groups. With the initial size of the category as the denominator, ten percent or fewer cases were added to the idiopathic categories or to the nonidiopathic generalized categories as a result of errors in initial diagnosis.

The most common reason for making a correction to a syndrome involved more specific information obtained from one or more subsequent EEGs. This highlights the importance of the EEG in the diagnosis of epilepsy and identification of the specific forms of epilepsy. Of note, while the EEG is invaluable in the diagnosis of epilepsy and identification of specific syndromes, its use over time must take into account that the activity recorded by the EEG is subject to modification in the presence of some antiepileptic drugs. Another issue to consider for the researcher interested in classifying syndromes is that the interictal EEG frequently provides limited information, and, in some patients, the ictal EEG may be more informative. Unfortunately for the researcher although fortunately for the patients, the majority of children and adults do not have sufficiently frequent seizures to justify a prolonged monitoring session. Even if they were monitored, it would, in a vast majority of cases be an unproductive exercise in newly diagnosed patients. Where it does contribute in some new (and old) cases is to establishing the diagnosis of epilepsy versus other non-epileptic conditions.

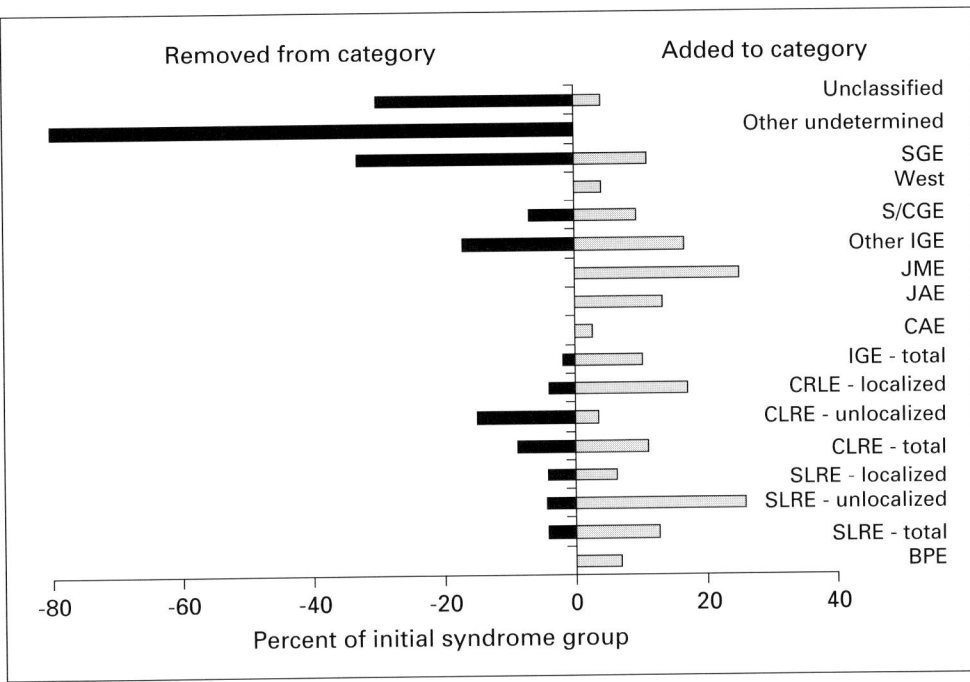

Figure 1. Cases added to and removed from each category after two years of follow-up as a proportion of cases initially in each category (SGE = symptomatic generalized epilepsy, S/CGE = symptomatic or cryptogenic generalized epilepsy, IGE-idiopathic generalized epilepsy, JME = juvenile myoclonic epilepsy, JAE = juvenile absence epilepsy, CAE = childhood absence epilepsy, CRLE = cryptogenic localization-related epilepsy, SRLE = symptomatic localization-related epilepsy, IPE = idiopathic partial epilepsy).

Finally, one must consider the philosophical and scientific question regarding the distinction made here between the evolution of a syndrome versus a missed diagnosis. For example, was a patient who was initially unclassified and later found to have a temporal lobe focus really misdiagnosed initially (i.e. he had temporal lobe epilepsy all along but it was missed) or has something altered in the underlying epilepsy causing it to become more localized?

Preliminary data from the review of all cases after five years of follow-up indicates that further changes will occur. The pattern of changes appears highly comparable to what was observed at two years: evolution of some syndromes, more specific diagnosis for partially or completely unclassified forms of epilepsy, errors in cases for whom information was initially of poor quality or highly confusing are later reclassified.

One may study relatively common, well-defined syndromes in this manner. Some of the rarer and more complex (and also severe) syndromes are hard to address in this context. It is unclear how well clinicians in the community diagnosis these rarer syndromes.

Consistency in use of the classification criteria

Within the Connecticut study, a high level of agreement was obtained between three independent child neurologists in the use of the classification of the epilepsies [14]. In this study, however, investigators addressed the ambiguous points in the classification and decided upon a set of "rules" for applying the classification. With those "rules", agreement was excellent. Disagreements were largely due to poor quality information or complicated cases with contradictory evidence.

Across studies, however, different "rules" have been applied by different teams of investigators. This is not entirely surprising as the wording of the 1989 document [2] leaves much to interpretation. For example, the definition of symptomatic localization-related has been variously interpreted as meaning strictly on the basis of etiology as well as on the basis of etiology or localization [9-12, 15, 19]. Extensive Talmudic reasoning has yet to resolve this issue. The most parsimonious approach is to cross-classify based on localization and etiology. In some cases, identification of specific syndromes has been based simply on seizure type [20]. The use of relatively nonspecific categories has also varied. One group classified all patients with normal EEGs and apparently generalized onset tonic-clonic seizures as "other" idiopathic generalized [21] although most other studies considered such cases as unclassified. For highly specific syndromes, there are published easily accessible and internationally accepted guidelines for identification of syndromes, at least in children and adolescents [17]. For the less specific categories some collaborative discussion is necessary.

Ultimately, for results to be useful and especially for them to provide a valid basis of comparison across studies, it is imperative that all investigators subscribe to the same criteria. To the extent that departures from these criteria occur, one should still provide the information necessary to reconcile approaches used in different studies.

Is early identification of the syndrome worthwhile?

Evidence would suggest the answer is "yes". The use of neuroimaging, initiation of treatment, and choice of specific medication is significantly influenced by the syndrome [10, 22-25]. For example, neuroimaging is used less in idiopathic forms of epilepsy. The determination of idiopathic relies heavily on the specific EEG findings. This assumes that physicians first use clinical and EEG information to identify the syndrome and then decide whether to order a neuroimaging study. In fact, this would be consistent with recent practice guidelines for evaluating a child with a first unprovoked seizure [26].

Initiation of treatment varied by syndrome, and the choice of specific drug largely reflected recommendations for treatment of specific syndromes. Thus, knowledge of the syndrome does appear to have some influence on evaluation and management, at least of children with epilepsy. For adults who have largely nonidiopathic forms of partial epilepsy, the specific syndrome (to the extent that we can currently identify specific nonidiopathic partial syndromes) may be less important to treatment and evaluation decisions. Unfortunately, with the exception of work done by the French investigators, little attention has given up to this point to classifying syndromes in adults.

Ideally early identification of the syndrome should aid in understanding prognosis. In fact, after an average of six years of follow-up in the Connecticut study, the outcomes of many of the highly specific syndromes (as identified at diagnosis) are very much what is expected *(figure 2)* [27, 28]. Recent studies have also examined the value of the syndromic approach for understanding patterns of mortality in people with epilepsy [29-31]. While the results suggest the approach may be very helpful, it is not yet clear whether it is useful above and beyond the association with seizure control, polypharmacy, and other factors shown to be associated with mortality. Regardless, early identification of the syndrome permits early knowledge about the likelihood of outcomes such as mortality even if this should turn out to be largely a function of the seizure outcome.

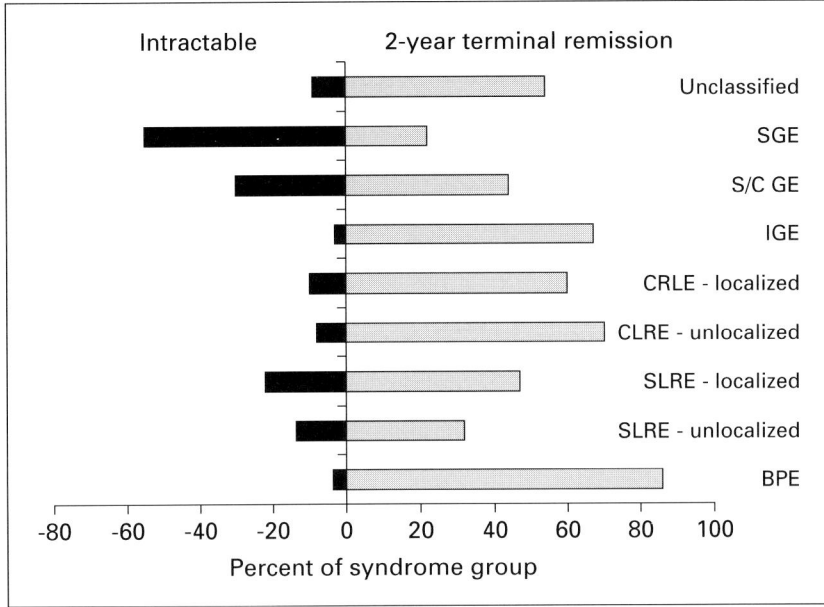

Figure 2. Proportion intractable and in two year remission after six years of follow-up according to type of epilepsy syndrome (SGE = symptomatic generalized epilepsy, S/CGE = symptomatic or cryptogenic generalized epilepsy, IGE-idiopathic generalized epilepsy, CRLE = cryptogenic localization-related epilepsy, SRLE = symptomatic localization-related epilepsy, IPE = idiopathic partial epilepsy).

Nonidiopathic partial epilepsy

The partial epilepsies deserve special attention both in terms of early identification and evolution of syndromes as they account for 30-50% of all epilepsy in children and ~ 90% of epilepsy in adults. Aside from the presence of a remote symptomatic etiology, it is not clear that the syndrome, as identified at initial diagnosis, is helpful in defining prognosis *(figure 3)*.

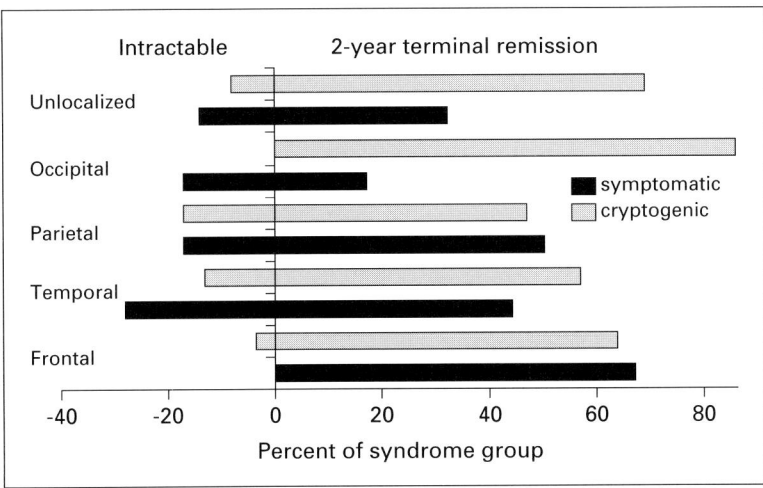

Figure 3. Proportion intractable and in 2-year remission after six years of follow-up for those with nonidiopathic localization-related epilepsy.

The temporal lobe group is particularly interesting in the context of a discussion of the variation of syndromes over time. Mesial temporal lobe epilepsy often with hippocampal sclerosis represents the single most common surgically treated form of epilepsy. Very little of this surgery is done in children [32], and almost all is done in adults. What is often not appreciated is that half or more of adults who have surgery for this type of epilepsy had their initial onset during childhood and adolescence, the same age of those prospectively followed in the Connecticut study. Their typical duration of epilepsy prior to surgery is often 20 years or longer [33-40]. In the Connecticut study, ~ 80% of children with seizures and EEG findings referable to the temporal lobe had a MRI, and only one had hippocampal atrophy characteristic of temporal lobe epilepsy. This suggests that either temporal lobe epilepsy of childhood onset seen in adults undergoing surgery is very rare or is not easily identified at onset.

The long delay typically seen between onset of epilepsy and surgery in adult surgical patients may not simply be a matter of putting off surgery for a protracted period but may be due a relatively benign initial course. In a recent series of surgical patients, the average time between onset of epilepsy and failure of the second medication (a rough marker for the appearance of intractable seizures) was on the order of about nine years [41]. This figure increased to 15 years in those with initial onset under the age of five. In addition, a large proportion of patients reported having had a period of at least 1 year of remission and 10% had experienced a remission of five or more years duration. Such remissions were much more common in adult patients whose epilepsy began during early childhood. Others have also reported histories of prolonged remissions in the histories of individuals with intractable temporal lobe epilepsy [42, 43].

These compiled observations suggest the rather sobering possibility that, in some forms of epilepsy, the evolution of the syndrome and its prognosis may occur over a very prolonged period of time. They also underscore how little is currently understood, from an epidemiological and clinical perspective, about the diversity, evolution and prognosis of non-idiopathic partial epilepsies. We may not, at present, know how to identify the specific syndrome of mesial temporal lobe epilepsy – of the type seen so often by neurosurgeons – at diagnosis or even a few years later. Prospective documentation of its progression from the point of diagnosis to development of intractability will require more than a decade of follow-up. Other than merely satisfying our curiosity about the time course of this syndrome's prognosis, we might have the possibility one day of understanding the mechanisms by which it becomes intractable and possibly even intervening in this process and preventing the development of some forms of intractable epilepsy. This could represent one of the ultimate accomplishments of the syndromic approach to the epilepsies.

Conclusions

1) The highly specific, common forms of childhood epilepsy are reasonably likely to be identified at onset. They are rarely diagnosed in error.

2) At initial diagnosis, a third or more of children can only be partially classified or are left completely unclassified. With time, many can be classified and frequently turn out to have a form of nonidiopathic partial epilepsy.

3) Very rare and serious forms of epilepsy are difficult to study in a community or population-based setting.

4) Even under ideal circumstances, there is expressed concern regarding the utility of the syndromic approach in adults where the vast majority of the epilepsy seems to be nonidiopathic partial. The current classification may therefore be of somewhat limited utility

in adult epilepsy, as we currently understand it. This can change as we learn to distinguish specific forms of partial epilepsy in both children and adults. There is absolutely no reason, however, to ignore what is know about clear, coherent syndromes that have been well-established just because we have not yet been able to fit all forms of epilepsy into highly specific syndromic categories.

5) The results of current and future research and time will tell whether there are specific syndromes in adults as well as in children that can be readily identified and meaningfully used in the treatment and management of epilepsy and in understanding – possibly one day altering – prognosis.

References

1. Commission on Classification and Terminology of the International League Against Epilepsy. Proposal for the International Classification of the Epilepsies. *Epilepsia* 1970; 11: 114-9.
2. Commission on Classification and Terminology of the International League Against Epilepsy. Proposal for revised classification of epilepsies and epileptic syndromes. *Epilepsia* 1989; 30: 389-99.
3. Engel J. A proposed diagnostic scheme for people with epileptic seizures and with epilepsy: Report of the ILAE Task Force on Classification and Terminology. *Epilepsia* 2001; 42: 796-803.
4. Bouma PA, Bovenkerk AC, Westendorp RG, Brouwer OF. The course of benign partial epilepsy of childhood with centrotemporal spikes: a meta-analysis. *Neurology* 1997; 48: 430-7.
5. Commission on Epidemiology and Prognosis, International League Against Epilepsy. Guidelines for epidemiologic studies on epilepsy. *Epilepsia* 1993; 34: 592-6.
6. Carole G. Délais évolutifs des syndromes épileptiques avant leur diagnostic: résultats descriptifs de l'enquête CAROLE. *Rev Neurol (Paris)* 2000; 156: 481-90.
7. Loiseau P, Loiseau J. Épilepsies. Vous avez dit épilepsie? *Rev Neurol (Paris)* 1999; 155: 193-8.
8. Osservatorio Regionale per L'Epilessia (OREp) L. ILAE classification of epilepsies: its applicability and practical value of different diagnostic categories. Osservatorio Regionale per L'Epilessia (OREp), Lombardy. *Epilepsia* 1996; 37: 1051-9.
9. Loiseau J, Loiseau P, Guyot M, Duche B, Dartigues JF, Aublet B. Survey of seizure disorders in the French southwest. I. Incidence of epileptic syndromes. *Epilepsia* 1990; 31: 391-6.
10. Jallon P, Loiseau P, Loiseau J. Newly diagnosed unprovoked epileptic seizures: presentation at diagnosis in CAROLE study. *Epilepsia* 2001; 42: 464-75.
11. Shinnar S, O'Dell C, Berg AT. Distribution of epilepsy syndromes in a cohort of children prospectively monitored from the time of their first unprovoked seizure. *Epilepsia* 1999; 40: 1378-83.
12. Callenbach PM, Geerts AT, Arts WF, van Donselaar CA, Peters AC, Stroink H, Brouwer OF. Familial occurrence of epilepsy in children with newly diagnosed multiple seizures: Dutch Study of Epilepsy in Childhood. *Epilepsia* 1998; 39: 331-6.
13. Berg AT, Shinnar S, Levy SR, Testa FM, Smith-Rapaport S, Beckerman B. How well can epilepsy syndromes be identified at diagnosis? A reassessment two years after initial diagnosis. *Epilepsia* 2000; 41: 1269-75.
14. Berg AT, Levy SR, Testa FM, Shinnar S. Classification of childhood epilepsy syndromes in newly diagnosed epilepsy: Interrater agreement and reasons for disagreement. *Epilepsia* 1999; 40: 439-44.
15. Berg AT, Shinnar S, Levy SR, Testa FM. Newly-diagnosed epilepsy in children: presentation at diagnosis. *Epilepsia* 1999; 40: 445-52.
16. Commission on Classification and Terminology of the International League Against Epilepsy. Proposal for revised clinical and electrographic classification of epileptic seizures. *Epilepsia* 1981; 22: 489-501.
17. Roger J, Bureau M, Dravet C, Dreifuss FE, Perret A, Wolf P. Epileptic syndromes in infancy, childhood, and adolescence. London: John Libbey, 1992.
18. Loiseau J, Picot MC, Jallon P, Dartigues JF, Loiseau P. Classification and incidence of epileptic syndromes in a prospective study: reliability and causes of change. *Epilepsia* 1998; 39 (suppl 6): 181.
19. Sillanpaa M, Jalava M, Shinnar S. Epilepsy syndromes in patients with childhood-onset seizures in Finland. *Pediatr Neurol* 1999; 21: 533-7.
20. Wirrell EC, Camfield CS, Camfield PR, Gordon KE, Dooley JM. Long-term prognosis of typical childhood absence epilepsy: remission or progression to juvenile myoclonic epilepsy. *Neurology* 1996; 47: 912-8.

21. Middeldorp CM, Geerts AT, Brouwer OF, Peters ACB, HS, van Donselaar CA, Arts WFM. Non-symptomatic generalized epilepsy in children under six: excellent prognosis but the classification should be reconsidered after followup: The Dutch study of epilepsy in childhood. *Epilepsia* in press.
22. Berg AT, Levy SR, Testa FT, Shinnar S. Treatment of newly diagnosed pediatric epilepsy: a community-based study. *Arch Pediatr Adol Med* 1999; 153: 1267-71.
23. Berg AT, Testa FM, Levy SR, Shinnar S. Neuroimaging in children with newly diagnosed epilepsy: a community-based study. *Pediatrics* 2000; 106: 527-32.
24. Carpay JA, Arts WFM, Geerts AT, Stroink H, Brouwer OF, Peters ACB, van Donselaar CA. Epilepsy in childhood: an audit of clinical practice. *Arch Neurol* 1998; 55: 668-73.
25. Groupe CAROLE. Traitement des crises epileptiques nouvellement diagnostiquees. Une experience francaise. *Revue Neurologique* 2001; 157: 1500-12.
26. Hirtz D, Ashwal S, Berg AT, Bettis D, Camfield C, Camfield P, Crumrine P, Elterman R, Schneider S, Shinnar S. Evaluating a first nonfebrile seizure in children: an evidence-based practice parameter. *Neurology* 2000; 55: 616-23.
27. Berg AT, Shinnar S, Levy SR, Testa F, Smith-Rapaport S, Beckerman B. Intractable epilepsy in children: a prospective study. *Neurology* 2001; 56: 1445-52.
28. Berg AT, Shinnar S, Levy SR, Testa FM, Smith-Rapaport S, Beckerman B. Two-year remission and subsequent relapse in children with newly diagnosed epilepsy. *Epilepsia* 2001; 42: 1553-62.
29. Loiseau J, M-C P, Loiseau P. Short-term mortality after a first epileptic seizure: a population-based study. *Epilepsia* 1999; 40: 1388-92.
30. Callenbach PMC, Westendorb RGJ, Geerts AT, Arts WFM, Peeters EAJ, van Donselaar CA, Peters ACB, Stroink H, Brouwer OF. Mortality in children with epilepsy: The Dutch study of epilepsy in childhood. *Pediatrics* 2001; 107: 1259-63.
31. Camfield CS, Camfield PR, Veugelers PJ. Death in children with epilepsy: a population-based study. *Lancet* 2002; http//image.thelancet.com/extras/01art3267web.pdf.
32. Mathern GW, Giza CC, Yudovin S, Vinters HV, Peacock WJ, Shewmon DA, Shields WD. Postoperative seizure control and antiepileptic drug use in pediatric epilepsy surgery patients: the UCLA experience, 1986-1997. *Epilepsia* 1999; 40: 1740-9.
33. Kilpatrick C, Cook M, Matkovic Z, O'Brien T, Kaye A, Murphy M. Seizure frequency and duration of epilepsy are not risk factors for postoperative seizure outcome in patients with hippocampal sclerosis. *Epilepsia* 1999; 40: 899-903.
34. Sperling MR, MJ OC, Saykin AJ, Plummer C. Temporal lobectomy for refractory epilepsy. *JAMA* 1996; 276: 470-5.
35. Zentner J, Hufnagel A, Wolf HK, Ostertun B, Behrens E, Campos MG, Solymosi L, Elger CR, Wiestler OD, Schramm J. Surgical treatment of temporal lobe epilepsy: clinical, radiological, and histopathological findings in 178 patients. *J Neurol Neurosurg Psychiatry* 1995; 1995: 666-73.
36. Walczak TS, Radtke RA, McNamara JO, Lewis DV, Luther JS, Thompson E, Wilson WP, Friedman AH, Nashold BS. Anterior temporal lobectomy for complex partial seizures: evaluation, results, and long-term follow-up in 100 cases. *Neurology* 1990; 40: 413-8.
37. Duncan JS, Sagar HJ. Seizure characteristics, pathology, and outcome after temporal lobectomy. *Neurology* 1987; 37: 405-9.
38. Dodrill CB, Wilkus RJ, Ojemann GA, Ward AA, Wyler AR, van Belle G, Tamas L. Multidisciplinary prediction of seizure relief from cortical resection surgery. *Ann Neurol* 1986; 20: 2-12.
39. Abou-Khalil B, Andermann E, Andermann F, Olivier A, Quesney LF. Temporal lobe epilepsy after prolonged febrile convulsions: Excellent outcome after surgical treatment. *Epilepsia* 1993; 34: 878-83.
40. Hufnagel A, Elger CE, Pels H, Zenter J, Wolf HK, Schramm J, Wiestler OD. Prognostic significance of ictal and interictal epileptiform activity in temporal lobe epilepsy. *Epilepsia* 1994; 35: 1146-53.
41. Berg AT, Langfitt J, Shinnar S, Vickrey BG, Sperling MR, Walczak T, Bazil C, Pacia SV, Spencer SS. How long does it take for partial epilepsy to become intractable? *Neurology* in press.
42. French JA, Williamson PD, Thadani VM, Darcey TM, Mattson RH, Spencer SS, Spencer DD. Characteristics of medial temporal lobe epilepsy: I. results of history and physical examination. *Ann Neurol* 1993; 34: 774-80.
43. Takenaka J, Kosaburo, Watanabe K, Okumura A, Negoro T. Transient remission in intractable localization-related epilepsy. *Pediatr Neurol* 2000; 23: 328-31.

Part 2
Prognosis of epilepsy syndromes

Prognosis of neonatal seizures

Perrine Plouin, Emmanuel Raffo, Talvany de Oliveira

The term neonatal seizures refers to seizures occurring in the first 28 days of life. We will focus on infants born at term (> 37 weeks gestational age) as very few data are available for small, premature infants. When epileptic seizures occur in neonates, they occur during the first week in more than 80% of cases. Most of these seizures are symptomatic of brain injury although in some cases they do represent a true epileptic condition. In most reports on neonatal seizures (the word convulsion is often used; however, seizure is the preferred term), the study series comes from a neonatal intensive care unit (NICU). On the other hand neonatologists and neuropediatricians have reported benign as well as severe epileptic conditions in neonates. Some of these conditions have been recognized as epilepsy syndromes by the International Classification of Epilepsies and Epilepsy Syndromes [1]. The occurrence of a subsequent epilepsy in infancy, childhood or adulthood depends on many factors, the most important being etiology of the neonatal seizures [NNS] [2].

In this paper we consider data from different medical services. It must be emphasised that there are various referral biases associated with recruiting patients from the three main sources for identifying NNS [NICU, neonatology and pediatric neurology]. In the NICU, one finds infants who are in a critical state and who often require ventilation. By contrast, in neonatology, benign conditions are more common. Infants who are seen in pediatric neurology are often referred there because of persistent and even intractable seizures.

Another issue to resolve is the definition of epileptic seizures in this population. Some authors report on clinical seizures, whereas others only consider seizures for which there is a clear electrographic correlation. Controversy remains about how to handle electrographic seizures [without a clinical component] and clinical manifestations with no EEG change [so called subtle seizures]. In this setting "convulsion" refers to events that have a motor component, and the term "seizure" includes events without a clear motor component such as complex partial seizures which definitely exist among neonates.

We will first report data on NNS, as they are the most frequently discussed in the literature. Next we will focus on epilepsy syndromes among neonates. Finally we will discuss our own data derived from a pediatric neurology unit.

Neonatal Seizures

Incidence

Methodology differs widely among the studies that have addressed the incidence of NNS. We have already mentioned the definitional issues surrounding neonatal seizures [inclusion or not of EEG data, or even video-EEG data]. Whether the studies are retrospective or prospective can also affect the results. Other factors to be considered include the target population, the duration of follow-up [between the first few days and the first month] and the time period during which cases were accrued as the numerous improvements in neonatal intensive care that have occurred since the 1960s and have influenced survival and other outcomes among neonates.

In 1998, Mizrahi and Kellaway [3], reviewed the reported incidence of NNS in different studies. The first data come from the National Collaborative Perinatal Project [50 000 pregnant women studied between 1959 and 1966]. This study found an incidence of NNS of 5.1/1 000 live births. Subsequent studies reported incidences ranging from 1.5/1 000 to 5.5/1 000 live births.

The two most recent studies provide an estimate of the incidence of 1.8/1 000 live births [4] and 2.6/1 000 live births [5] respectively. The first one reports on the population of infants born between 1992 and 1994 in Harris County, Texas who presented with clinical seizures. There were 207 cases identified among 116 048 live births. The incidence was clearly higher in infants who weighed less than 1500 g [19.1/1 000] and decreased with increasing birth weight. There was no significant difference in incidence by ethnicity. The incidence of NNS was lower in this study than among some previous studies: 3.5/1 000 [Fayette County, Kentucky, for 1985-1989], or 2.5/1 000 [New foundland, Canada, 1990-1995], but higher than the incidence estimated from Rochester, Minnesota, for 1935-1984 [1/1 000 live births]. In a prospective 5-year study by Ronen *et al.* [1999], the incidence was estimated as 2.6/1 000 live births. Again in this population the birthweight was an important factor, the incidence being 13.5/1 000 in infants with a birthweight < 2500 g. The incidence was higher in preterm compared with full-term neonates (11.1/1 000 versus 2/1 000).

Mortality

Many authors have reported the rate of mortality and morbidity, between 1954 and 1997 and, although the quality of care has tremendously changed, this rate has not changed substantially *(table I)*. The more recent publications still show a high percentage of death, between 25% and 50% in the 1990s.

Prognosis

Are seizures per se responsible for long-term neurological and cognitive sequelae as well as for subsequent epilepsy in neonates? Numerous clinical and animal based studies of the effect of seizures on the developing brain have tried to answer this important question, but there is still no consensus. On the other hand, there is a general agreement that etiology and resulting brain dysfunction are the over-riding factors in determining prognosis.

Table I. Outcome of NNS reported by various investigators [Mizrahi and Kellaway, 1998]

Investigators	Year	Patient number	Mortality %	Morbidity %	Normal %
Burke	1954	46	38	17	
Cadilhac *et al.*	1959	90	20	20	
Craig	1960	374	42	3	35
Harris and Tizard	1960	41	20	27	44
Prichard	1964	278	23	27	50
Keith	1964	56	32	36	33
Schulte	1966	57	26	45	29
Massa and Niedermeyer	1968	82	10	28	59
McInerny and Schubert	1969	95	19	25	30
Rose and Lombroso	1970	137	20	29	52
Kuromori *et al.*	1976	130	33	24	43
Dennis	1978	50	22	36	44
Holden *et al.*	1982	277	35	30	
Lombroso	1983	117	16	35	48
Bergman *et al.*	1983	131		42	39
Mizrahi and Kellaway	1987	82	17	45	38
Andre *et al.*	1988	71	21	21	58
Clancy and Legido	1991	40	33	38	30
Siber *et al.*	1993	92	50	27	23
Ortibus *et al.*	1996	81	29	49	22
Bye *et al.*	1997	32	25	31	38

Animal Investigations

In adult animals, it has been clearly demonstrated that brain damage can be the consequence of seizures through the excessive release of excitatory amino acids [6]. During seizures, a sequence of intracellular biochemical reactions leads to generation of potentially toxic metabolites and cell death due to necrosis and apoptosis [7]. But this type of brain damage is age dependent and the immature brain seems to have a significantly decreased vulnerability to such injury.

More recent data suggest that the neonatal brain may be more susceptible to develop seizures, but that the immature brain may also be more resistant to develop subsequent seizures after an initial seizure [8].

In terms of the possible consequence of NNS on brain growth and development, it has been shown that prolonged seizures result in an increase in energy utilization leading to a profound inhibition of DNA synthesis. But these findings are transient and are followed by a period of "catch-up" brain growth [8]. Recent findings indicate that seizures in the immature brain do not result in significant alterations of learning, memory, or activity levels [9].

Clinical outcome measures

Neurological outcome has been evaluated in different ways. Some studies have included only the neurological examination at the time of hospital discharge. For those studies that have considered various neurological abnormalities, many issues remain ill-defined. It may be that the timing of the neurological evaluation is most critical. Specifically, the older the children at the time of evaluation, the more reliable are the data.

Developmental assessment scales have also been used in this clinical population. Again, the more reliable data are obtained from older children.

The Relationship between NNS and subsequent epilepsy has rarely been studied [10, 11]. Numerous factors may affect this association. These include the underlying pathology, the degree of brain damage, the specific antiepileptic drugs that are used, and the extent to which neurodevelopmental processes have been interrupted. Consequently, it may be difficult to predict precisely which child will develop subsequent epilepsy after having had NNS.

Factors predicting the outcome

Etiology is the most important determinant of outcome *(table II)*; however, gestational age, age at onset of seizures, seizure type and duration, neurological status, and ictal and interictal EEG patterns also have to be taken into account.

Prognosis is slightly worse in premature infants. In those who have NNS, mortality is as high as 50% compared with 40% in full-term infants [12]. In survivors, neurological sequelae are present in 65% of infants.

In cases associated with anoxic-ischemic encephalopathy, it seems that the earlier the seizures start, the better is the prognosis. The relation between prognosis and the type of seizures is not clear, although subtle seizures are more severe. Persistence of seizures over a period of three or more days as well as status epilepticus are associated with poorer outcomes.

Since the 1970s, the prognostic value of the interictal EEG has been clearly demonstrated. Findings presaging a poor outcome include low voltage plus theta, paroxysmal and suppression-burst patterns. On the other hand, if there is a clear correlation between electrographic evidence of seizures and the clinical events and the interictal tracing is normal or only moderately abnormal, then the prognosis is favorable [13].

Epilepsy syndromes in neonates

Benign Familial Neonatal Seizures [BFNS]

By definition an idiopathic syndrome does not have any identifiable etiology. This is the case for BFNS. Nevertheless when seizures occur in neonates it seems necessary to exclude any other etiology, particularly anoxic-ischemic, metabolic or infectious. For this reason, a full work-up including a lumbar puncture should be done in any neonate presenting with seizures. One can consider the diagnosis of BFNS as a diagnosis by exclusion reinforced by the familial history of neonatal seizures. In 80% of cases, seizures start on the second or third day of life, although occasionally, infants start having seizures later, during the first month of life and even up to three months. Ronen *et al.* [1993], in their extensive family, report that two of the individuals in whom seizures started at one month of age,

Table II. Morbidity and mortality by various investigators according to etiology [Mizrahi and Kellaway, 1998]

	Year	Patients	Dead		Neurological deficit		Normal	
			%	n	%	n	%	n
Asphyxia								
Harris and Tizard	1960	17	12	2	29	5	59	10
Schulte	1966	57	9	2	41	9	36	8
McInerny and Schubert	1969	31	19	6	42	13	19	6
Rose and Lombroso	1970	10	20	2	70	7	10	1
Bergman et al.	1983	28			57	16	39	11
Lombroso	1983	51	22	11	57	29	22	11
Mizrahi and Kellaway	1986	16	25	4	44	7	31	5
Andre et al.	1988	34	12	4	26	9	62	21
Ortibus et al.	1996	30	33	10	60	18	7	2
Infection								
Schulte	1966	4	75	3	25	1	0	0
McInerny and Schubert	1969	9	56	5	33	3	11	1
Rose and Lombroso	1970	15	40	6	33	5	27	4
Bergman et al.	1983	16	–	–	44	7	56	9
Lombroso	1983	20	25	5	40	8	35	7
Mizrahi and Kellaway	1986	5	0	0	60	3	40	2
Andre et al.	1988	6	50	3	33	2	17	1
Ortibus et al.	1996	20	15	3	40	1	45	9
Hemorrhage								
Harris and Tizard	1960	3	33	1	33	1	33	1
Rose and Lombroso	1970	14	21	3	21	3	57	8
Lombroso	1983	30	20	6	50	15	30	9
Mizrahi and Kellaway	1986	6	0	0	17	1	83	5
Andre et al.	1988	6	50	3	33	2	17	1
Ortibus et al.	1996	20	15	3	40	1	45	9
Congenital abnormalities								
Harris and Tizard	1960	4	75	3	25	1	0	0
McInerny and Schubert	1969	4	100	4	0	0	0	0
Rose and Lombroso	1970	11	64	7	36	4	0	0
Bergman et al.	1983	5	0	0	100	5	0	0
Lombroso	1983	19	32	6	63	12	5	1
Mizrahi and Kellaway	1986	1	0	0	100	1	0	0
Ortibus et al.	1996	5	60	3	40	2	0	0
Hypoglycemia								
Harris and Tizard	1960	1	0	0	0	0	100	1
McInerny and Schubert	1969	6	17	1	33	2	50	3
Rose and Lombroso	1970	7	0	0	43	3	57	4
Bergman et al.	1983	7	–	–	29	2	71	5
Lombroso	1983	19	5	1	21	4	74	14
Mizrahi and Kellaway	1986	1	0	0	0	0	100	1
Ortibus et al.	1996	4	0	0	50	2	50	2
Unknown								
Harris and Tizard	1960	5	0	0	0	0	100	5
Schulte	1966	6	9	1	18	2	36	4
McInerny and Schubert	1969	12	8	1	33	4	33	4
Rose and Lombroso	1970	38	11	4	29	11	61	23
Bergman et al.	1983	16	–	–	25	4	75	12
Lombroso	1983	54	6	3	26	14	69	37
Infarction								
Mannino and Trauner	1983	4	0	0	50	2	50	2
Clancy et al.	1985	7	0	0	27	2	73	5
Levy et al.	1985	7	0	0	86	6	14	1
Mizrahi and Kellaway	1986	3	0	0	33	1	66	2
Ortibus et al.	1996	20	15	3	40	8	45	9

were premature. Premature infants could not be able to have seizures before having reached full-term neurological state. Thus gestational age must be taken into account when considering the strict age-dependence of this syndrome.

No longitudinal study has been published about BFNS. When reviewing the literature [14] we found that infants with BFNS have a 5% risk of febrile seizures which is not very different from the risk in the general population. The risk of subsequent epilepsy, on the other hand, is about 11%, many times higher than what is seen in the general population. It should be noted, however, that no case of severe epilepsy was reported in this group. In a family with 9 cases of BFNS, Takebe *et al.* reported one case of benign epilepsy with centro-temporal spikes (BECTS) associated with a moderate psychomotor delay [15]. Mami *et al.* in 1999 reported a family with 4 cases of BFNS, one of them with BECTS at age 10 years [16]. In 1999, Maihara *et al.* reported two siblings with BFNS who later developed BECTS. Both stopped having seizures with carbamazepine, and had a normal developmental course [17]. No case of psycho-motor retardation or mental impairment has been reported among published cases of BFNS.

More recently Beaussart [personal communication] retrospectively found 12 cases of BFNS among a series of children presenting with BECTS.

Benign Idiopathic Neonatal Seizures (BINS)

BINS were first reported in 1977 and recognized as an epilepsy syndrome in 1989 [18]. BINS may represent anywhere from four to 38% of all NNS. This large range in estimates probably reflects differences in patient referral and recruitment patterns from NICUs, maternity clinics, neonatology, and pediatric neurology. A rate of 38% probably overestimates the true prevalence of BINS, whereas the 4% figure is in good agreement with the 2 to 7% range [14].

There tends to be a preponderance of boy [62%]. North *et al.* [1989] report 20% excess of boys among their 94 cases [19].

In all cases the convulsions occurred between the first and seventh days of life including 90% between D4 and D7 and 97% between D3 and D7. This syndrome must be isolated with regard to all clinical and paraclinical elements which compose it including the EEG interictal pattern. However the "théta pointu alternant" EEG pattern is present in only 60% of cases and is not specific. Accurate diagnosis of BINS allows one to predict a favorable neurological outcome.

Finally, the long-term favorable outcome must be confirmed by more extensive studies of larger numbers of patients. The 90 cases reported by Pryor *et al.* [1981] [20] have not been followed beyond the neonatal period. The 92 cases reported by the French authors were followed from 6 months to 6 years: in five cases a transitory psychomotor retardation was noted which resolved by the end of the first year. One child had a simple febrile convulsion, and another had an afebrile convulsion at the age of three. In six other children spike foci were present on the EEG between the ages of two and a half and six years, but none had any evidence of clinical seizures [21].

Among the 94 cases reported by North *et al.* [1989], 33 [38%] have been followed to between six months and two years of age. In half of these 33 infants, the authors found abnormalities: febrile convulsions [2 cases], convulsions without fever [2 cases], developmental delay [6 cases], microcephaly [2 cases], and minor neurological impairment [3 cases]. One infant had hypothyroidism, and another had a ventricular septal defect. In 1996, 23 cases were reported including 10 cases of BINS and 13 cases of BFNS [22]. Clinical outcome was normal in 22 of them. EEG showed centro-temporal spikes in two cases without any clinical seizure.

BECTS and Benign Neonatal Seizures (BNS)

Among a large population of children referred for [BECTS], Beaussart [personal communication] has pointed out the frequency of history of BNS. Among 3438 patients with epilepsy, 324 presented with BECTS. Seventeen of these 324 patients [5.25%], had a history of BINS [12 cases] or BFNS [5 cases in 2 families]. The clinical presentation of these cases was entirely typical for both BNS and BECTS. It could be of great interest to look back into populations of benign epilepsies [generalized or focal] for BNS preceeding these syndromes *(table III)*.

Table III. Patients with BECTS and BNS [familial or not]

	Age	NNS [days]	FS	BECTS 1st Seizure [years]	BECTS Last seizure	EEG	Clinical Outcome
1°	42	5		6	14	CTS	Normal
2°	47	5		11	11		Normal
3	39	9		7	7	CTS	Normal
4	33	1		6	7	CTS	Mild Retardation
5	36	1		10	10	CTS	?
6	42	7		3	13	CTS	Mild Retardation
7*	38	3	+	6	6	CTS + SW ILS	Normal
8*	36	3	+	5	9	CTS + SW ILS	Normal
9*	31	3					DC 5 days
10	40	1		8	12	CTS	Normal
11	36	45		7	7	CTS	Mild Retardation
12	39	1		12	12	CTS	Normal
13	36	1		3	6	CTS	Normal
14	41	1		3	5	CTS + OSW	Mild Retardation
15	32	20		2	4	CTS + OSW	Normal
16	54	11		8	10	CTS	?
17	30	1		2	?	CTS	Psychosis
18	40	22		7	11	CTS	Normal

°, *: same families.
NNS – neonatal seizures.
FS – febrile seizures.
BECTS – benign epilepsy with centro-temporal spikes.
CTS: Centro Temporal Spikes.
OSW: Occipital Spikes and Waves.

Ohtahara Syndrome

More than 100 cases of Ohtahara syndrome have been reported. The clinical outcome was first reported to be extremely severe by Ohtahara in 1982. Subsequent reports have not been able to provide a more optimistic outlook. Among 61 cases published in 7 series, the authors report 23 deaths before the age of one year [38%] [23-29]. The majority of surviving children have severe epilepsy, epileptic spasms being the most frequent type of seizure. The hypsarrhythmic pattern immediately follows the initial suppression-burst pattern. Four children have had surgery, two for focal cortical dysplasia and two for hemimegalencephaly. In all cases there was a dramatic clinical improvement with all four becoming seizure-free [24, 28, 30-32]. In two of our own cases a transitory clinical improvement was obtained with new AEDs. ACTH and ketogenic diet may be a useful form of treatment for children with this condition.

Early Myoclonic Encephalopathy

This syndrome is defined by the occurrence during the first month of life, of myoclonic seizures, erratic myoclonia, and focal seizures. The neurological state is always abnormal. No etiology has been found, except for glycine encephalopathy. From the first publication [33], the prognosis has been reported as very severe, with mortality reaching 50% before the age of two years. In the surviving 50% of cases, none is neurologically normal. Epilepsy in these children is also very severe. Since 1990, 20 cases have been reported, half of whom died before one year of age [34-46].

Neonatal seizures in a department of pediatric neurology

In a retrospective study we reviewed 45 children with an onset of seizures in the first month of life and recorded their seizures with EEG. An etiology could be found in 44.5%. The remaining 55.5% of cases were cryptogenic *(table IV)*. No difference was found between the two groups with respect to the clinical outcomes except that, the cryptogenic cases were twice as likely to have severe epilepsy In 82% of cases, seizures started during the first week of life. The interictal EEG was also correlated with the clinical outcome and subsequent epilepsy *(table V)*.

Table IV. Etiology in the group of patients of a neuropediatric department (n = 45)

	N	%
Cryptogenic	25	55.5
Symptomatic	20	44.5
Hemimegalencephaly	6	13.3
FCD	6	13.3
Acute foetal desease	2	6.6
Miscellaneous	5	11.3

FCD – focal cortical dysplasia.

Table V. Interictal EEG, clinical outcome and secondary epilepsy

Neonatal EEG	Clinical outcome					Epilepsy			
	n	nl	mild	moderate	severe	death	absent	controlled	severe
Normal	1	1	–	–	–	–	1	–	–
Subnormal	9	3	5	–	–	1	1	6	2
Abnormal patterns	8		1	–	2	2	–	2	6
S-B	9	1		3	4	2	–	2	4
Discontinuous	18	2	1	2	11	4	2	7	12

S-B: Suppression Burst.

This series of NNS referred to a department of pediatric neurology specializing in infantile epilepsy, is mostly composed of cryptogenic cases and cases with brain malformations. The outcome is severe in 69% of cases [including deaths]. In 60% of cases, severe epilepsy persists. Moreover, 80% of children with subsequent epilepsy have severe mental retardation *(table VI)*. Interictal EEG was found to be a good predicitive tool. A suppression-burst pattern and a discontinuous tracing after the first week were associated with a poor outcome *(table V)*. Epileptiform activity on the EEG was associated with an increased risk of severe epilepsy. When clinical seizures were recorded without an electrographic correlate, 100% of cases had a poor outcome.

Table VI. Secondary epilepsy and clinical outcome

Epilepsy	Clinical outcome					
	n	nl	mild	moderate	severe	death
Absent	4	4	–	–	–	–
Controlled	14	3	6	4	1	–
Severe	27	–	1	1	16	9

In summary, in symptomatic NNS prognosis is largely determined by etiology *(table II)*. Anoxic-ischemic encephalopathy remains the most frequent cause and is associated with a high mortality and frequent neurological sequelae, including epilepsy, among survivors. NNS secondary to intracranial infections share the same gloomy prognosis. On the other hand, NNS do not seem to worsen the favorable prognosis in stroke. Long-term studies are missing for benign as well as for severe neonatal epilepsy syndromes. The prognosis of NNS referred to pediatric neurologists has a very severe prognosis with respect to both neurological outcomes and epilepsy.

Thanks to Dr Marc Beaussart, for his data about BNS followed by BECTS.

References

1. Commission on classification and terminology of the international league against epilepsy: proposal for revised classification of epilepsies and epileptic syndroms. *Epilepsia* 1989; 30: 389-99.
2. Plouin P. Benign neonatal convulsions. In: Wasterlain CG, Vert P, ed. *Neonatal Seizures* New York: Raven Press, 1990: 51-9.

3. Mizrahi EM, Kellaway P. *Diagnosis and management of neonatal seizures.* Philadelphia: Lippincott-Raven, 1998: 181.
4. Saliba RM, *et al.* Incidence of neonatal seizures in Harris County, Texas, 1992-1994. *Am J Epidemiol* 1999; 150: 763-9.
5. Ronen GM, Penney S, Andrews W. The epidemiology of clinical neonatal seizures in Newfoundland: a population-based study. *J Pediatr* 1999; 134: 71-5.
6. Choi DW. Glutamat toxicity and diseases of the nervous system. *Neuron* 1988; 1: 623-4.
7. Sloviter RS, *et al.* Apoptosis and necrosis induced in different hippocampal neuron populations by repetitive perforant path stimulation in the rat. *J Comp Neurol* 1996; 366: 516-33.
8. Wasterlain CG. Neonatal seizures and brain growth. *Neuropädiatrie* 1978; 9: 213-28.
9. Holmes GL, *et al.* Consequences of neonatal seizures in the rat: morphological and behavioral effects. *Ann Neurol* 1998; 44: 845-57.
10. Ellenberg JH, Hirtz DG, Nelson KB. Age at onset of seizures in young children. *Ann Neurol* 1984; 15: 127-34.
11. Watanabe K, *et al.* Neonatal seizures and subsequent epilepsy. *Brain Dev* 1982; 4: 341-6.
12. Scher MS, *et al.* Ictal and interictal electrographic seizure durations in preterm and term neonates. *Epilepsia* 1993; 34: 284-8.
13. Monod N, Pajot N, Guidasci S. The neonatal EEG: statistical studies and prognostic value in full-term and pre-term babies. *Electroencephalogr Clin Neurophysiol* 1972; 32: 529-44.
14. Plouin P. Benign idiopathic neonatal convulsions (familial and non-familial). In: Roger JJ, ed. *Epileptic syndromes in infancy, childhood and adolescence.* London: John Libbey, 1992: 3-11.
15. Takebe Y, Chiba C, Kimura S. Benign familial neonatal convulsions. *Brain Dev* 1983; 5: 319-22.
16. Mami C, *et al.* Neonatal familial benign convulsions. *Arch Fr Pediatr* 1993; 50: 31-3.
17. Maihara T, *et al.* Benign familial neonatal convulsions followed by benign epilepsy with centrotemporal spikes in two siblings. *Epilepsia* 1999; 40: 110-3.
18. Dehan M, *et al.* Convulsions in the fifth day of life: a new syndrome? *Arch Fr Pediatr* 1977; 34: 730-42.
19. North KN, Storey GNB, Handerso-Smart DJ. Fifth day fits in the newborn. *Austr Paediatr J* 1989; 25: 284-7.
20. Pryor DS, Don N, Macourt DC. Fifth day fits: a syndrome of neonatal convulsions. *Arch Dis Child* 1981; 56: 753-8.
21. Dehan M, *et al.* Quelques précisions sur le syndrome des convulsions du cinquième jour de vie. *Arch Fr Pediatr* 1982; 39: 405-7.
22. Gonzalez Ipina M, *et al.* Benign neonatal convulsions. Review of 23 cases. *Neurologia* 1996; 11: 51-5.
23. Clarke M, *et al.* Early infantile epileptic encephalopathy with suppression burst: Ohtahara syndrome. *Dev Med Child Neurol* 1987; 29: 520-8.
24. Martinez Bermejo A, *et al.* Early infantile epileptic encephalopathy. *Rev Neurol* 1995; 23: 297-300.
25. Chakova L. On a rare form of epilepsy in infants-Ohtahara syndrome. *Folia Med* 1996; 38: 69-73.
26. Verrotti A, *et al.* Early infantile epileptic encephalopathy: a long-term follow-up study. *Childs Nerv Syst* 1996; 12: 530-3.
27. Campistol J, *et al.* The Ohtahara's syndrome: a special form of age-dependent epilepsy. *Rev Neurol* 1997; 25: 212-4.
28. Fusco L, *et al.* Video/EEG aspects of early-infantile epileptic encephalopathy with suppression-bursts (Ohtahara syndrome). *Brain Dev* 2001; 23: 708-14.
29. Yamatogi Y, Ohtahara S. Early-infantile epileptic encephalopathy with suppression-bursts, Ohtahara syndrome; its overview referring to our 16 cases. *Brain Dev* 2002; 24: 13-23.
30. Pedespan JM, *et al.* Surgical treatment of an early epileptic encephalopathy with suppression-bursts and focal cortical dysplasia. *Epilepsia* 1995; 36: 37-40.
31. Komaki H, *et al.* Surgical treatment of a case of early infantile epileptic encephalopathy with suppression-bursts associated with focal cortical dysplasia. *Epilepsia* 1999; 40: 365-9.
32. Komaki H, *et al.* Surgical treatment of early-infantile epileptic encephalopathy with suppression-bursts associated with focal cortical dysplasia. *Brain Dev* 2001; 23: 727-31.
33. Aicardi J, Goutieres F. Neonatal myoclonic encephalopathy (author's transl). *Rev Electroencephalogr Neurophysiol Clin* 1978; 8: 99-101.

34. Ando M, *et al.* A longitudinal study of clinical and electroencephalographic findings in a female infant with early myoclonic encephalopathy. *No To Hattatsu* 1991; 23: 389-94.
35. Du Plessis AJ, Kaufmann WE, Kupsky WJ. Intrauterine-onset myoclonic encephalopathy associated with cerebral cortical dysgenesis. *J Child Neurol* 1993; 8: 164-70.
36. Spreafico R, *et al.* Burst suppression and impairment of neocortical ontogenesis: electroclinical and neuropathologic findings in two infants with early myoclonic encephalopathy. *Epilepsia* 1993; 34: 800-8.
37. Muranaka H, Takebe Y. A case of early myoclonic encephalopathy accompanied with central respiratory dysfunction. *No To Hattatsu* 1994; 26: 428-33.
38. Bado M, *et al.* Early myoclonic encephalopathy and spinal muscular atrophy type I. *Minerva Pediatr* 1995; 47: 233-8.
39. Nishikawa M, *et al.* A case of early myoclonic encephalopathy with the congenital nephrotic syndrome. *Brain Dev* 1997; 19: 144-7.
40. Bruel H, *et al.* Early myoclonic epileptic encephalopathy and non-ketotic hyperglycemia in the same family. *Arch Pediatr* 1998; 5: 397-9.
41. Wang PJ, *et al.* The controversy regarding diagnostic criteria for early myoclonic encephalopathy. *Brain Dev* 1998; 20: 530-5.
42. Hirabayashi S, *et al.* A neurodegenerative disorder with early myoclonic encephalopathy, retinal pigmentary degeneration and nephronophthisis. *Brain Dev* 2000; 22: 24-30.
43. Chen PT, *et al.* Early epileptic encephalopathy with suppression burst electroencephalographic pattern – an analysis of eight Taiwanese patients. *Brain Dev* 2001; 23: 715-20.
44. Kalra V, *et al.* West syndrome and other infantile epileptic encephalopathies – Indian hospital experience. *Brain Dev* 2001; 23: 593-602.
45. Tendero Gormaz A, *et al.* Neonatal EEG trace of burst suppression. Etiological and evolutionary factors. *Rev Neurol* 2001; 33: 514-8.
46. Castro-Gago M, *et al.* Early mitochondrial encephalomyopathy due to complex IV deficiency consistent with Alpers-Huttenlocher syndrome: report of two cases. *Rev Neurol* 1999; 29: 912-7.

Prognosis of infantile spasms

Marja-Liisa Granström

Infantile spasms (IS) is an age-dependent epileptic syndrome with multiple etiology characterized by epileptic spasms and interictal epileptiform activity that may be focal or diffuse [1]. Epileptic spasms start during the first year of life, usually between 4 and 7 months. Interictally most infants show hypsarrhythmia or multiple independent spikes on EEG [2].

The commission on Pediatric Epilepsy of ILAE held a special workshop on infantile spasms in 1991. The definitions agreed upon in the workshop have been published in Epilepsia 1992 [3]. It was important to distinguish the seizure type (spasms or epileptic spasms) and the epilepsy syndrome of infantile spasms. The term West syndrome was suggested for those patients with documented hypsarrhythmia in combination with epileptic spasms, whereas infantile spasms could be used for all infants with epileptic spasms and interictal epileptiform activity. The workshop also suggested that atypical features of interictal epileptiform activity should be described instead of using the term of modified hypsarrhytmia.

Epileptic spasm are brief axial muscular contractions and occur most often in clusters [3, 4]. They start more slowly and last longer (usually 1-2 s) than myoclonic jerks but are more rapid and shorter than tonic seizures [5]. Asymmetric and subtle variants have been described [5-8]. Dulac and coworkers [9] and Fusco and Vigevano [10] separated "independent spasms" where hypsarrhytmia reappears between spasms and "clustering spasms" where no hypsarrhythmia is seen between spasms. Fusco and Vigevano found that independent spasms may predict a better outcome than spasm clusters. This was not, however, observed in other studies [2, 11]. The motor pattern of spasms do not have any prognostic significance but partial seizures and asymmetrical spasms are strongly associated with symptomatic etiology [10, 11]. The ictal EEG phenomena associated with infantile spasms include fast "spindle-like" or paroxysmal fast activity (PFA), high voltage spikes, spike-waves, slow waves, and attenuation [5]. PFA seems to be the most consistent ictal EEG signature of spasms. In the study of Gaily *et al.* [2] PFA without a slow wave was typical of subtle spasm variants, whereas motor spasms were usually associated with slow wave, with or without PFA.

4-hour video-EEG recordings containing wake, sleep, and awakening are usually sufficient to detect spasms [2]. Video-EEG recordings are necessary to diagnose or exclude spasms before treatment in infants with multifocal spikes on interictal EEG and developmental delay or cerebral palsy, even if no spasms are clinically observed or reported by care-takers.

Treatment may modify ictal behavior from motor spasms to subtle variants, which are difficult to recognize without video-EEG recordings [2]. Eradication of spasms often precedes the disappearance of hypsarrhythmia and multifocal spikes on EEG. Persisting multifocal spikes are, however, usually associated with continuing spasms which may be subtle. Although most newly diagnosed infants have hypsarrhythmia at least in sleep on their first EEG recordings, more than one third show only multifocal independent spikes with normal or nearly normal background [2, 12]. Asymmetrical interictal EEG is significantly associated with symptomatic etiology [2, 5, 11].

Etiology

The etiology of infantile spasms has been divided into symptomatic, cryptogenic, and idiopathic. In most earlier studies, the symptomatic group included infants with known etiologies and infants with developmental delay or with other signs of brain damage at onset of spasms [13]. Within the symptomatic group, the etiologies for infantile spasms have traditionally been divided into prenatal, perinatal, and postnatal causes. Most studies identify prenatal etiologies as the most common, accounting for almost 50% of symptomatic cases [14] although perinatal causes have been reported to be on the rise [15, 16]. Prenatal causes include intrauterine insults and infections, malformations of cortical development, neurocutaneous syndromes, metabolic disorders, and other genetic or chromosomal defects. The list of specific genetic causes connected to infantile spasms in addition to the most common Down syndrome and tuberous sclerosis has increased remarkably [17, 18]. The perinatal group consists primarily of hypoxic-ischemic encephalopathy, obstetric trauma, and other labor complications. Postnatal etiologies include infection, trauma, hypoxic-ischemic insults, and tumors [13, 16]. The cryptogenic group includes infants with normal development and without any signs of brain damage before onset of spasms and without any known etiology. An idiopathic category previously was either not recognized or was synonymous with the cryptogenic group.

The ILAE revised classification of epilepsies [4] included infantile spasm syndromes in the symptomatic and cryptogenic group. It defines cryptogenic etiology as probably symptomatic but with unknown cause, whereas idiopathic epilepsies typically are attributed to a known or presumed genetic predisposition with generally favorable prognoses. The ILAE workshop on infantile spasms (1991), however, introduced an idiopathic group consisting of infants with normal development at onset, normal examination and neuroimaging, positive family history for epilepsy and recurrence of hypsarrhythmia between consecutive spasms of a cluster and without focal EEG epileptiform abnormalities [3, 9, 10].

Although the list of specific diseases potentially causing infantile spasms is enormous, history and physical examination alone may identify the majority of symptomatic etiologies [19]. MRI allows more specific classification into various etiology groups. It is especially helpful in differentiating between prenatal and perinatal etiologies. FDG-PET shows global and focal cortical hypometabolism in children with infantile spasms [20, 21]. Findings by neuroimaging during the first year of life may, however, change in later follow-up studies. Delayed myelination may be visible only at a certain age and focal hypometabolism on PET may be transient [20, 21].

Epidemiology

Incidence rates of infantile spasms have usually varied between 2,5 and 4,5 per 10 000 live births among different studies [22-27]. The lifetime prevalence of infantile spasms at age 10 years has been estimated to be 1.5 to 2 per 10 000 children in two American studies [23, 26]. IS is an uncommon epilepsy syndrome; the mean annual incidence was 2,86 in 100 000 children younger than 15 years in a Finnish study [27]. Lower prevalence than incidence rates of IS are mainly explained by the relatively high mortality associated with infantile spasms, the evolution of spasms into other seizure types, and incomplete ascertainment of older children in population-based studies [13].

The percentage of IS cases classified as symptomatic has risen during the last decades. In the early 1980s, most studies identified symptomatic etiologies in approximately 45-60% of patients [28, 29]. Improved sensitivity of diagnostic testing, especially of neuroimaging studies has increased the percentage of IS infants with symptomatic etiology up to 70-80% in later studies [25, 27, 30].

The incidence of IS and the proportion of different etiologies has been studied since 1960 in the Uusimaa county with a population of 1,36 million in southern Finland *(table I)*. Raili Riikonen [22, 31] published the incidence rates between 1960 and 1990. The latest incidence rates have been calculated from the patients treated at the Epilepsy Unit of the Department of Neuropediatrics at Helsinki University Central Hospital between 1994 and 1999. The incidence varied between 0.41 and 0,50 per 10 000 live births. In contrast to other studies, the percentage of infants with cryptogenic etiology has not changed during these four decades.

Table I. Incidence rate and etiology of IS in the county of Uusimaa between 1960 and 1999

Year of diagnosis	1960-76*	1977-90*	1994-99
Total number of infants with IS – with cryptogenic etiology (%) – with symptomatic etiology (%)	107 19 (17,7%) 88 (82,3%)	102 19 (18,6%) 83 (81,4%)	55 11 (20%) 44 (80%)
Incidence of IS	0,41/1 000	0,43/1 000	0,51/1 000**

* Riikonen R [31].
** Infantile spasms diagnosed in 56 infants born during 1994-1999 in the Uusimaa County (with a population of 1,36 milj 31.12.1998).

Treatment response

Definitions and documentation of the treatment response

The immediate goal of treatment of IS is complete suppression of spasms. The other goals are lasting seizure control and improved intellectual outcome. Cessation of spasms observed by parents or hospital personnel has commonly used as treatment response in several studies [28, 32, 33]. This may sometimes be misleading as subtle spasms and even motor spasms of multihandicapped children are often very difficult to recognize [34]. Interictal EEG changes other than complete normalization during treatment may also be difficult to interpret.

Treatment responses in different studies are difficult to compare without video-EEG confirmation, which is superior to all observation methods [6, 34-36]. Many studies also report relapses after treatment, which means that spasms are again recognized after a short period of weeks or a couple of months [28, 30, 32]. During partial response, infants may experience days without spasms. Therefore very short periods could not be accepted as a treatment response. In our own study, only total disappearance of spasms for at least one month was accepted as response [34], and no spasm relapses were observed.

For almost 50 years, results achieved by ACTH have offered a golden standard for treatment results in IS. Initial response rates to steroids or ACTH have varied between 50% and 90% in different studies [28, 30, 32, 37-39]. The response rates of IS infants with cryptogenic etiology have been higher than of those with symptomatic etiology [32, 33, 37, 40]. ACTH has been considered either as equally effective as oral steroids [41] or as more effective [39, 40]. Although the highest response rates have been observed in the studies using high dose ACTH treatment [38-40] no difference in response rates was observed in a prospective study of Hrachovy *et al.* between a high (150 IU/m2/day) and a low (20-30 IU/day) dose of ACTH [42]. Side effects are common during ACTH treatment and they may be serious especially at high doses [33, 42-44].

Chiron *et al.* [45] were the first authors to observe that vigabatrin (VGB) was effective against intractable IS. During the last 10 years, VGB has also been used in treatment of newly diagnosed IS, with response rates between 23 and 68% [46-50]. In a placebo-controlled, double-blind study, 43% of infants treated with VGB (50-150 mg/kg) were spasm free after five days compared to 15% of those treated with placebo [51]. In the European Retrospective Survey, 90% of the infants responded within 7 days to a mean dose of 105 mg/kg/day (range, 25-400 mg/kg/day), but a relapse was seen in 21% of responders after a mean period of 4 months, in 77% of them by 3 months [46]. Although the response rate for VGB treatment has been higher for infants with cryptogenic etiology, the best response rate has been observed in IS infants with tuberous sclerosis [52]. In a prospective study, where VGB and ACTH were compared, more infants responded to ACTH (74%) than to VGB (48%), but more relapses and difficult side-effects were seen after ACTH treatment [47].

In contrast to ACTH, VGB does not have any life threatening side effects. However, visual field defects (VFDs) have been found up to 40% of the adults after VGB treatment [53, 54]. Although the risk of VFDs seems to be lower in children and adolescents, VGB treatment in children should always be accompanied with regular VF assessments if possible [55]. Because children with IS are unable to co-operate in quantitative perimetry, a regular clinical age appropriate assessment of visual function and visual fields should be included in follow-up.

Since 1994, all newly diagnosed IS infants in our hospital have first received VGB treatment (50-150 mg/kg). If spasms continued more than 2 weeks, add-on ACTH treatment (3-12 U/kg) was offered [34]. Some multihandicapped infants were not treated by ACTH because of the risk of side-effects. In 1994-1999 21 (38%) of the infants responded to VGB within two weeks. Responses were more common among infants with cryptogenic etiology (64%) than among those with symptomatic etiology (31%). All infants with cryptogenic etiology responded to our treatment protocol, but 36% of the infants with symptomatic etiology still continued to have spasms after it *(table II)*.

Of older antiepileptic drugs, only valproate (VPA) and benzodiazepines have been effective in reducing of spasms, but total cessation has occurred later and less commonly than with steroid treatment [56, 57]. High dose of pyridoxine (100 to 300 mg/kg/day) has also been effective in some children [58] and pyridoxin has been the most common first drug in Japan [59]). Only small number of treatment trials have been conducted by new drugs [60, 61].

Hrachovy *et al.* [36] studied patients, who were treated before steroid or ACTH treatment was available. Spontaneous remission of spasms was observed within three months in 5%

Table II. Treatment response of infants with newly diagnosed IS in Uusimaa county 1994-1999

Etiology	No of infants treated by VGB	Response to VGB	No of infants treated by ACTH	Response to ACTH	Response to other AEDs	Infants without response to IS treatment protocol
All	55	21 (3 late)	22	13 responded	1 responded to VPA	16 (29%)
		4 no response		9 no response	4 responded (3 VPA, 1 LGT)	
				12 not treated		
Cryptogenetic	11	7 responded	4	4 responded		0
		4 no response				
Symptomatic	44	14 responded (3 late)	18	9 responded	1 responded to VPA	16 (36%)
		30 no response		9 no response	4 responded (3 VPA, 1 LGT)	
				12 not treated		
Unknown	11	4 responded (2 late)	5	2 responded	1 responded to VPA	3 (27%)
		7 no response		3 no response		
				2 not treated		
Hypoxic-ischemic injury*	14	3 responded (1 late)	4	4 responded	1 responded to VPA	4 (29%)
		11 no response		7 not treated	3 responded (2 to VPAja 1 to LGT)	
Dysgenetic lesion	9	1 responded	6	1 responded		7 (78%)
		8 no response		5 no response		
				2 not treated		
Tuberous sclerosis	5	4 responded	1	1 no response		1 (20%)
		1 no response				
Down syndrome*	4	2 responded	2	2 responded		0
		2 no response				
Progressive disease	1	1 no response	0			1 (100%)

* One infant with Down syndrome and hypoxic-ischemic injury has been grouped in this group.

and within 12 months in 25% of the patients. For comparison, cessation of spasms has been achieved with VGB and ACTH treatment protocols in 50-80% of the infants with even symptomatic etiology.

Outcome

Mortality

The mortality rate of infants with IS during the first years of life has varied between 4 and 11% [25, 27, 31]. It increased to 19% by the age of 10 years and to 31% by adulthood [62]. However, during the last four decades, the mortality rate of the first three years of life has remained unchanged in the county of Uusimaa *(table III)*.

Table III. The outcome of children with IS from Uusimaa county treated during 1960-76 and 1994-99

Time	1960-1976	1994-1999
Number of infants	214	55
Died before the age of 3 years	22 (11%)	7 (13%)
Normal or nearly normal development	43 (20%) had IQ > 68	10 (18%) had IQ or DQ > 70
Mental retardation	139 (65%) had IQ < 51	36 (65%) had IQ or DQ < 50
Cessation of spasms	At least 29 (14%) continued to have spasms after 3 years of age. In addition the time of cessation of spasms was unknown for 26 patients.	At least 5 (9%) had still spasms at the age of 3 years. In addition 6 might have had some spasms still at the same age
Epilepsy	56 (26%) have been seizure-free > 2 years	13 (24%) without epilepsy or epilepsy treatment at the age of 3 years
Severe epilepsy	?	6 (11%) has refractory epilepsy with frequent seizures and many seizure types ("Lennox-like") at the age of 3 years

Epilepsy

Some infants with symptomatic etiology may show partial seizures already before the onset of spasms. After cessation of spasms, many children continue to have other seizures. The percentage of children with IS evolving to Lennox-Gastaut Syndrome (LGS) have varied between 23 and 50% [26, 28, 32]. Rantala and Putkonen discovered that 27% of infants with IS evolved to LGS. The mean time interval from the beginning of IS to the beginning of LGS was 2,8 years (range 0,4-8.8 years) [27]. Forty percent of LGS-patients in that study had previous IS. In the study conducted in Atlanta, USA, half of IS patients evolved to LGS [26]. In both studies, infants have been followed up to the age of 10 years. Refractory epilepsy was found at the age of three years in six out of 49 living children from the Uusimaa county treated at our Unit during 1994-1999 *(table III)*. The figure is similar to the data of the other Finnish study [27].

Table IV. Outcome of infants in different etiology and treatment response groups at the age of 3 years

Etiology		No of infants and their IS treatment response		Died	With spasms	With epilepsy or AED treatment	Cognitive outcome**
		Responder	11				
Cryptogenetic				7	0	1	10 normal, 1 mild MR
Symptomatic	All		44	7	5 yes, 5?	32 (6 severe epilepsy), ?	8 mild MR, 29 MR
	Responder		28	5	1?	18 (2 severe epilepsy)	7 mild MR, 16 MR
	Non responder		16	2	5 yes, 5?	14 (4 severe epilepsy), ?	1 mild MR, 13 MR, ?
Unknown	All		11	0	1 yes, 1?	7 (2 with severe epilepsy)	3 mild MR, 8 MR
	Responder		8	0	0	4	3 mild MR, 5 MR
	Non responder		3	0	1 yes, 1?	3 (2 with severe epilepsy)	3 MR
Hypoxic-ischemic injury*	All		14	5	1 yes, 1?	8 (2 with severe epilepsy)	1 mild MR, 8 MR
	Responder		10	3	1?	6 (2 with severe epilepsy)	7 MR
	Non responder		4	2	1 yes	3	1 mild MR, 1 MR, 1?
Dysgenetic lesion	All		9	0	2 yes, 2?	9 (1 with severe epilepsy)	1 mild MR, 8 MR
	Responder		2	0	0	2	1 mild MR, 1 MR
	Non responder		7	0	2 yes, 2?	7 (1 with severe epilepsy)	7 MR
Tuberous sclerosis	All		5	0	1 yes	5 (1 with severe epilepsy)	3 mild MR 2 MR
	Responder		4	0	0	4	3 mild MR 1 MR
	Non responder		1	0	1 yes	1 (1 with severe epilepsy)	1 MR
Down syndrome	Responder		4	2	0	2	2 MR
Progressive disease	Non responder		1	0	1?	1?	1 MR

* One infant with Down syndrome and hypoxic-ischemic injury has been grouped in this group.
** Cognitive outcome was normal if IQ values or DQ values have been assessed over 70, mildmentally retarded (MR) if between 50 and 70 and retarded if below 50.

Cognitive outcome

Only 9 to 28% of infants with IS have later shown normal or nearly normal cognitive development [14, 25, 30, 37]. The most important factor in predicting developmental outcome is etiology. Infants with cryptogenic etiology have more often (38 to 79%) normal or nearly normal cognitive development than infants with symptomatic etiology (2 to 18%). Although children with symptomatic infantile spasms generally have a poor prognosis, neurofibromatosis and Down syndrome may be associated with a relatively benign course [18, 63]. Other favourable prognostic signs include normal neurological examination and development at onset, absence of other seizure types at onset, older age of onset, short duration of spasms, and early effective treatment of spasms [13, 31].

In the 1960-76 Uusimaa study [31], 69% of children with cryptogenic etiology (20/29) were normal or nearly normal. Etiology predicted the outcome of children treated in 1994-99 even better: 91% (10/11) children with cryptogenic etiology showed normal or nearly normal development. On the other hand, in the older study still 11% (20/185) infants with symptomatic etiology showed normal or nearly normal development compared to none (0/ 44) children in the recent study *(table IV)*. Infants with symptomatic etiology had poor cognitive outcome especially it they did not respond to our treatment protocol *(table IV)*. The cessation of spasms was also associated with improvement of cognition and behaviour in children with tuberous sclerosis treated by VGB [64].

Infants with cryptogenic etiology in our recent series probably represent patients with the idiopathic form of IS [9, 10]. Their cognitive outcome in general is good, although some of them may later show specific cognitive deficits or mild learning disabilities [64].

Conclusions

Incidence of infantile spasms has not changed during last decades. Outcome in general is poor but highly dependent on etiology. Increased mortality, refractory epilepsy and mental retardation with other handicaps are common among infants with symptomatic etiology. Outcome is clearly predicted by specific etiology and obviously dependent on size and location of brain injury or malformation or on natural course of the disease causing IS. Outcome of children with cryptogenic etiology is good and usually already predictable at the onset of spasms.

All infants with cryptogenic etiology respond to treatment, but one third of infants with symptomatic etiology seem to be refractory. Some of those patients may later present with Lennox-Gastaut syndrome. Surgical treatment helps some children but the proportion of surgical candidates might be low.

Effective treatment of spasms and other epileptic seizures is important because cognitive development continues only after cessation of spasms and frequent seizures. Although the treatment response to ACTH may be better, VGB often is the only option for multihandicapped children because of the high risk of serious or life threatening side effects of ACTH. Long term efficacy of VGB treatment and the risk of visual field defects needs further study.

References

1. Roger J, Dulac O. West syndrome: history and nosology. In: Dulac O, Chugani HT, Dalla Bernardina B, eds. *Infantile spasms and West syndrome*. London: Saunders, 1992: 6-11.

2. Gaily E, Liukkonen E, Paetau R, Rekola M, Granström ML. Infantile spasms: diagnosis and assessment of treatment response by video-EEG. *Dev Med Child Neur* 2001; 43: 658-67.
3. Commission on Pediatric Epilepsy of the International League Against Epilepsy. Workshop on infantile spasms. *Epilepsia* 1992; 33: 195.
4. Commission on Classification and Terminology of the International League Against Epilepsy. Proposal for revised classification of epilepsies and epileptic syndromes. *Epilepsia* 1989; 30: 389-99.
5. Fusco L, Vigevano F. Ictal clinical electroencephalographic findings of spasms in West syndrome. *Epilepsia* 1993; 34: 671-8.
6. Kellaway P, R.A. Hrachovy RA,, J.D. Frost JD, Zion T. Precise characterization and quantification of infantile spasms. *Ann Neurol* 1979; 6: 214-8.
7. Donat JF, Wright FS. Unusual variants of infantile spasms. *J Child Neurol* 1991; 6: 313-8.
8. Gaily EK, Shewmon DA, Chugani HT, Curran JG. Asymmetric and asynchronous infantile spasms. *Epilepsia* 1995; 36; 873-82.
9. Dulac O, Plouin P, Jambaque I. Predicting favourable outcome in idiopathic West syndrome. *Epilepsia* 1993; 34: 747-56.
10. Vigevano F, Fusco L, Cusmai R, Claps D, Ricci S, Milani L. The idiopathic form of West syndrome. *Epilepsia* 1993; 34: 743-6.
11. Haga Y, Watanabe K, Negoro T, Aso K, Kasai K, Ohki T, Natume J. Do ictal, clinical, and electroencephalographic features predict outcome in West syndrome? *Ped Neur* 1995; 13: 226-9.
12. Watanabe K, Negoroso T, Aso K, Matsumoto A. Reappraisal of interictal electroencephalograms in infantile spasms. *Epilepsia* 1993; 34: 679-85.
13. Wong M, Trevathan E. Infantile spasms. *Pediatr Neurol* 2001; 24: 89-98.
14. Ohtahara S, Ohtsuka Y, Yamatogi Y, Oka E, Yoshinaga H, Sato M. Prenatal etiologies of West syndrome. *Epilepsia* 1993; 34: 716-22.
15. Watanabe K. West syndrome: Etiological and prognostic aspects. *Brain Dev* 1998; 20: 1-8.
16. Cusmai R. Ricci S, Pinard JM, Plouin P, Fariello G, Dulac O. West syndrome due perinatal insults. *Epilepsia* 1993; 34: 738-42.
17. Somer M. Diagnostic criteria and genetics of the PEHO syndrome. *J Med Genet* 1993; 30: 932-6.
18. Motte, J Billard C, Fejerman N, Sfaello Z, Arroyo H, Dulac O. Neurofibromatosis type one and West syndrome: a relatively benign association. *Epilepsia* 1993; 34: 723-6.
19. Trasmonte JV, Barron TF. Infantile spasms: A proposal for a staged evaluation. *Pediatr Neurol* 1998; 19: 368-71.
20. Natsume J, Watanabe K, Maeda N, Kasai K, Negoro T, Aso K, Nakasihima S, Masanori T. Cortical hypometabolism and delayed myelination in West syndrome. *Epilepsia* 1996; 37: 1180-84.
21. Metsähonkala L, Gaily E, Rantala H, Salmi E, Valanne L, Äärimaa T, Liukkonen E, Holopainen I, Granström ML, Erkinjuntti M, Grönroos T, Sillanpää M. Focal and global cortical hypometabolism in patients with newly diagnosed infantile spasms. *Neurology* 2002; 58: 1646-51.
22. Riikonen R, Donner M. Incidence and aetiology of infantile spasms from 1960 to 1976: A population study in Finland. *Dev Med Child Neurol* 1979; 21: 333-43.
23. Cowan LD, Bodensteiner JB, Leviton A, Doherty L. Prevalence of the epilepsies in children and adolescents. *Epilepsia* 1989; 30: 94-106.
24. Ludvigsson P, Olafsson E, Siguroardottir S, Hauser WA. Epidemiologic features of infantile spasms in Iceland. *Epilepsia* 1994; 35: 802-5.
25. Sidenvall R, Eeg-Olofsson O. Epidemiology of infantile spasms in Sweden. *Epilepsia* 1995; 36: 572-4.
26. Trevathan E, Murphy CC, Yeargin-Allsopp M. The descriptive epidemiology of infantile spasms among Atlanta children. *Epilepsia* 1999; 40: 748-51.
27. Rantala H, Putkonen T. Occurrence, outcome, and prognostic factors of infantile spasms and Lennox-Gastaut syndrome. *Epilepsia* 1999; 40: 286-9.
28. Lombroso CT. A prospective study of infantile spasms: clinical and therapeutic correlations. *Epilepsia* 1983; 24: 135-58.
29. Matsumoto A, Watanabe K, Negoro T, Sugiura M, Iwase K, Hara K, Miyazaki S. Long-term prognosis after infantile spasms: A statistical study of prognositic factors in 200 cases. *Dev Med Child Neurol* 1981; 23: 51-65.

30. Koo B, Hwang PA, Logan WJ. Infantile spasms: outcome and prognostic factors of cryptogenic and symptomatic groups. *Neurology* 1993; 43: 2322-7.
31. Riikonen R. Decreasing perinatal mortality: unchanged infantile spasm morbidity. *Dev Med Child Neur* 1995; 37: 232-8.
32. Riikonen R. A long-term follow-up study of 214 children with the syndrome of infantile spasms. *Neuropediatrics* 1982; 13: 14-23.
33. Heiskala H, Riikonen R, Santavuori P, et al. West syndrome: individualized ACTH therapy. *Brain Dev* 1996; 18: 456-60.
34. Granstrom ML. Gaily E. Liukkonen E. Treatment of infantile spasms: results of a population-based study with vigabatrin as the first drug for spasms. *Epilepsia* 1999; 40: 950-7.
35. Hrachovy RA, Kellaway P, Zion T. Quantitative analysis and characterization of infantile spasms. *Epilepsia* 1978; 19: 273-82.
36. Hrachovy RA, Glaze DG, Frost JD. A retrospective study of spontaneous remission and long-term outcome in patients with infantile spasms. *Epilepsia* 1991; 32: 212-4.
37. Glaze DG, Hrachovy RA, Forst JD, Kellaway P, Zion TE. Prospective study of outcome of infants with infantile spasms treated during controlled studies of ACTH and prednisone. *J Pediatr* 1988; 112: 389-96.
38. Snead OC, Benton JW, Hosey LC, et al. Treatment of infantile spasms with high dose ACTH: efficacy and plasma levels of ACTH and cortisol. *Neurology* 1989; 39: 1027-30.
39. Baram TZ, Mitchell WG, Tournay A, Snead OC, Hanson RA, Horton EJ. High-dose corticotropin (ACTH) versus prednisone for infantile spasms: a prospective, randomized, blinded study. *Pediatrics* 1996; 97: 375-9.
40. Snead OC, Benton JW, Myers GJ. ACTH and prednisone in childhood seizure disorders. *Neurology* 1983; 33: 966-70.
41. Hrachovy RA, Frost JD, Kellaway PR, Zion TE. Double-blind study of ACTH vs prednisone therapy in infantile spasms. *J Pediatr* 1983; 103: 641-5.
42. Hrachovy RA, Frost I, Glaze DG. High dose, long-duration versus low-dose, short-duration corticotropin therapy for infantile spasms. *J Pediatr* 1994; 124: 803-6.
43. Riikonen R, Donner M. ACTH therapy in infantile spasms: side effects. *Arch Dis Child* 1980; 55: 664-72.
44. Nolte R, Christen HJ, Doerrer J. Preliminary report of a multicenter study on the West syndrome. *Brain Dev* 1988; 10: 236-42.
45. Chiron C, Dulac O, Beamont D, et al. Therapeutic trial of vigabatrin in refractory infantile spasms. *J Child Neurol* 1991; 6 (Suppl 2): 52-9.
46. Aicardi J, Sabril IS Investigator and Peer Review groups, Mumford JP, Dumas C, Wood S. Vigabatrin as initial therapy for infantilespasms: a European retrospective survey. *Epilepsia* 1996; 37: 618-24.
47. Vigevano F, Cilio MR. Vigabatrin versus ACTH as first-line treatment for infantile spasms. *Epilepsia* 1997; 38: 1270-4.
48. Wohlrab G, Boltshauser E, Schmitt B. Vigabatrin as a first-line drug in West syndrome: clinical and electroencephalographic outcome. *Neuropediatrics* 1998; 29: 133-6.
49. Cossette P, J.J. Riviello JJ Carmant L. ACTH versus vigabatrin therapy in infantile spasms: A retrospective study. *Neurology* 1999; 52: 1691-4.
50. Elterman RD, Shields WD, Mansfield KA, Nakagawa J and US Infantile Spasms Vigabatrin Study Group. Randomized trial of vigabatrin in patients with infantile spasms. *Neurology* 2001; 57: 1416-21.
51. Appleton RE, Peters ACB, Mumford JP, Shaw DE. Randomised, placebo-controlled study of vigabatrin as first-line treatment of infantile spasms. *Epilepsia* 1999; 40: 1627-33.
52. Chiron C, Dumas C, Jambaque I, Mumford J, Dulac O. Randomized trial comparing vigabatrin and hydrocortisone in infantile spasmsdue to tuberous sclerosis. *Epilepsy Res* 1997; 26: 389-95.
53. Krauss GL, Johnson MA, Miller NR. Vigabatrin-associated retinal cone system dysfunction: electroretinogram and ophtalmologic findings. *Neurology* 1998; 50: 614-8.
54. Kälviainen R, Nousiainen I, Mäntyjarvi M, Nikoskelainen E, Partanen J, Partanen K, Riekkinen P Sr. Vigabatrin, a gabaergic antiepileptic drug, causes concentric visual field defects. *Neurology* 1999; 53: 922-6.
55. Vanhatalo S, Nousiainen I, Eriksson K, Rantala H, Riikonen R, Vainionpää L, Mustonen K, Äärimaa T, Alen R, Byring R, Aine MR, Hirvasniemi A, Nuutila A, Walden T, Ritanen-Mohammed UM, Karttunen-Lewandowski P, Pohjola LM, Kaksonen S, Pekka J, Granström ML. Visual Field Constriction in 91 Finnish children treated with vigabatrin. *Epilepsia* 2002; 43: 748-56.

56. Siemens H, Spohr HL, Michael T, Nau H. Therapy of infantile spasms with valproate: results of a prospective study. *Epilepsia* 1988; 29: 553-60.
57. Dreifuss F, Farwell J, Holmes G, *et al.* Infantile spasms: comparative trial of nitrazepam and corticotropin. *Arch Neurol* 1986; 43: 1107-10.
58. Pietz J, Benninger C, Schäfer H, Sontheimer D, Mittermaier G, Rating D. Treatment of infantile spasms with high-dosage vitamin B6. *Epilepsia* 1993; 34: 757-63.
59. Ito M. Antiepileptic drug treatment of West syndrome. *Epilepsia* 1998; 39 (Suppl 5): S38-41.
60. Suzuki Y, Imai K, Toribe Y, Ueda H, Yanagihara K, Shimono K, Okinaga T, Ono J, Nagai T, Matsuoka T, Tagawa T, Abe J, Morita Y, Fujikawa Y, Arai H, Mano T, Okada S. Long-term response to zonisamide in patientsd with West syndrome. *Neurology* 2002; 58: 1556-9.
61. Glauser TA, Clark PO, McGee K. Long-term response to topiramate in patients with West syndrome. *Epilepsia* 2000; 41 (Suppl 1): S91-4.
62. Riikonen R. Long-term outcome of West syndrome: a study of adults with a history of infantile spasms. *Epilepsia* 1996; 37: 367-72.
63. Stafstrom CE, Konkol RJ. Infantile spasms in children with Down syndrome. *Dev Med Child Neurol* 1994; 36: 576-85.
64. Jambaque I, Chiron C, Dumas C, Mumford J, Dulac O. Mental and behavioural outcome of infantile epilepsy treated by vigabatrin in tuberous sclerosis patients. *Epilepsy Res* 2000; 38: 151-60.
65. Gaily E, Appelqvist K, Kantola-Sorsa E, Liukkonen E, Kyyronen P, Sarpola M, Huttunen H, Valanne L, Granstrom ML. Cognitive deficits after cryptogenic infantile spasms with benign seizure evolution. *Dev Med Child Neurol* 1999; 41; 660-4.

Prognosis of febrile seizures

Anne T. Berg

Definition and epidemiology

Febrile seizures* are the single most common type of seizure disorder and occur in 2-5% of children in the US and Western Europe. Estimates from Japan are higher as are estimates from areas in the developing world [1]. Febrile seizures follow a very predictable pattern. Onset is in infancy and young childhood with a median age at onset of 18 months. Roughly 90 percent of children who have febrile seizures have the first by the time they are three years old and 95%-99% by the time they are 5-7 years old. There is no official upper age limit for when a febrile seizure can occur. Although the ILAE guidelines define febrile seizures as occurring in "childhood", many investigators and clinicians prefer to set an upper limit of 5 years. This is a convention, however, and is not based on scientific evidence that febrile seizures in an older child are substantively different from those in a younger child. Without solid scientific evidence to provide a basis for an absolute age cutoff (and most things in biology are not so absolute), one can understand the clinician's reticence to diagnosis (say) a twelve year old as having a simple benign febrile seizure as well as the researcher's reluctance to include such a case within a series of children who are mostly under three years of age. This is an area very much open for exploration. Regardless of the exact cutoff used, febrile seizures are believed to occur during a developmental window of susceptibility which is generally over by age five.

Most studies find a preponderance of boys among children with febrile seizures although this may simply be due to an increased susceptibility to illness and not to febrile seizure per se [2]. A family history of febrile seizures and often of epilepsy is found more often in children who have febrile seizures [2-7]; however, most of this latter effect is largely due to the influence of a family history of febrile seizures [2]. Apart from these fundamental risk factors, children who are developmentally compromised may be at increased risk of febrile seizures [6, 7]. Finally, the height of fever during an illness appears to influence the

---

* Supported by Grant RO1 NS 31146 from the National Institutes of Neurological Disorders and Stroke.

likelihood that a febrile seizure will occur during that illness [2]. Contrary to a popularly held belief in the past, there is no sound evidence that the rapid onset of fever is the precipitating factor in causing a febrile seizure [8].

The majority of febrile seizures are simple: brief, generally < 10 or < 15 minutes, generalized in onset, and occurring only once during an illness episode. Up to a third of febrile seizures may have one or more complex features (prolonged, focal onset, multiple seizures within a single illness episode). The consequences of these different types of febrile seizures are considered below.

Prognosis

In the past, febrile seizures were thought to be the beginning of epilepsy or the cause of epilepsy. Based upon inadequately designed studies, children who had febrile seizures were thought to have an extremely high risk of developing epilepsy and of cognitive difficulties. Febrile seizures were also implicated as the cause of hippocampal sclerosis and resulting intractable temporal lobe epilepsy [9, 10]. Much of this misunderstanding was clarified with the appearance of two key epidemiological studies of febrile seizures [11, 12] and a superb systematic review of published studies [13]. These studies showed that in population-based or birth cohorts, the prognosis of febrile seizures was almost always benign. Furthermore the earlier view of febrile seizures as being such a strong determinant of epilepsy and other neurological problems was based upon referral samples and not unselected series of children. This has served to underscore the overriding importance of study design and methods in investigations into the natural history of a disorder.

This chapter will address three aspects of the prognosis of febrile seizures:
1) the prognosis for recurrent febrile seizures,
2) the intellectual outcomes associated with febrile seizures,
3) the association between febrile seizures and subsequent unprovoked seizures or epilepsy.

Recurrent febrile seizures

Approximately 30-40% of children who have a first febrile seizure experience recurrent febrile seizures during subsequent illnesses [11, 14-18]. Of those who experience a second, approximately half experience a third febrile seizure and about half of those will have a fourth. Roughly ten percent of children will have three or more recurrences.

Time course of recurrences: First recurrences tend to happen within a year of the initial seizure and subsequent recurrences within a year of the previous recurrence. The risk drops with time, perhaps in part, because the brain matures out of the developmental window of susceptibility. It is very rare to see a recurrence after the age of about ten.

Well-established risk factors for recurrence: Three well documented factors are associated with the risk of recurrent febrile seizures: age, family history of febrile seizures, and temperature at the time of the initial febrile seizure.

Age at onset

Virtually every study that has examined age at onset has found a striking effect of age. The younger a child is during the developmental window of susceptibility, the greater the opportunity to have another febrile seizure while still within that window of susceptibility [14-16, 19-27]. The risk drops off with increasing age at onset [16, 27]. In a pooled analysis of five different studies, Offringa *et al.* found that what was most important was attained age and not age at the time of the seizure [16]. The risk decreased with increasing age of the child. For example, two children, one of whom had the first febrile seizure at 12 months of age and the other at 24 months, would, assuming no recurrences before age 3 years, have the same risk of recurrence at three years of age.

Family history of febrile seizures

A history of febrile seizures in a first degree relative is a factor that most investigators find to be associated with recurrence of febrile seizures [14, 16, 17, 28]. The risk may be doubled in children with such a history. Of interest, a family history of epilepsy does not appear to be a consistent or strong predictor of recurrent febrile seizures and probably should not, at this time, be considered a risk factor for recurrence.

Temperature at time of the initial febrile seizure

Children who seize with a lower degree of fever (often < 40° C) are at increased risk of subsequent febrile seizures [16, 20, 21, 24, 27, 29]. This fits well with a threshold interpretation. Children who seize with a relatively small fever challenge will require less provocation in the future to seize compared to children who require a relatively high challenge. Fever, however, is neurologically regulated. Recent discoveries about the role of the immune response to an infectious illness may require rethinking of how these associations are interpreted [30].

Other factors

Aside from these three factors, there are some others that have been examined in a limited number of studies or in several studies but with inconsistent results. Rate of recognized fever onset was, in the past, thought to be a precipitating factor in causing febrile seizures; however, this belief is not supported by any credible evidence [8, 30]. One study did find that children whose seizures occurred within a very short period of recognized onset of fever had an increased risk of recurrent febrile seizures [17]. Although this was a very dramatic effect, the significance of this effect is not clear and it remains to be tested and replicated in other studies.

Complex features, neurodevelopmental abnormalities, and a family history of febrile seizures have all been implicated in at least one or more studies as risk factors for recurrence. Other studies have not found them to be associated with recurrent febrile seizures. Overall, there is little evidence that any of these is a strong reliable predictor of recurrent febrile seizures although some small effect cannot be ruled out. Their importance lies in their association with later epilepsy.

With combined information about age at first seizure (< 18 months), positive family history of febrile seizures, and temperature (< 40° C), the risk of a recurrence is only about 15% in those with none of these risk factors and up to 65% in those with all three factors present. The average risk is about 30% in those with only one risk factor and about 40% in those with two.

Intellectual outcomes

An early twin study reported relatively poorer performance in 47 children with febrile seizures compared with twin controls [31]. It is not clear if all children were free of neurodevelopmental abnormalities prior to their initial febrile seizure. Very few of the

350 individual comparisons made were actually statistically significant, and the interpretation of the data was based on more comparisons favoring the non-affected co-twin than the affected twin. Thus, the authors had to conclude that the differences were very subtle, and one must question their clinical significance.

Despite frequent concerns in the past, there is now ample evidence to show that, in neurologically normal children, a history of febrile seizures is not associated with significant or important intellectual deficits. Some of the most definitive work in this area comes from two large studies from the United States [32] and the United Kingdom [33]. Both of these were large birth cohort studies and were highly representative of the populations from which they were drawn. The American study examined 431 children with febrile seizures who, during the course of the followup period had not developed unprovoked seizures and for whom a sibling control was available. In children known to be neurologically normal prior to the initial febrile seizure, there was no difference in full scale IQ scores between index cases and their sibling controls. Even in those who were deemed neurologically abnormal prior to the onset of the first febrile seizures, the mean IQ was lower by only 5.7 points. No difference was found in those pairs in which the febrile seizure case had had a complex febrile seizure (including status epilepticus), nor was there any effect of the total number of febrile seizure recurrences. The main limitation of this study is that the measure of intellectual outcome used, full scale IQ, does not permit analysis of specific cognitive functions and educational or behavioral outcomes.

In the British study, 381 children who were neurologically normal prior to their initial febrile seizure were compared to the rest of the population-based cohort with respect to 102 different measures of intelligence, behavior, and academic performance. The study reported significant differences on only four tests between children with febrile seizures and the rest of the cohort, a finding consistent with chance. The number of recurrent febrile seizures and type of seizures (simple versus complex) did not influence the measures examined. This study had much more detailed information regarding specific cognitive domains and still found nothing suggestive of deficits in those children with a history of prior febrile seizures.

A recent population-based Taiwanese study actually found evidence of slightly better memory function in children with prior febrile seizures compared to population-based controls [34]. Memory was of particular interest because of the concern over the association between febrile seizures and hippocampal atrophy.

As a final note, randomized clinical trials have demonstrated that treatment prevents recurrent febrile seizures but that decreasing recurrences is not associated with any advantage or disadvantage in intellectual outcomes [35]. In fact, treatment with phenobarbital, although effective in preventing recurrent febrile seizures is itself associated with a significant depression in measures of cognitive performance [36]. These disadvantages associated with treatment outlast the treatment although it is not clear for how long.

Given the findings that there are few if any intellectual, behavioral, or academic differences between children with and without febrile seizures, and given the concerns over the potentially deleterious effects of continuous prophylaxis with phenobarbital, it would seem the wisest course would be not to treat.

Unprovoked seizures and epilepsy

In large population-based or relatively representative samples of children with febrile seizures, the risk of developing at least one unprovoked seizure is on the order of 2-7%. This represents a several-fold increase over what is seen in the population-based or birth cohort studies [18, 19, 37]. Factors frequently associated with subsequent unprovoked seizures include pre-existing neurological abnormalities in the child, family history of febrile seizures and of epilepsy, characteristics of the febrile seizures, and the number of recurrent febrile seizures.

Pre-existing neurological abnormalities

Children with neurological or developmental abnormalities predating the initial febrile seizure are at substantially increased risk of developing subsequent unprovoked seizures and epilepsy [12, 18, 19, 38, 39]. In children with no prior abnormalities the risk of an unprovoked seizure is only on the order of 3-5% and of epilepsy (recurrent unprovoked seizures) only about 1-3%. By contrast, in those with neurodevelopmental abnormalities, the risk may be as high as 30% or even greater.

Complex features

Focal, prolonged (> 10 or > 15 minutes) and multiple seizures within a single illness episode are virtually always implicated as risk factors for subsequent epilepsy [12, 19, 37-39]. The retrospective Rochester study suggested that the effects of the different complex features were additive: the more features present, the greater the risk [12]. A separate prospective study, however, did not find this to be the case [38]. The association between complex febrile seizures and subsequent epilepsy appears to be strongest in children with pre-existing neurodevelopmental abnormalities [19, 38].

Family seizure history

Children who have a first degree relative with epilepsy are about two times more likely to develop unprovoked seizures or epilepsy although this finding is not always statistically significant [11, 12, 37-39]. A family history of febrile seizures, although a strong risk factor for recurrent febrile seizures, does not appear to be associated with the risk of subsequent unprovoked seizures [38, 39].

Recurrent febrile seizures

Some association between febrile seizure recurrence and epilepsy is frequently reported, although the effect is often limited to subgroups of the study sample. For example, Nelson and Ellenberg found the risk of epilepsy to increase with the number of febrile seizure recurrences but only in children with neurodevelopmental abnormalities [19]. A separate study found the number of recurrences was important regardless of the child's neurodevelopmental status [38]. Annegers *et al.* reported that the number of recurrences increased the risk for subsequent generalized – but not partial – onset unprovoked seizures [12]. Two other studies reported findings, one suggesting an increased risk associated with the number of recurrent febrile seizures [18], the other finding no association whatsoever [39]. Overall, the number of recurrences does indeed seem to be associated with some increased risk of subsequent unprovoked seizures; however, the magnitude of the risk and whether it applies primarily to a specific subgroup is unclear.

Other factors

Temperature at the time of the initial febrile seizure does not appear to be associated with risk of subsequent unprovoked seizures [38]. On the other hand, children whose initial seizure occurred immediately or within a very short time of the onset of fever were at increased risk of later unprovoked seizures. Such findings require independent replication studies before they can be accepted as widely applicable.

Prophylactic treatment of febrile seizures was, in the past, justified on the grounds that the prevention of recurrent febrile seizures would decrease the risk of subsequent epilepsy. The notion that treatment can alter the outcome of febrile seizures by preventing recurrent febrile seizures and in doing so reducing the risk of subsequent epilepsy has been dispelled. From randomized clinical trials, it is reasonably clear that treatment can be highly effective in reducing the risk of a recurrent febrile seizure [40-42]. It is, however, equally clear that children who are treated for febrile seizures have the same risk of subsequent unprovoked seizures as those who received placebo or no treatment [35, 43, 44]. Currently, none of the available evidence supports a policy of treating febrile seizures in order to prevent the occurrence of subsequent unprovoked seizures.

A paradox

Across the literature, there in an apparent paradox in that factors that seem to be associated with recurrent febrile seizures are not associated with the risk of epilepsy, yet the risk of epilepsy appears to be somewhat higher in those who have experienced recurrent febrile seizures. One study found that, in those children who were at high risk of recurrent febrile seizures (family history of febrile seizures, young age at first febrile seizures, relatively lower degree of fever), having recurrences was not associated with an increased risk of subsequent epilepsy. It was only in those at low risk of febrile seizure recurrence who, if they had recurrences, experienced an increased risk of subsequent unprovoked seizures [38]. A summary of the association between the risk factors discussed above and each of the seizure outcomes is provided in *table I*.

Table I. Summary of risk factors for recurrent febrile and subsequent unprovoked seizures

	Associated with an increased risk of	
	Recurrent febrile seizures	*Subsequent unprovoked seizures*
Young age at first febrile seizure	↑↑***	Ø**
First degree relative with history of febrile seizures	↑↑***	Ø**
First degree relative with history of epilepsy	Ø***	↑↑***
Low degree of fever at time of first febrile seizure	↑↑***	Ø*
Brief duration of fever prior to initial febrile seizures	↑↑*	↑↑*
Complex features of febrile seizure	Ø?***	↑↑***
Neurodevelopmental abnormalities	Ø**	↑↑***

↑↑ Substantial increase in risk associated with factor.
Ø No substantial or significant risk associated with factor.
* Needs further examination in other studies.
** Documented in at least 2 or 3 studies..
*** Consistently documented in multiple studies, high level of agreement across studies.
? Some minor effect cannot be fully ruled out.

Epilepsies associated with febrile seizures

Because only a few percent of children with febrile seizures go on to have epilepsy, it is very difficult to study in detail the association between febrile seizures and specific types of epilepsy. Annegers examined risk factors for partial- versus generalized-onset seizures in 32 children who developed unprovoked seizures [45]. Some very salient differences were seen. Factors associated with generalized- but not partial-onset unprovoked seizures were the number of febrile seizures and family history. By contrast, complex features were strongly correlated with development of partial but not generalized onset seizures. This study was done before the wide-spread acceptance of epilepsy syndromes and therefore is hard to interpret with respect to the modern understanding of epilepsy currently in force today.

A different approach, used by some teams, has been to examine the characteristics of epilepsy associated with febrile seizures in children with newly diagnosed epilepsy. Roughly 15% of children with newly diagnosed epilepsy or new onset seizures have a history of febrile seizures [46-49]. In children with epilepsy, compared to those with no preceding history of febrile seizures, those who had febrile seizures tended to have a younger age at onset and were more likely to have a family history of both febrile seizures and of epilepsy [46]. Children with preceding complex febrile seizures had a younger age at onset and were more likely to have a first degree relative who also had febrile seizures. Children with preceding simple febrile seizures were more likely to have a family history of both first as well second degree and higher order relatives with febrile seizures as well as a family history of epilepsy. Absence seizures (largely reflecting childhood and juvenile absence epilepsy) were uncommon in children with any type of febrile seizure.

Although most studies have tried to identify a link between febrile seizures and partial epilepsy and temporal lobe epilepsy in particular, studies of newly diagnosed patients fail to provide much evidence of any specific link. This seems somewhat peculiar because data from adult epilepsy series indicate a very strong association between a history of febrile seizures and medial temporal lobe epilepsy [50]. The relationships between prior febrile seizures and type of epilepsy were examined in one of the prospective studies *(table II)* [46]. There was no evidence to suggest that nonidiopathic epilepsy localized to the temporal lobe was more likely than other nonidiopathic partial epilepsy to be preceded by febrile seizures or specifically complex or recurrent febrile seizures. Children with idiopathic syndromes, however, were slightly less likely to have a history of febrile seizures, several times less likely to have had recurrent febrile seizures, and those with idiopathic generalized epilepsy were substantially less likely to have a history of complex febrile seizures.

As previously discussed [51] some of these associations do not appear at first but may become evident with time. The implications for this are that prospective studies will have to plan on prolonged follow-up and analyses will have to be focused on a specific syndrome and not all epilepsy at once.

Other areas

Although the epidemiological evidence provides ample basis for assuaging the concerns of most parents, we cannot ignore the fact that, in a few rare instances, febrile seizures in fact presage the onset of some of the most severe forms of epilepsy identified. Severe myoclonic epilepsy of infancy is one such syndrome [52, 53]. and there may well be others. Because they are so rare, epidemiological studies have not been able to shed much light on such serious disorders.

Table II. History of febrile seizures in children according to type of epilepsy as classified two years after initial diagnosis [52]

Type of Epilepsy	N*	Any FSz** n (%)	> 1 FSz n (%)	Complex FSz n (%)	Prolonged FSz (> 10 min) n (%)	Focal FSz n (%)	Multiple Fsz (> 1/illness) n (%)
Idiopathic partial epilepsy	66	7 (11)	2 (3)	3 (5)	0	3 (5)	0
S/C*** partial, unlocalized	117	16 (14)	10 (9)	7 (6)	2 (2)	2 (2)	5 (4)
S/C partial, localized, non-temporal	84	15 (18)	6 (7)	5 (6)	3 (4)	2 (2)	2 (2)
S/C partial, temporal	96	14 (15)	10 (10)	8 (8)	2 (2)	3 (3)	6 (6)
Idiopathic generalized epilepsy	134	10 (7)	3 (2)	3 (2)	0	3 (2)	0
S/C generalized epilepsy	59	5 (8)	2 (3)	3 (5)	2 (3)	1 (2)	2 (3)
Undetermined/unclassified	52	9 (17)	5 (10)	6 (12)	1 (2)	3 (6)	6 (12)

* Based on N = 609, 4 children missing history of febrile seizures.
** FSZ – febrile seizures.
*** S/C – symptomatic or cryptogenic.

The EEG, while essential in the determination of epileptic syndromes (syndromes involving unprovoked seizures), has not been shown to be a great help in evaluating children with febrile seizures. Occasional findings of interest from selected clinical samples are no more than that until they can be tested in representative series of patients and their true prevalence and significance examined in appropriately conducted studies. The current practice in the United States and probably throughout most of the world is not to perform EEGs routinely in children with febrile seizures. This creates both financial as well as practical problems for those who would do such a study of EEG in children with febrile seizures on a large scale.

Recent and continuing developments in genetics and neuroimmunology, and an increased understanding of the neurophysiological events underlying fever and seizures are, on a daily basis, changing our understanding of this common seizures disorder [54]. Tremendous heterogeneity within what are called febrile seizures is undoubtedly present. It has yet to be sufficiently described and understood to be readily applicable for clinical or epidemiological purposes at this point in time. We may be approaching the point where we stop referring to febrile seizures as a single entity.

References

1. Stafstrom CE. The incidence and prevalence of *Febrile seizures*. In: Baram TZ, Shinnar S, eds. Febrile Seizures. San Diego: Academic Press, 2001: 1-26.
2. Berg AT, Shinnar S, Shapiro ED, Salomon ME, Crain EF, Hauser WA. Risk factors for a first febrile seizure: a matched case-control study. *Epilepsia* 1995; 36: 334-41.
3. Nelson KB, Ellenberg JH. Prenatal and perinatal antecedents of febrile seizures. *Ann Neurol* 1990; 27: 127-31.

4. Forsgren L, Sidenvall R, Blomquist HK, Heijbel J, Nystrom L. An incident case-referent study of febrile convulsions in children: genetical and social aspects. *Neuropediatrics* 1990; 21: 153-9.
5. Zhao F, Emoto SE, Lavine L, Nelson KB, Wang CC, Li SC, Cheng XM, Bolis CL, Schoenberg BS. Risk factors for febrile seizures in the People's Republic of China: a case control study. *Epilepsia* 1991; 32: 510-4.
6. Bethune P, Gordon K, Dooley J, Camfield C, Camfield P. Which child will have a febrile seizure? *Am J Dis Child* 1993; 147: 35-9.
7. Huang CC, Wang ST, Chang YC, Huang MC, Chi YC, Tsai JJ. Risk factors for a first febrile convulsion in children: a population study in southern Taiwan. *Epilepsia* 1999; 40: 719-25.
8. Berg AT. Are febrile seizures provoked by a rapid rise in temperature? *Am J Dis Child* 1993; 147: 1101-3.
9. Falconer MA, Serafetinides EA, Corsellis JAN. Etiology and pathogenesis of temporal lobe epilepsy. *Arch Neurol* 1964; 10: 233-48.
10. Van Lierde A, Mira L. Aetiological role of febrile convulsive atacks in limbic epilepsy. In: Avanzini G, Beaumanoir A, Mira L, eds. *Limbic Seizures in Children*. London: John Libbey & Co, 2001: 159-65.
11. Nelson KB, Ellenberg JH. Prognosis in children with febrile seizures. *Pediatrics* 1978; 61: 720-7.
12. Annegers JF, Hauser WA, Shirts SB, Kurland LT. Factors prognostic of unprovoked seizures after febrile convulsions. *N Engl J Med* 1987; 316: 493-8.
13. Ellenberg JH, Nelson KB. Sample selection and the natural history of disease: studies of febrile seizures. *JAMA* 1980; 243: 1337-40.
14. Annegers JF, Blakley SA, Hauser WA, Kurland LT. Recurrence of febrile convulsions in a population-based cohort. *Epilepsy Res* 1990; 5: 209-16.
15. Verity CM, Butler NR, Golding J. Febrile convulsions in a national cohort followed up from birth. I-prevalence and recurrence in the first five years of life. *Br Med J* 1985; 290: 1307-10.
16. Offringa M, Derksen-Lubsen G, Bossuyt PM, Lubsen J. Seizure recurrence after a first febrile seizure: a multivariate approach. *Dev Med Child Neurol* 1992; 34: 15-24.
17. Berg AT, Shinnar S, Darefsky AS, Holford TR, Shapiro ED, Salomon ME, Crain EF, Wa H. Predictors of recurrent febrile seizures: a prospective cohort study. *Arch Pediatr Adolescent Medicine* 1997; 151: 371-8.
18. MacDonald BK, Johnson AL, Sander JWAS, Shorvon SD. Febrile convulsions in 220 children – neurological sequelae at 12 years followup. *Eur Neurol* 1999; 41: 179-6.
19. Nelson KB, Ellenberg JH. Predictors of epilepsy in children who have experienced febrile seizures. *N Engl J Med* 1976; 295: 1029-33.
20. Al-Eissa YA. Febrile seizures: rate and risk factors of recurrence. *J Child Neurol* 1995; 10: 315-9.
21. Laditan AAO. Seizure recurrence after a first febrile convulsion. *Ann Trop Paediatr* 1994; 14: 303-8.
22. Airede AI. Febrile convulsions: factors and recurrence rate. *Trop Geogr Med* 1992; 44: 233-7.
23. van den Berg BJ. Studies on convulsive disorders in young children III. Recurrence of febrile convulsions. *Epilepsia* 1974; 15: 177-90.
24. El-Radhi AS, Withana K, Banajeh S. Recurrence rate of febrile convulsion related to the degree of pyrexia during the first attack. *Clinical Pediatrics* 1986; 25: 311-3.
25. Knudsen FU. Recurrence risk after a first febrile seizure and effect of short-term diazepam prophylaxis. *Arch Dis Child* 1985; 60: 1045-9.
26. van Stuijvenberg M, Jansen NE, Steyerberg EW, Derek-Lubsen G, Moll HA. Frequency of fever episodes related to febrile seizure recurrence. *Acta Paediatr* 1999; 88: 52-5.
27. Berg AT, Shinnar S, Hauser WA, Alemany M, Shapiro ED, Salomon ME, Ef C. A prospective study of recurrent febrile seizures. *N Engl J Med* 1992; 327: 1122-7.
28. Offringa M, Bossuyt PMM, Lubsen J, Ellenberg JH, Nelson KB, Knudsen FU, Annegers JF, El-Radhi ASM, Habbema JDF, Derksen-Lubsen G, Hauser WA, Kurland LT, Banajeh SMA, Larsen S. Risk factors for seizure recurrence in children with febrile seizures: a pooled analysis of individual patient data from five studies. *J Pediatr* 1994; 124: 574-84.
29. El-Radhi AS. Lower degree of fever at the intial febrile convulsion is associated with an increased risk of subsequent convulsions. *Eur J Paediatr Neurol* 1998; 2: 91-6.
30. Gatti S, Vezzani A, Barfati T. Mechanisms of fever and febrile seizures: putative role of the interleukin-1 system. In: Baram TZ, Shinnar S, eds. Febrile Seizures. San Diego: Academic Press, 2002: 169-88.
31. Schiottz-Christensen E, Bruhn P. Intelligence, behavior and scholastic achievement subsequent to febrile convulsions: an analysis of discordant twin-pairs. *Develop Med Child Neurol* 1973; 15: 565-75.

32. Ellenberg JH, Hirtz DG, Nelson KB. Do seizures in children cause intellectual deterioration? *N Engl J Med* 1986; 314: 1085-8.
33. Verity CM, Greenwood R, Golding J. Long-term Intellectual and Behavioral Outcomes of Children with Febrile Convulsions. *New Engl J Med* 1998; 388: 1723-8.
34. Chang Y, Guo N, Wang S, Huang C, Tsai J. Working memory of school-aged children with a history of febrile convulsions. *Neurology* 2001; 57: 37-42.
35. Knudsen FU, Paerregaard A, Andersen R, Andresen J. Long term outcome of prophylaxis for febrile convulsions. *Arch Dis Child* 1996; 74: 13-8.
36. Farwell JR, Lee YJ, Hirtz DG, Sulzbacher SI, Ellenberg JH, Nelson KB. Phenobarbital for febrile seizures-effects on intelligence and on seizure recurrence. *N Engl J Med* 1990; 322: 364-9.
37. Verity CM, Golding J. Risk of epilepsy after febrile convulsions: a national cohort study. *Br Med J* 1991; 303: 1373-6.
38. Berg AT, Shinnar S. Unprovoked seizures in children with febrile seizures: short-term outcome. *Neurology* 1996; 47: 562-8.
39. Tsai ML, Hung KL. Risk factors for subsequent epilepsy after febrile convulsions. *J Formos Med Assoc* 1995; 94: 327-31.
40. Knudsen FU. Effective short-term diazepam prophylaxis in febrile convulsions. *J Pediatr* 1985; 106: 487-90.
41. Wolf SM. The effectiveness of phenobarbital in the prevention of recurrent febrile convulsions in children with and without a history of pre-, peri- and postnatal abnormalities. *Acta Paediatr Scand* 1977; 66: 585-7.
42. Rosman NP, Colton T, Labazzo J, Gilbert PL, Gardella NB, Kaye EM, Van Bennekom C, Winter MR. A controlled trial of diazepam adminstered during febrile illnesses to prevent recurrence of febrile seizures. *N Engl J Med* 1993; 329: 79-94.
43. Wolf SM, Forsythe A. Epilepsy and mental retardation following febrile seizures in childhood. *Acta Paediatr Scand* 1989; 78: 291-5.
44. Rosman NP, Labazzo J, Colton T. Factors predisposing to afebrile seizures after febrile convulsions and preventive treatment. *Ann Neurol* 1993; 34: 452.
45. Annegers JF, Hauser WA, Elveback LR, Kurland LT. The risk of epilepsy following febrile convulsions. *Neurology* 1979; 29: 297-303.
46. Berg AT, Shinnar S, Levy SR, Testa FM. Childhood-onset epilepsy with and without preceding febrile seizures. *Neurology* 1999; 53: 1742-8.
47. Camfield P, Camfield C, Gordon K, Dooley J. What types of epilepsy are preceded by febrile seizures? A population-based study of children. *Dev Med Child Neurol* 1994; 36: 887-92.
48. Sofijanov N, Sadikario A, Dukovski M, Kuturec M. Febrile convulsions and later development of epilepsy. *Am J Dis Child* 1983; 137: 123-6.
49. Shinnar S, Berg AT, Moshe SL, Petix M, Maytal J, Kang H, Goldensohn ES, Wa H. The risk of seizure recurrence following a first unprovoked seizure in childhood: a prospective study. *Pediatrics* 1990; 85: 1076-85.
50. Hamati-Haddad A, Abou-Khalil B. Epilepsy diagnosis and localization in patients with antecedent childhood febrile convulsions. *Neurology* 1998; 50: 917-22.
51. Berg AT. Identification of epilepsy syndroms at diagnosis and modification with time. In: Jallon P, ed. *Prognosis of the Epilepsies*. Paris: John Libbey Eurotext, 2002: 185-96.
52. Dravet C, Bureau M, Guerrini R, Giraud N, Roger J. Severe myoclonic epilepsy in infants. In: Roger J, Bureau M, Dravet C, Dreifuss FE, Perret A, Wolf P, eds. *Epileptic syndromes in infancy, childhood, and adolescence*. London: John Libbey, 1992: 75-88.
53. Chiron C. Prognosis of severe myoclonic epilepsy in infancy (Dravet syndrome). In: Jallon P, ed. *Prognosis of epilepsies*. Paris: John Libbey Eurotext, 2002: 239-48.
54. Baram TZ, Shinnar S. *Febrile Seizures*. San Diego: Academic Press, 2001: 397.
55. Berg AT, Shinnar S, Levy SR, Testa FM, Smith-Rapaport S, Beckerman B. How well can epilepsy syndromes be identified at diagnosis? A reassessment two years after initial diagnosis. *Epilepsia* 2000; 41: 1269-75.

Prognosis of myoclonic-astatic epilepsy

Olivier Dulac and Anna Kaminska

Myoclonic-astatic epilepsy (MAE) is a recently identified type of potentially severe idiopathic epilepsy. The nosological limits are still not clearly delineated, mainly because the description of the syndrome was developed on the basis of two distinct concepts that developed within two distinct schools of epileptology. A clear definition therefore must be established that distinguishes MAE from both the Lennox-Gastaut syndrome and from other kinds of myoclonic epilepsy occurring in early childhood. This has not been done in most epidemiologic studies. In addition, many antiepileptic compounds are likely to aggravate the condition. This is particularly true of some of the first and second generation drugs. Consequently, prognostic data drawn from old series are likely to overestimate the pharmacoresistance of MAE.

In this chapter, we will define MAE as a syndrome from a historical perspective; delineate it nosologically and identify the various patterns of its evolution and outcome; describe the specific associated pattern of cognitive and motor dysfunction; discuss the potential drug-induced worsening that may occur; identify the drugs from which patients may benefit; and identify the factors that are related to prognosis, both with respect to seizures and to cognitive functions. We will then elaborate on a hypothesis regarding the neurobiological basis for the variation in severity seen in this condition.

Definition

Myoclonic-astatic epilepsy is a severe form of epilepsy that begins in early childhood, usually before the age of five years, in children who, up until the onset of the disorder, experienced normal development, although a mild speech delay may be present in a small proportion. Drop attacks, generalized spike-waves on the EEG, frequent episodes of status epilepticus, together with cognitive deterioration are all features that MAE shares with the Lennox-Gastaut syndrome. Myoclonic seizures are commonly the main seizure type in many of the severe epilepsies of early childhood. Conditions comprising myoclonic seizure as the major seizure type include progressive diseases due to inborn errors of metabolism, epilepsies affecting the course of nonprogressive encephalopathies, as well as several forms of idiopathic epilepsies [1]. In both nonprogressive encephalopathies and idiopathic epilepsies, the occurrence of very frequent myoclonic seizures is often linked to cognitive and motor deterioration. This often raises the diagnostic suspicion of an inborn error of metabolism. As a result, many of these children undergo large but useless metabolic work-ups that could have been avoided had the clinical pattern of the condition been recognized and properly understood. The complexity of the condition, however, does present considerable diagnostic challenges to the clinician.

In order to understand the apparent contradictions that have paved the way to the identification of MAE, one has to imagine Europe before Europe. Two major schools of epileptology have contributed to our recognition and understanding of MAE. The German school with, among others, Janz for adults [2] and Doose for children [3] made considerable efforts to clarify the genetic basis of epilepsy. Fine neurophysiological analysis played a major role, particularly in children. Doose identified the correlation between several EEG patterns and familial antecedents of epilepsy, namely theta rhythms, generalized spike-waves, either spontaneously occurring or triggered by hyperventilation, and photosensitivity [for a review, see 3]. This allowed him to identify a whole range of epilepsy conditions occurring in early childhood that were believed to be the result of a genetic predisposition with polygenic inheritance. He called this group "centrencephalic myoclonic-astatic petit mal" [4]. The main theoretical interest for the identification of this group was to show that children with severe epilepsy involving the whole brain did not all have Lennox-Gastaut syndrome, most, if not all, of which is caused by some kind of brain lesion. Instead such patients could have genetically inherited epilepsy, distinct from inborn errors of metabolism. Patients within the "centrencephalic myoclonic-astatic petit mal" spectrum exhibit a whole range of different seizures: tonic-clonic, myoclonic, myoclonic-astatic, tonic, absence, and status epilepticus, with both myoclonic and tonic components. Doose, however, distinguished within this group various patterns, with various outcomes [5]. Patients who only exhibit generalized myoclonic seizures usually had a good outcome. Those with tonic-clonic seizures starting in the first year of life experienced poor outcomes. In this group the occurrence of prolonged clonic status epilepticus contrasted with the occurrence of very few if any spike-waves on the EEG. A poor outcome is also typical in patients who develop frequent tonic seizures in sleep as well as in patients who have episodes of myoclonic status and who evidence a rapid global deterioration in cognitive function. The usual onset in such cases is after the second year of life. However, other patients with onset after two years of age may completely recover despite having experienced tonic seizures and daily drop attacks for weeks and an EEG with a very active spike and wave pattern. Thus the group seems totally heterogeneous in terms of clinical presentation, EEG characteristics and outcome. The entity identified by the German school is by no means a syndrome, but an etiologic concept: difficult to treat generalized epilepsy secondary to a genetic predisposition.

In the meantime, the Marseille school developed the concept of epilepsy syndromes following the observation that patients with epilepsy experience a range of outcomes from total recovery to pharmacoresistance accompanied by a major impact on cognitive and motor functions. This variability is not related solely to the specific etiology which can be identified in only a quarter of the patients. Within an etiological group (including no identified etiology) considerable variation in outcome may occur. Many patients exhibit more than one type of seizure. Therefore it is not meaningful either to distinguish patients based on seizure type alone. Other salient clinical features that vary among patients include the age of onset, the neurological condition prior to the onset of seizures and the interictal pattern on the EEG. It became clear that there were groups of patients who shared constellations of clinical features, particularly age of onset, seizure types, interictal EEG pattern and outcome, hence syndromes.

This concept of syndromes appeared soon after the development of the modern EEG. The identification of two major EEG patterns each linked to distinct clinical presentations and patterns provided the neurophysiological basis for identifying syndromes. These two EEG patterns were the "petit mal" and the "petit mal variant" pattern associated with absence epilepsy and the "hypsarrhythmic" pattern associated with infantile spasms. This approach to the separation of various epilepsy patterns with distinct outcomes was further developed and enlarged by the Marseille school. Among patients with drop attacks, a group with unusually pharmacoresistant epilepsy and in whom cognitive and motor functions were severely affected, the Lennox-Gastaut syndrome could be distinguished, in part based on the relative rarity of myoclonic seizures which, by contrast, represent the predominant seizure-type in other severe generalized epilepsies occurring in young children. Among the latter, when they began in infancy and were not caused by an inborn error of metabolism, two groups, severe and benign, could be further distinguished.

It was not until the 1990s that it became clear that these two patterns were included in the series of patients designated as having "centrencephalic myoclonic-astatic petit mal" epilepsy, although Doose's series was not restricted to these two patterns. A major difficulty then remained: to distinguish from the Lennox-Gastaut syndrome those patients of the Doose group who started after the age of two years. The usual approach, expressed by Aicardi, was that there was a whole range, from Lennox-Gastaut to myoclonic epilepsy, the myoclonic-astatic epilepsy being a link between these two extremes [6]. This concept of a continuum was similar to that of the Montreal school regarding idiopathic generalized epilepsy, expressed by Berkovic [7]. Patients in these groups had a similar age of onset (2 to 5 years), multiple seizure types including absences and drop attacks, generalized spike-waves on the EEG, and severe cognitive impairments. Given the large number of characteristics that had to be considered, it was impossible simply to look at the array of information and discern meaningful patterns and groups. Computer-implemented mathematical models have greatly helped in this regard. One method, "multiple correspondence analysis" [8], has been applied to this specific problem. This method is able to identify within a heterogeneous group of items, clusters of items shared by a subgroup and to identify the members of this subgroup [9]. When applying this method to patients with various types of generalized seizures and various patterns of generalized spike-waves including either 3Hz spike-waves (SW) or slow spike-waves, normal brain imaging, and who had their first seizures between one and ten years of age, it was possible to distinguish three groups:

– The first cluster contained patients with onset between two and five years of age who had mainly myoclonic and tonic-clonic seizures with 3Hz SW. There was a high incidence of familial antecedents suggesting a genetic predisposition. There was an excess of male patients. Frequent tonic-clonic seizures usually preceded the occurrence of myoclonic-astatic seizures. One third of these patients had tonic seizures as shown by ictal EEG recording, a feature not previously observed in patients who had done well. This first group tended to have a favorable outcome.

– The second group also had an onset between two and five years. In addition to the features observed in the first group, these patients had tonic and absence seizures as well as episodes of myoclonic status. On the EEG, both SW and slow SW were evident. Although the incidence of genetic predisposition was slightly lower than in the first group, it remained significant. The incidence of tonic and absence seizures in this group was significantly higher than in the previous group. Most patients in this group experienced very prolonged episodes of myoclonic and tonic status epilepticus, and later clusters of vibratory tonic seizures in sleep prior to awakening persisted for many years. This group tended to have a poor outcome.

– In the third group, the age at onset was somewhat older than in the first two groups with a peak between five and seven years. The predominant seizure types in this group were tonic and absence seizures, and the characteristic EEG finding was slow SW along with an excess of focal abnormalities. Males and females were equally represented. The outcome in this group was poor.

One possible explanation for these 3 groups was indeed that there was a continuum from the first group, which would represent part of the "centrencephalic myoclonic-astatic petit mal" syndrome, to the third group, which would correspond to the Lennox-Gastaut syndrome. Variants in between these two extremes would be generated by various factors including treatment. An alternative was however much more consistent with additional findings. When restricting the study to features observable during the first year of the disorder, only two groups could be identified, and the distinction between the first and second groups of the first analysis disappeared. Thus, it was some feature that appeared during the course of the disorder that resulted in the distinction between the first two groups. Patients in these two groups shared myoclonus, 3Hz SW and a genetic predisposition expressed by the high incidence of familial antecedents of epilepsy. It was possible to conclude that the first two groups were genetically determined, and indeed they had the characteristics identified by Doose in his "centrencephalic myoclonic-astatic petit mal" group, for patients whose epilepsy began after infancy. The third group corresponded to the Lennox-Gastaut syndrome. In this group, there was no increase in familial predisposition, but there was an excess of focal EEG abnormalities consistent with some brain damage not disclosed by conventional imaging. In addition, although the second and third groups were distinct from onset, during the course of the disorder they were both associated with the occurrence of tonic and absence seizures, and both exhibited slow SW on the EEG.

Nosology

Thus, it becomes possible to define myoclonic-astatic epilepsy (MAE) as a condition that begins between two and five years of age, usually first presenting with repeat tonic-clonic seizures and then later with various types of generalized seizures, particularly myoclonic-astatic seizures, as well SW on the EEG. The outcome is variable, ranging from very favorable – total recovery within a few months –, to very unfavorable – typically associated with the occurrence of myoclonic status. The long term course of patients with an unfavorable outcome is characterized by the persistence, many years later, even by the beginning of the third decade, of clusters of tonic seizures prior to awakening.

Pattern of cognitive and motor dysfunction

Ataxia, together with abnormal fine movements due to dyspraxia, and speech difficulties are the main findings in patients who experience a mild impact of the disease. Many patients suffer from an attentional deficit with hyperkinesia that may persist for many months after the end of the seizure themselves. Those who undergo prolonged episodes of myoclonic status tend to suffer progressive cognitive deterioration best characterized as dementia [10].

Potential for drug induced worsening

Drug induced worsening has been reported by a number of research groups [for review, see 11]. Carbamazepine was long considered as the drug of choice for children with epilepsy, and this still remains the case for a number of physicians. It is now clear that this compound has a pronounced tendency to aggravate MAE. Kaminska *et al.* reported carbamazepine-related seizure exacerbation in over half the patients in their case series [8]. It is of course difficult to give precise likelihood of carbamazepine associated seizure aggravation due to the lack of controlled data.

Phenytoin is also known to aggravate seizures in MAE although this compound is less often administered to children. Phenytoin is, however, an excellent drug for the treatment of status epilepticus which many of these patients tend to have. Unfortunately, it is then tempting to switch from the IV to the oral formulation of this drug.

Although the use of vigabatrin has been restricted due to its potential retinal toxicity, it remains an excellent compound for infants and children with some forms of pharmacoresistant epilepsy. Vigabatrin, however, is likely to worsen seizures in patients with MAE [12].

The risk related to the administration of phenobarbital is not as clear. Given the high incidence of absence seizures in this type of epilepsy and the ability of phenobarbital to precipitate nonconvulsive status epilepticus, this compound clearly represents a theoretical risk for seizure exacerbation.

Effective therapies

Valproate has some beneficial effect on tonic-clonic, absence and myoclonic seizures. Ethosuximide is helpful for absences and myoclonic seizures. Benzodiazepines are indicated for the treatment of status epilepticus, but the benefit of long term everyday administration is less clear for two reasons: these compounds may increase the incidence of tonic seizures or even precipitate tonic status epilepticus, and the chronic administration of the compound may reduce the potential of these compounds to interrupt status epilepticus.

The introduction of lamotrigine represents a revolution in the treatment of MAE as over three quarters of patients treated with this drug experience more than a 75% decrease in seizure frequency and many experiencing a complete cessation of seizures altogether [13]. Topiramate is effective, reducing seizure frequency by 50% in over half the cases [14]. Levetiracetam seems very promising, provided moderate doses are administered at onset (Chiron *et al.*, unpublished personal experience).

Ketogenic diet is useful in the context of an acute worsening of seizure frequency (Villeneuve *et al.*, in prep).

Prognostic features

Mental retardation and persisting seizures are the two major features that impede social integration in these patients. In fact, our study shows that mental retardation and persisting seizures were strongly linked ($p < 0.001$) [8]. The major factors for developing mental retardation were the lack of familial antecedents and short 3Hz SW bursts, as shown with univariate analysis of electroclinical vaiables. Analysis using multiple logistic regression further identified the presence of tonic and absence seizures at onset as additional major risk factors (p = 0.01). On follow up, univariate analysis showed that the main factors associated with mental retardation were the duration of epilepsy for over three years (p < 0.001), the presence of vibratory tonic seizures (p < 0.001) and of myoclonic status epilepticus (p = 0.02).

Mechanism of intractability and cognitive troubles

The statistical distinction of three groups among severe generalized epilepsy requires careful consideration and interpretation as different groups share common features at different stages of the disorder. The first two groups appear to be genetically determined and share myoclonic and tonic-clonic seizure with onset before five years as well as having generalized bursts of 3Hz SW on the EEG. Thus they seem to be mainly determined by genetic factors occurring early in life. These are also features seen at various ages in the idiopathic generalized epilepsies and supposedly involve the thalamo-cortical loop, the rhythmicity being generated by the thalamic reticular system and the cortical contribution mainly involving the rolandic strip to generate myoclonus. On the other hand, both groups with unfavorable outcome share similar features in the second half of the first decade. These mainly include tonic seizures, atypical absences and slow SW on the EEG. These are signs of epiletogenic encephalopathy, clearly related to brain maturation, which, at that age, primarily involves the frontal lobes. These findings are probably due to secondary bilateral synchrony through the corpus callosum between the frontal lobes which are highly excitable during rapid maturation of this part of the brain. However, the latter two groups also have either a genetic predisposition (the MAE group) or some suspected focal or multifocal brain damage (the LGS group). Therefore, whereas the MAE group with favorable outcome results solely from a genetic predisposition, the one with an unfavorable outcome results from factors related to maturation of the brain, in addition to the genetic predisposition.

It is this combination of two epileptogenic factors that may lead to pharmacoresistance. This is clearly the case for LGS. It seems likely also for the second group of unfavourable cases with MAE, although the etiologic features are partly different from those of LGS. The combination could also explain the long lasting episodes of myoclonic status epilepticus: the interaction of two distinct, more or less rhythmic activities, at 2 and 3Hz could generate irregular and synchronous spike and slow wave activity resembling hypsarrhythmia. The continuous spiking and slow wave discharges would explain the drowsiness of these patients, the interference of the 2Hz activity with the 3Hz rhythm would interfere with the expression of massive myoclonus and instead result in erratic myoclonus. The predominance of the latter in the perioral and tongue areas and in distal parts of the upper limbs is consistent with the involvement of pyramidal pathways, since these areas are those mainly represented in the rolandic strip.

Neuropsychological findings are also consistent with this undersanding of pathophysiology: major features are dysarthria and apraxia, in addition to ataxia which is often linked to myoclonus. Dysarthria and apraxia both involve areas of the cortex that are adjacent to the rolandic strip. Cases with a poor outcome also exhibit slowness and attentional deficits, and eventually may also have additional features of frontal lobe dysfunction. The latter is seen in patients with LGS, although to a more severe extent, probably as a result of the underlying brain insult.

What is the precise contribution of genetic predisposition?

The identification of a specific genetic predisposition to Dravet syndrome may open an alternate understanding of the differences between cases with favorable and unfavorable outcome. In particular, a specific monogenic predisposition could apply only to unfavorable cases [15]. The slightly lower incidence of familial antecedents of epilepsy in unfavorable cases would be consistent with this hypothesis. However, it is also consistent with the hypothesis previously mentioned of a combination of genetic and maturational features. In the case of Dravet syndrome, one study showed that the characteristic pattern in patients with the mutation in SCNA1 can be recognized from the beginning of the disorder because of the occurrence of unilateral clonic seizures (Nabbout *et al.*, submitted). Resolution of the questions raised about the neurobiological basis of the various aspects of MAE will require extensive research into the molecular basis in this disorder combined with very precise phenotyping.

Conclusions

This is a particularly important model for understanding the roles of the three major categories of factors predisposing to epilepsy: lesions, genetic predisposition and maturation of the brain. In addition, this model contributes to the understanding of some factors of intractability in childhood epilepsy. Finally, it has provided an opportunity to apply a mathematical method, MCA, which is particularly useful for distinguishing discrete groups of patients with epilepsy based upon an array of complex clinical features. To the clinician these groups may appear to represent a continuum, but in fact, they result from discrete etiologic factors and thus from distinct neurobiological mechanisms. The impression of a continuum is given by the combination of several factors in some patients. In addition, recent findings regarding the genetic predisposition to epilepsy suggest that the genetic predisposition is heterogeneous, due to several monogenic conditions. Thus this heterogeneity also contributes to the impression of a continuum. Modulating genetic factors yet to be identified could also increase the clinical variability, thus further contributing to the impression of a continuum.

References

1. Dulac O, Plouin P, Shewmon A. Myoclonus and epilepsy in childhood: 1996 Royaumont meeting. *Epilepsy Res* 1998; 30: 91-106.
2. Janz D, Christian W. Impulsive-Petit mal. *Nervenheilk* 1957; 176: 346-86.
3. Doose H. Epilepsien im Kindes- und Jugendalter (11. Auflage). Flensburg: Desitin Arzneimittel, 1998.
4. Doose H, Gerken H, Morstmann T, Völtzke. Centrencephalic myoclonic-astatic petit mal. *Neuropediatrics* 1970; 2: 59-78.
5. Doose H. Myoclonic astatic epilepsy of early childhood. In: Roger J, Bureau M, Dravet C, Dreifuss F, Perret A, Wolf P, eds. *Epileptic syndromes in infancy, childhood and adolescence (2nd edition)*. London, Paris, Rome: John Libbey, 1992: 103-14.
6. Aicardi J. Myoclonic epilepsies difficult to classify as either Lennox-Gastaut or myoclonic-astatic epilepsy. In: Wallace S, ed. *Epilepsy in children*. London: Chapman and Hall, 1995: 271-3.
7. Berkovic SF, Andermann F, Andermann E, Gloor P. Concepts of absence epilepsies: discrete syndromes or biological continuum? *Neurology* 1987; 37: 993-1000.
8. Kaminska A, Ickowicz A, Plouin P, Bru MF, Dellatolas G, Dulac O. Delineation of cryptogenic Lennox-Gastaut syndrome and myoclonic astatic epilepsy using multiple correspondence analysis. *Epilepsy Res* 1999; 36: 15-29.

9. Benzecri JP. *Handbook of correspondance analysis*. New York: Dekker, 1992.
10. Kieffer-Renaux V, Kaminska A, Dulac O. Cognitive deterioration in Lennox-Gastaut syndrome and Doose epilepsy. In: Jambaqué I, Lassonde M, Dulac O, eds. *Neuropsychology of childhood epilepsy*. New York: Kluwer Academic-Plenum Publisher, 2001: 185-90.
11. Perucca E, Gram L, Avanzini G, Dulac O. Antiepileptic drugs as a cause of worsening seizures. *Epilepsia* 1998; 39: 5-17.
12. Lortie A, Chiron C, Mumford J, Dulac O. The potential for increasing seizure frequency, relapse, and appearance of new seizure types with vigabatrin. *Neurology* 1993; 43 (11 Suppl 5): S24-7.
13. Kaminska A. New antiepileptic drugs in childhood epilepsies: indications and limits. *Epileptic Disord* 2001; 3 (Spec no 2): SI37-46.
14. Wheless JW. Use of topiramate in childhood generalized seizure disorders. *J Child Neurol* 2000; 15 (Suppl 1): S7-13.
15. Claes L, Del-Favero J, Ceulemans B, Lagae L, Van Broeckhoven C, De Jonghe P. De novo mutations in the sodium-channel gene SCN1A cause severe myoclonic epilepsy of infancy. *Am J Hum Genet* 2001; 68: 1327-32.

Prognosis of severe myoclonic epilepsy in infancy (Dravet syndrome)

Catherine Chiron

Most severe forms of infantile myoclonic epilepsy fall into the category of severe myoclonic epilepsy in infancy (SMEI) or Dravet syndrome, the topic of this chapter. Other severe infantile epilepsies with myoclonia are very rare and do not constitute identifiable populations with the exception of specific metabolic disorders such as ceroid lipofuscinosis, Menkes disease, pyridoxine-dependency, Alpers disease and some mitochondriopathies. Any cerebral lesion and Angelman syndrome may also occasionally induce epileptic myoclonia during infancy. Dalla Bernardina identified a particular form in infants with non-progressive encephalopathy who experience myoclonic status epilepticus that may go unrecognized and which can be so prolonged that it may simulate a progressive encephalopathy [1].

Dravet syndrome is a remarkably homogeneous syndrome, nosologically and etiologically. Its electroclinical pattern is stereotyped enough to permit an early and accurate diagnosis in most cases, and a genetic mutation of sodium channel has recently been identified. Prognosis is also unfortunately stereotyped: it is invariably poor. Among severe childhood epilepsies, Dravet syndrome is one of the most malignant epilepsy syndromes reported in the syndromic classification of the International League Against Epilepsy [2]. Dravet syndrome is probably the only epilepsy syndrome in which 100% of the patients experience an unfavorable outcome, for seizures as well as for cognition. This pattern is all the more remarkable as all patients appear to have normal mental development before the first seizures occur. Therefore, the patients undergo a process of deterioration. Studying the underlying mechanisms of this disorder will provide the only hope for improving what is currently a catastrophic outcome.

Description of the syndrome

Dravet syndrome is, along with infantile spasms, the most frequent and the most severe epilepsy syndrome with generalized seizures that occur during the first year of life. Its exact incidence is not known but has been estimated to be about 1/40 000 in the general population [3]. It represents about 3% of the infantile epilepsies referred to a representative epilepsy center [4].

Characteristics of the syndrome have been described for the first time by Dravet *et al.* in Marseille [5, 6] and included in the syndromic classification of the International League against Epilepsy [2]. The first seizures always occur during the first year of life, between 2 and 9 months of age. They are convulsive tonic-clonic or clonic seizures, either generalized or affecting alternatively each side of the body. The rare seizures recorded at this age consisted in discharges of rapid spikes which could be generalized, unilateral hemispheric, or even multifocal from onset. The initial seizures are often prolonged. Most patients experience recurrent convulsive status epilepticus lasting over 30 minutes and even over one hour. A postictal unilateral deficit may be the only signature of a hemispheric seizure. This deficit may last anywhere from a few minutes to a few hours. Seizures are often provoked by fever, although only a moderate increase of the temperature may be observed. As a result and depending on the vaccination schedule, more than half of the children with SMEI have their first seizure after a DPT vaccination [7]. Afebrile seizures also occur.

Children with SMEI typically have a normal perinatal history. In the initial stages of the disorder, they present with normal psychomotor development, normal neurological examination and normal EEG between seizures. Structural neuroimaging (either CT scan or MRI), is also normal. These characteristics are similar to those seen in children with idiopathic generalized epilepsy.

The pattern changes, however, from the second year on. Tonic-clonic or clonic seizures persist with the same characteristics, but additional seizure types usually occur. These include massive or parcellar myoclonia or both, atypical absences, and partial seizures. Generalized nonconvulsive status with prolonged obtundation and erratic myoclonia may appear. Generalized spike and waves (SW) or polySW are observed during sleep and massive myoclonia while background activity becomes slow during the awake state. Photosensitivity is frequent. Patients develop ataxia, hyperactivity and mental retardation. The MRI remains normal although in adolescents, diffuse and nonspecific cortico-subcortical atrophy may be observed.

Because of the remarkably stereotyped clinical characteristics at onset, diagnosing SMEI is usually feasible early in the course of the disorder. The diagnosis should be suspected in any infant experiencing recurrent prolonged seizures with only moderate fever and can usually be confirmed as soon as afebrile seizures occur. Based on these criteria, SMEI can be diagnosed before the age of 1 year in more than 75% of the cases [8, 9]. Later on, the occurrence of atypical absences or complex partial seizures strongly supports the diagnosis of SMEI even though myoclonia may not yet be evident. Finally, most cases are diagnosed before the age of 3 years.

SMEI is easy to distinguish from febrile convulsions. The early age of onset, the long lasting seizures, the postictal deficits, the moderate increase of temperature, and the occurrence of afebrile seizures are useful in distinguishing between the two syndromes. One feature alone should be enough to raise sufficient suspicion of SMEI to justify initiation of antiepileptic treatment starting with the first febrile seizure. The differential diagnosis between SMEI and cryptogenic localization related epilepsy is perhaps the most difficult. Repeat focal seizures and persisting spike focus are the earliest and most reliable signs of localization related epilepsy, whereas alternating seizures, generalized myoclonus, and/or spike waves appear before the end of the 1st year in most infants with severe myoclonic epilepsy [9].

The genetic component of Dravet syndrome has been suspected for a long time. Observations of monozygotic twins have supported this concept [10]. SMEI was included in the cohort of severe idiopathic generalized epilepsy with generalized tonic-clonic seizures isolated by Doose because of its high probability to be genetically determined [11]. Patients with SMEI have a significantly increased incidence of febrile convulsions and idiopathic generalized epilepsy in their relatives [12]. Families have been described in which cases of both SMEI and GEFS+ (generalized epilepsy with febrile seizures plus, a form of epilepsy with afebrile generalized tonic-clonic seizures and febrile seizures persisting beyond six years of age) have occurred. GEFS+ is associated with molecular defects in three sodium channel subunit genes [13, 14]. Molecular defects of one of these genes, SCN1A, have been recently identified in seven patients with SMEI. They are severe truncation mutations arising de novo [15]. The authors therefore suggest that SMEI could be the most severe phenotype in the GEFS+ spectrum [16].

Prognosis

All authors agree that Dravet syndrome carries a very poor prognosis. SMEI is considered to be a type of epileptic encephalopathy, intractable epilepsy, as well as a form of catastrophic epilepsy [17-19]. Relatively few studies, however, have focused on long-term outcome of patients with SMEI.

Epilepsy prognosis

SMEI is one of the few epilepsy syndromes whose the refractoriness is truly predictable [17]. Among the 63 cases of Dravet's series, of those followed through adulthood, none was seizure free [6]. Similar results were obtained in a series of 14 patients followed for up to 16 years with a mean of 10 years [20]. During the follow up, each patient exhibited three or four different types of seizures, but the pattern of appearance and disappearance of each seizure type varied considerably among the patients. Tonic-clonic convulsions, either generalized or unilateral, were seen most consistently through the entire course and continued to the end of follow up in 11 patients (79%). On the other hand, myoclonic seizures, complex partial seizures, and atypical absences often disappeared and reappeared repeatedly throughout the course of the disorder. Similar findings were obtained in another Japanese series of 10 patients, aged 2-11 years at the last evaluation. No patient was seizure free. Generalized tonic-clonic seizures, partial seizures, and status epilepticus were all still present; however, myoclonic seizures and atypical absences had diminished in conjunction with a clear-cut decrease in generalized abnormalities on the EEG in 4 cases older than seven years [21].

Prognosis seems to be better in patients who have only generalized tonic-clonic (GTC) seizures without the occurrence of myoclonia as described by the Japanese authors [22]; however, this epilepsy probably represents a syndrome different from SMEI. The same applies to the 50 patients included in Doose's series, who had GTC seizures alone of whom 11% were seizure free for at least 2 years at final examination [11]. Such patients represented 15% of the 20 children who met diagnosis criteria for SMEI during the first year of life in a retrospective French pediatric series [8].

Generalized nonconvulsive status epilepticus has also been described as part of Dravet syndrome. This consists of long-lasting atypical absences or "obtundation status" and is often associated with erratic myoclonia in the context of a myoclonic status. Diagnosis of such status epilepticus depends on the ictal EEG demonstrating diffuse slow waves with irregular spikes and sometimes generalized spikes, polyspikes and spike and waves corresponding to myoclonia. In a personal series of 29 myoclonic epilepsies with generalized nonconvulsive status, four patients presented with Dravet syndrome, four with nonprogressive encephalopathy and 21 with myoclono-astatic epilepsy. Nonconvulsive status epilepticus occurred the latest in SMEI (at an average of 7 years) compared to myoclonic-astatic epilepsy (4 years) and nonprogressive encephalopathy (9 months). Cumulative duration of status was higher in SMEI (51 months) than in myoclonic-astatic epilepsy (26 months).

Simple as well as complex partial seizures may also occur in 40% and 75% (respectively) of patients with SMEI. Intermittent focal sharp waves occurred in 26% of Dooses's series [11]. A case of partial nonconvulsive status has even been reported. Such a partial component is multifocal and is rarely observed from the onset of SMEI when most features tend to be either generalized or unilateral (6% of partial seizures at onset in Dravet's series).

Sudden death and SUDEP (unexplained sudden death) seem to be especially high in SMEI, although they did not appear in most epidemiological studies, probably because of the low incidence of this epilepsy syndrome in the population [23]. Dravet reported 10 cases of death including 2 SUDEP among 63 patients [6]. The number of SUDEP could have been underestimated in this series, particularly in adults. In a therapeutic trial of 41 patients with SMEI, 2 had SUDEP [24]. Doose reports a mortality rate of 9% among 101 children with severe idiopathic generalized epilepsy in infancy with GTC seizures, an entity that includes SMEI [11].

Cognitive outcomes

All patients with SMEI ultimately experience severe cognitive delays. In a series of 20 children with SMEI who underwent a neuropsychological evaluation in Centre Saint Paul in Marseille, the developmental quotient (DQ) was between 20 and 40 in the 11 patients who were older than six years at the time of testing *(figure 1)* [25]. There was global retardation involving motor, linguistic and visual abilities. In as far as visuo-constructive functions were concerned, the global mode of organizing visual information was more affected than the sequential approach to construction. The authors suggested that the right

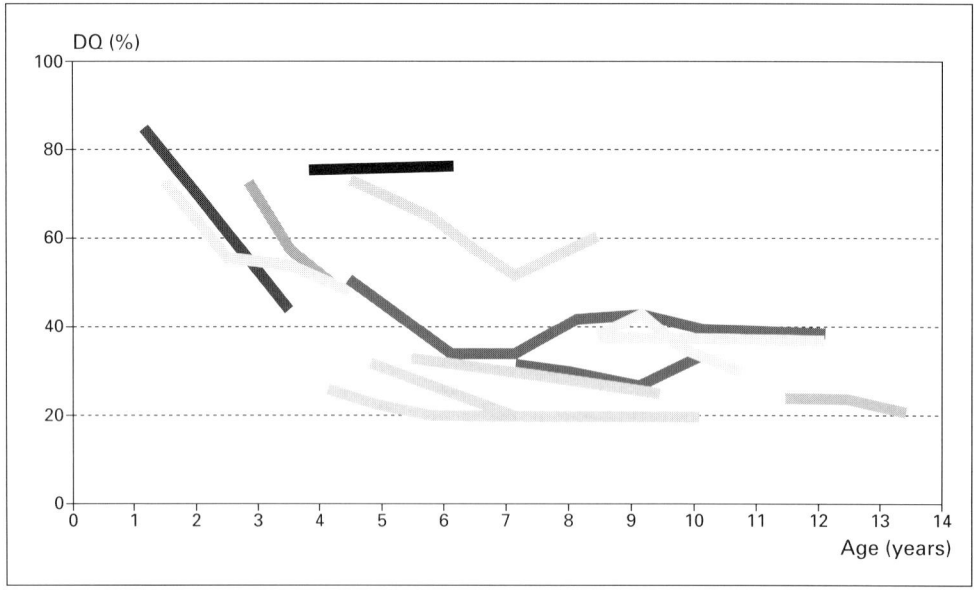

Figure 1. SMEI: Neuropsychological Data First Evaluation (N = 20)
Each line represents the developmental quotient (DQ) of each patient at the first evaluation.
DQ was in normal range before 3 years of age and was dramatically decreased after 3.

hemisphere was functionally more impaired than the left. In addition, all the patients presented with behavioral disorders consisting of hyperkinesia, psychotic and sometimes autistic traits. By contrast, the 4 patients who were under two years of age at the time they were tested had a mean DQ of 75. Two of these children had a DQ of 85 at 11 and 18 months. There was a clear slowing down starting at the end of the second year, and DQ remained relatively stable after the age of 4 years *(figure 2)*. The age of onset of deterioration and its magnitude was related to the frequency and the duration of seizures. The 3 patients with the best cognitive development corresponded either to cases with milder epilepsy or who experienced a marked decrease in convulsive seizures later on.

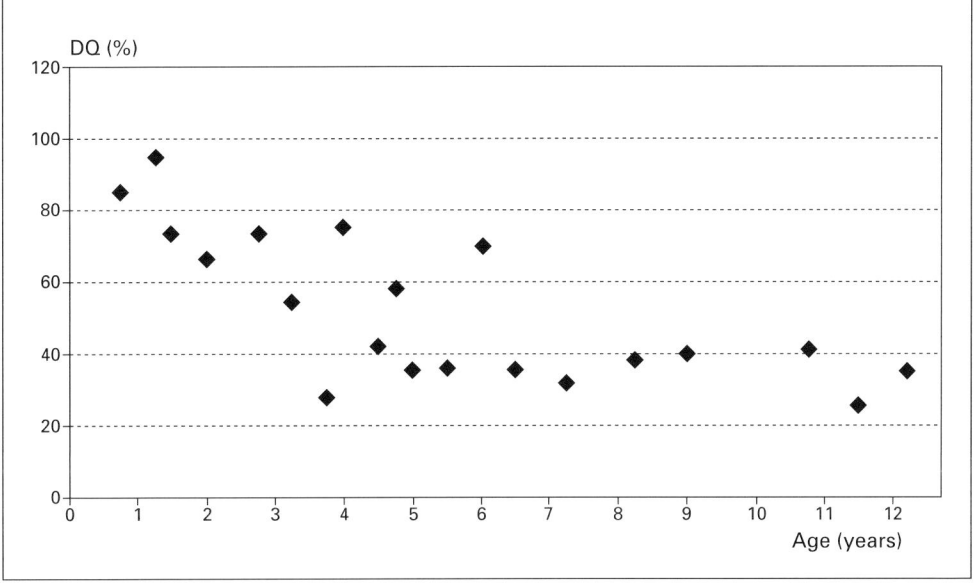

Figure 2. SMEI: Neuropsychological Data Follow up (N = 13)
Each point represents the course of the developmental quotient (DQ)
in the 13 patients in whom it was longitudinally assessed.
It dramatically decreased between 1 and 3-4 years of age and it remained low from the age of 4 years
(except for the 2 patients who had experienced the less numerous prolonged seizures in infancy).

In a personal series, neuropsychological evaluation and functional cerebral imaging using SPECT (Single Photon Emission Computed Tomography) and 133-Xenon were performed at the same time in 10 cases of SMEI with ages ranging from 6 months to 13 years [26]. Mental status was normal in the 2 youngest patients whereas the others had global mental retardation with a mean DQ of 53: there was a significant negative correlation between DQ and age *(figure 3)*. Mean cerebral blood flow (mCBF) (which reflects the neuronal cortical function) was positively correlated with DQ *(figure 4)*. Predominant troubles involved language (globally in 1, limited to the articulation of speech in 3). Some patients also had praxic disorders (dyspraxia in 1, difficulties in graphism in 1, visuospatial disability in 1). Most children exhibited behavioral disorders (hyperkinesia in 3, psychotic tendencies in 4). Focal hypoperfused areas were detected on SPECT in all patients but the 2 youngest. Their distribution was patchy but corresponded to the main neuropsychological troubles observed: frontal or Broca's areas were hypoperfused in the four patients with language disorders, temporo-occipital area in 2 of the 3 patients with visuopraxic disorders, and frontal area in the 3 psychotic patients.

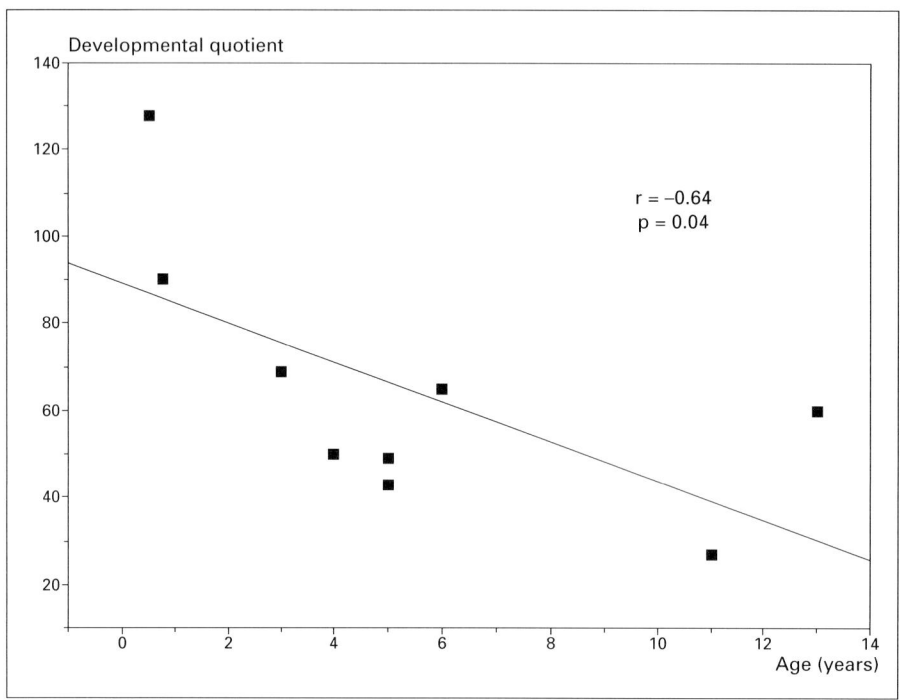

Figure 3. SMEI: relationship between DQ and age

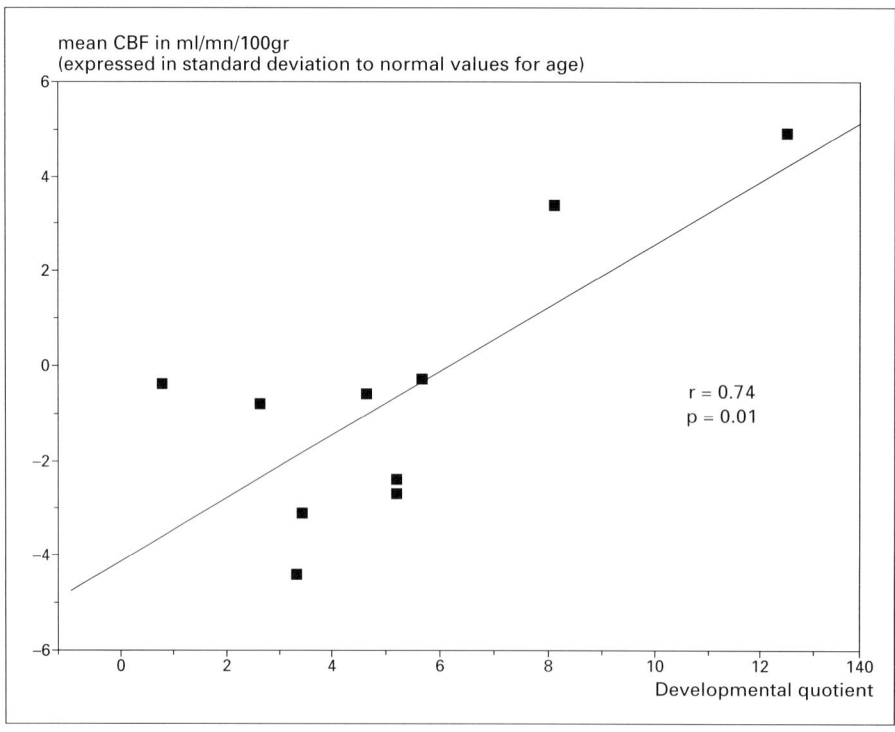

Figure 4. SMEI: relationship between mean Cerebral Blood Flow and DQ

Response to treatment

Most authors agree about the disappointing response to the conventional antiepileptic drugs (AEDs). Valproate and benzodiazepines may decrease the frequency and the duration of afebrile convulsive seizures, but the effect is only moderate. Some investigators associate phenobarbital, phenytoin or ethosuximide with poor results [6].

Paradoxically, some AEDs can aggravate seizures in SMEI. Lamotrigine induced worsening in 80% of 20 patients recruited in 3 epilepsy centers [27]. GTC seizures were more often exacerbated (40%) compared to myoclonic seizures (33%). Clear-cut worsening appeared within 3 months in most patients but was insidious in some, resulting in stopping lamotrigine after a mean of 14 months treatment. Improvement followed withdrawal in 95% of cases. Potential aggravation of seizures was also described with carbamazepine and vigabatrin [28].

In a personal series of 46 patients, 8 of 12 who received lamotrigine experienced a worsening of their seizures. Nine of 14 who received vigabatrin and and 17 of 28 who received carbamazepine also experienced an exacerbation of their seizures [29]. Six (26% of those having received this drug) also exhibited worsening after having received intravenous phenobarbital for convulsive status epilepticus and resulting in intoxication in 2 because of a mistake in doses administered; the two developed global and definitive cerebral atrophy with dramatic neurological worsening. Intravenous barbiturates seem inappropriate in status epilepticus of SMEI. Indeed, they recently proved to be ineffective and occasionally worsened seizures in patients with refractory epilepsy [30].

Occasional improvements of myoclonia were reported using Zonisamide [31]; our initial experiences with the ketogenic diet and vagal nerve stimulation have been disappointing.

By contrast, two new drugs could be helpful for treating patients with Dravet syndrome, stiripentol and topiramate. Stiripentol (STP) is a new antiepileptic drug (AED) whose mechanism of action mainly lies on pharmacokinetic interactions with other antiepileptic drugs. STP inhibits the cytochrome P450 system in the liver, resulting in an increased plasma concentration of concomitant AEDs, particularly clobazam [24]. The efficacy and tolerability of STP as an add-on therapy in children were first assessed on more than 200 patients with refractory epilepsy receiving STP in an open add-on trial [32]. Among the 20 children with SMEI entered in the trial, 10 experienced more than a 50% decrease in seizure frequency when STP was used in combination with valproate and clobazam. To confirm these results, 41 children with SMEI were included in a randomized placebo-controlled trial of stiripentol added to valproate and clobazam [24]. Fifteen (71%) patients were responders for tonic-clonic seizures on stiripentol (including nine who became seizure free) whereas there was only one partial responder (5%) on placebo. The percentage of change from baseline was higher on stiripentol (- 69%) than on placebo (+ 7%), p < 0.0001. 21 patients on stiripentol had moderate side-effects (drowsiness, loss of appetite) compared with eight on placebo, but side-effects disappeared when the dose of the other drug was decreased in 12 of the 21 cases. This controlled trial therefore demonstrated the short-term efficacy of add-on stiripentol in children with SMEI. To study its long term efficacy and to clarify its usefulness in infants, we retrospectively studied our exhaustive cohort of patients with SMEI treated with STP in combination with valproate and clobazam [29]. Among the 46 patients, none remained seizure free after a median follow up of three years; however, the frequency and the duration of seizures was significantly reduced (p < 0.001) as was the number of episodes of convulsive status epilepticus. Ten patients were dramatically improved (seizures significantly decreased in number [p = 0.002] and duration [p = 0.002] and status disappeared), 20 were moderately improved (seizures significantly decreased in duration [p = 0.001] and status epilepticus was less frequent), 4 had no response and the efficacy could not be evaluated in 12 mainly because of adverse events. Efficacy was better in the youngest patients. The most frequent adverse events were loss of appetite and loss of weight. These effects could be so severe in patients over 12 years that the stiripentol dosage could not be increased to 50 mg/kg/j. Stiripentol therefore maintains its efficacy at long term in children with SMEI. It should be introduced in polypharmacy as early as possible in order to prevent convulsive status epilepticus.

Topiramate has not been as extensively studied in SMEI. One open study included 18 patients in whom topiramate was administered as an add-on regimen to a maximum of 6-8 mg/kg/d [33]. After a mean of 11 months, 10 patients (56%) were considered to have responded favorably including three who were seizure free. Side-effects were observed in nine. These side effects were generally mild and transient, and related to rapid dosage titration. In the French and Italian experience, TPM was administered in 27 children with SMEI at a mean age of 11 years and added to valproate in 22, to benzodiazepines in 23, to stiripentol in 11 (unpublished data). Eighty-five percent were responders for GTC seizures, including five who became seizure free, at a dose over 3 mg/kg/d. As a result, behavior improved in six patients. Tolerability was acceptable, although 8 patients lost weight due to loss of appetite.

Conclusion

Dravet syndrome carries a very well-defined prognosis as it is characterized by an early deterioration followed by stagnation, in patients who were apparently normal before the onset of the first seizures. Although mental retardation is common in epileptic children (about 25%), mental deterioration is relatively rare (about 2% in a general epilepsy center) [34]. It can result from two mechanisms: (1) as the result of generalized and continuous EEG abnormalities which interfere with the development of specific cognitive functions at specific ages as is the case with infantile spasms, Lennox-Gastaut syndrome or continuous spike-waves during slow sleep, the so called epileptic encephalopathies; (2) as the sequelae of severe seizures. Dravet syndrome appears to involve the second mechanism. Deterioration can be objectively demonstrated through neuropsychological testing and confirmed by functional imaging and EEG. More than the absolute frequency or duration of seizures during the whole course, the frequency and long duration of seizures at the onset appears to play a key role in the poor outcome of this syndromes. AEDs that prove to affect these parameters could therefore improve not only the seizures but also the cognitive prognosis and should be administered as soon as the diagnosis is suspected, that is in the first year of life for most cases. The numerous episodes of status epilepticus experienced by these patients starting in the first year of life result in a rapid and global mental deterioration which then plateaus after a few years. The notion that there is a metabolic disorder underlying Dravet syndrome is therefore unlikely. Of note, there is no evidence of hippocampal atrophy in any patient, although Dravet syndrome often presents with prolonged febrile seizures during infancy. Synaptic reorganization due to excessive plasticity of cortical pathways at such an early stage of development is more likely to contribute to the persistence and refractoriness of seizures as well as the mental deterioration. Animal models would be useful for studying these neurobiological mechanisms. Using intact hippocampal structures from immature rats (1 to 12 postnatal days) maintained in a low magnesium environment, we recently obtained a promising model that demonstrated most of the major characteristics of seizures of severe infantile epilepsy in humans [35].

Aknowledgements

We thank Dr Marcus Wolf who permitted us to reproduce his data *(figures 1 and 2)* presented at the 24th International Epilepsy Congress in Buenos Aires in 2001 and reported as an abstract in Epilepsia 2001, 42, S61.

References

1. Dalla BB, Fontana E, Sgro V, Colamaria V, Elia M. Myoclonic epilepsy ("myoclonic status epilepticus") in the nonprogressive encephalopathies. In: Roger J, Bureau M, Dravet C, Dreifuss FE, Perret A, Wolf P, eds. *Epileptic syndromes in infancy, children and adolescence (2nd edition)*. London: John Libbey & Company Ltd, 1992: 89-96.
2. Proposal for revised classification of epilepsies and epileptic syndromes. Commission on Classification and Terminology of the International League Against Epilepsy. *Epilepsia* 1989; 30: 389-99.
3. Hurst DL. Epidemiology of severe myoclonic epilepsy of infancy. *Epilepsia* 1990; 31: 397-400.
4. Caraballo R, Cersosimo R, Galicchio S, Fejerman N. Epilepsies during the first year of life. *Rev Neurol* 1997; 25: 1521-4.
5. Dravet C, Roger J, Bureau M, Dalla BB. Myoclonic epilepsies in childhood. In: Akimoto H, ed. *Advances in epileptology, the XIIIth EIS*. New York: Raven Press, 1982: 135-40.
6. Dravet C, Bureau M, Guerrini R, Giraud N, Roger J. Severe myoclonic epilepsy in infants. In: Roger J, Bureau M, Dravet C, Dreifuss FE, Perret A, Wolf P, eds. *Epileptic syndromes in infancy, children and adolescence (2nd edition)*. London: John Libbey & Company Ltd, 1992: 75-88.
7. Nieto-Barrera M, Lillo MM, Rodriguez-Collado C, Candau R, Correa A. Severe myoclonic epilepsy in childhood. Epidemiologic analytical study. *Rev Neurol* 2000; 30: 620-4.
8. Yakoub M, Dulac O, Jambaque I, Chiron C, Plouin P. Early diagnosis of severe myoclonic epilepsy in infancy. *Brain Dev* 1992; 14: 299-303.
9. Sarisjulis N, Gamboni B, Plouin P, Kaminska A, Dulac O. Diagnosing idiopathic/cryptogenic epilepsy syndromes in infancy. *Arch Dis Child* 2000; 82: 226-30.
10. Fujiwara T, Watanabe M, Takahashi Y, Higashi T, Yagi K, Seino M. Long-term course of childhood epilepsy with intractable grand mal seizures. *Jpn J Psychiatry Neurol* 1992; 46: 297-302.
11. Doose H, Lunau H, Castiglione E, Waltz S. Severe idiopathic generalized epilepsy of infancy with generalized tonic-clonic seizures. *Neuropediatrics* 1998; 29: 229-38.
12. Benlounis A, Nabbout R, Feingold J, *et al*. Genetic predisposition to severe myoclonic epilepsy in infancy. *Epilepsia* 2001; 42: 204-9.
13. Escayg A, MacDonald BT, Meisler MH, *et al*. Mutations of SCN1A, encoding a neuronal sodium channel, in two families with GEFS+2. *Nat Genet* 2000; 24: 343-5.
14. Sugawara T, Tsurubuchi Y, Agarwala KL, *et al*. A missense mutation of the Na+ channel alpha II subunit gene Na(v)1.2 in a patient with febrile and afebrile seizures causes channel dysfunction. *Proc Natl Acad Sci USA* 2001; 98: 6384-9.
15. Claes L, Del Favero J, Ceulemans B, Lagae L, Van Broeckhoven C, De Jonghe P. De novo mutations in the sodium-channel gene SCN1A cause severe myoclonic epilepsy of infancy. *Am J Hum Genet* 2001; 68: 1327-32.
16. Singh R, Andermann E, Whitehouse WP, *et al*. Severe myoclonic epilepsy of infancy: extended spectrum of GEFS+? *Epilepsia* 2001; 42: 837-44.
17. Arroyo S, Brodie MJ, Avanzini G, *et al*. Is refractory epilepsy preventable? *Epilepsia* 2002; 43: 437-44.
18. Dulac O. Epileptic encephalopathy. *Epilepsia* 2001; 42 (Suppl 3): 23-6.
19. Shields WD. Catastrophic epilepsy in childhood. *Epilepsia* 2000; 41 (Suppl 2): S2-S6.
20. Ohki T, Watanabe K, Negoro T, *et al*. Severe myoclonic epilepsy in infancy: evolution of seizures. *Seizure* 1997; 6: 219-24.
21. Wang PJ, Fan PC, Lee WT, Young C, Huang CC, Shen YZ. Severe myoclonic epilepsy in infancy: evolution of electroencephalographic and clinical features. *Zhonghua Min Guo Xiao Er Ke Yi Xue Hui Za Zhi* 1996; 37: 428-32.
22. Kanazawa O. Refractory grand mal seizures with onset during infancy including severe myoclonic epilepsy in infancy. *Brain Dev* 2001; 23: 749-56.

23. Camfield CS, Camfield PR, Veugelers PJ. Death in children with epilepsy: a population-based study. *Lancet* 2002; 359: 1891-5.
24. Chiron C, Marchand MC, Tran A, *et al.* Stiripentol in severe myoclonic epilepsy in infancy: a randomised placebo-controlled syndrome-dedicated trial. STICLO study group. *Lancet* 2000; 356: 1638-42.
25. Casse-Perrot C, Wolf M, Dravet C. Neuropsychological aspects of severe myoclonic epilepsy in infancy. In: Jambaque I, Lassonde M, Dulac O, eds. *Neuropsychology of childhood epilepsy.* New York: Kluwer Academic/Plenum Publishers, 2001: 131-40.
26. Dulac O, Plouin P, Shewmon A. Myoclonus and epilepsy in childhood: 1996 Royaumont meeting. *Epilepsy Res* 1998; 30: 91-106.
27. Guerrini R, Dravet C, Genton P, Belmonte A, Kaminska A, Dulac O. Lamotrigine and seizure aggravation in severe myoclonic epilepsy. *Epilepsia* 1998; 39: 508-12.
28. Lortie A, Chiron C, Mumford J, Dulac O. The potential for increasing seizure frequency, relapse, and appearance of new seizure types with vigabatrin. *Neurology* 1993; 43: S24-S7.
29. Nguyen Thanh T, Chiron C, Dellatolas G, Rey E, Pons G, Vincent J, Dulac O. Long term efficacy and tolerability of stiripentol in severe myoclonic epilepsy of infancy (Dravet syndrome). *Arch Ped* (in press).
30. Rintala A, Saukkonen A, Remes M, Uhari M. Efficcay of five days barbiturate anesthesia in the treatment of intractable epilepsies in children. *Epilepsia* 1999; 40: 1775-9.
31. Wallace SJ. Myoclonus and epilepsy in childhood: a review of treatment with valproate, ethosuximide, lamotrigine and zonisamide. *Epilepsy Res* 1998; 29: 147-54.
32. Perez J, Chiron C, Musial C, *et al.* Stiripentol: efficacy and tolerability in children with epilepsy. *Epilepsia* 1999; 40: 1618-26.
33. Nieto-Barrera M, Candau R, Nieto-Jimenez M, Correa A, del Portal LR. Topiramate in the treatment of severe myoclonic epilepsy in infancy. *Seizure* 2000; 9: 590-4.
34. Oka E, Sanada S, Asano T, Ishida T. Mental deterioration in childhood epilepsy. *Acta Med Okayama* 1997; 51: 173-8.
35. Quilichini PP, Diabira D, Chiron C, Ben-Ari Y, Gozlan H. A persistent epileptiform activity induced by the activation of NMDA receptors in intact immature brain structures. *Eur J Neurosci* 2002; 16: 850-60.

Prognosis of idiopathic absence epilepsies

Jérôme Guiwer, Maria Paula Valenti, Ahmed Bourazza, Édouard Hirsch, Pierre Loiseau

Definitions

In the international classification of epilepsies [1] absence epilepsies are included in idiopathic generalized epilepsies and defined as follows:

Chilhood absence epilepsy (CAE)

Pyknolepsy occurs in children of school age (peak manifestation age 6-7 years); with a strong genetic predisposition; in otherwise normal children, more frequently in girls than in boys; with very frequent (several to many per day) absences; absence seizures associated in the EEG with a bilateral, synchronous symmetrical spike-waves, usually 3 Hz on a normal background activity; during adolescence, generalized tonic-clonic seizures often develop. Otherwise, absence seizures may remit or, more rarely, persist as the only seizure type [1].

Juvenile absence epilepsy (JAE)

It begins in a different age range (peak at 12 to 13 years), but this feature is not sufficient, because JAE may start before 10 years of age, and CAE may start in teenagers [3]. Less frequent absence seizures (AS) (less than 10 per day) and generalized tonic-clonic seizures as a presenting seizure are important clues. EEG is misleading, because of 3-Hz SW discharges in early JAE, and the classical 4-Hz SW discharges recorded later.

Absence seizures in juvenile myoclonic epilepsy (JME)

In a cohort of 81 children diagnosed as CAE in the province of Nova Scotia between 1977 and 1985, 15 per cent were considered in 1994-1995 to have progressed to JME [4].

Absence seizures may appear simultaneously with myoclonic jerks but also one to nine years before the myoclonus, i.e. in children [5-7]. When, later, myoclonia begin, diagnosis is not CAE evolving to JME, but JME with AS as the presenting seizure.

Myoclonic absences

AS characterized clinically by rhythmic jerks of the proximal muscles of the upper limbs are a rather rare condition. They are usually associated with impaired mental development and are resistant to treatment. They have been designated as an epilepsy syndrome. Its homogeneity is not clear: children otherwise fitting all CAE criteria have AS with sustained myoclonic jerks [8].

Others syndromes related to childhood absence epilepsy

Absence epilepsy of early childhood

A syndrome of absence epilepsy of early childhood was proposed in the sixties. It was characterized by an onset before the age of 5 years, possible occurrence, at the onset or later, of GTCS and/or myoclonic-astatic seizures, irregular 2-3 Hz SW discharges on the EEG, and an often unfavorable prognosis. Later, its heterogeneity was identified [9]. Age at onset artificially covers various idiopathic generalized epilepsies with a polygenic inheritance. Absence epilepsies of early childhood includes early onset CAE and other absence epilepsies in which more important environmental factors explain the frequency of GTCS and a less favorable outcome. The "intermediate petit mal" described by the Bologna school [10] probably corresponds to this condition.

Eyelid myoclonia with absences (Jeavons' syndrome)

The syndrome of eyelid myoclonia with absences was first described by Jeavons in 1977 as a form of photosensitive epilepsy [11] and was confirmed by other investigators [12]. It is considered more a myoclonic than an absence syndrome [13]. The following definition was proposed by Panayiotopoulos [7]. Eyelid myoclonia with absences is manifested with frequent typical absences with onset earlier than CAE (2-5 years). AS are brief (3-6 s), occur after eye-closure and demonstrate marked rhythmic eyelid myoclonias consisting of fast jerks of the eyelids (clearly different from the eyelid blinking-like, random or rare unsustained rhythmic movements of CAE) and retropulsion of the eyeballs with an associated tonic component of the involved muscles. Impairment of consciousnes may be mild and certainly not as severe as in CAE and JAE. AS do not occur without eyelid myoclonia. EEG ictal manifestations consist mainly of 3-5 generalised polyspike and slow-wave discharges, which are more likely to be induced by eye-closure in an illuminated room (total darkness abolishes the eye-closure abnormalities). All patients are highly photosensitive and self-induction may occur in some patients. GTCS, induced by flickering lights or other seizure precipitants, are probably inevitable in all patients. They are usually infrequent with appropriate medication. Eyelid myoclonia with absences is resistant to treatment and does not remit in adulthood. AS may become less frequent with age, and mild eyelid myoclonia may exist without any impairment of consciousness, as well as without EEG discharge. Eye-closure abnormalities may persist without demonstrable photosensitivity [14]. Family history of epilepsy is common with a high concordance for the syndrome.

Perioral myoclonia with absences

Panayiotopoulos reported that AS associated with marked perioral myoclonia may constitute a new epilepsy syndrome which he defined as follows: "Perioral myoclonus with absences is a syndrome of idiopathic generalized epilepsy with onset in childhood or adolescence, characterized by frequent typical absences with variable severity of impairment of consciousness and ictal localized rhythmic myoclonus of the perioral facial muscles (lip myoclonus) or occasionally of the masticatory muscles (jaw myoclonus)" [15]. AS duration is usually brief, ranging from 2 to 10 seconds. Ictal EEG shows generalized discharges of spikes, more often irregular polyspikes and slow waves at 3-5 Hz. They are not associated with eye-closure and photosensitivity. Absence status is not rare. GTCS always occur either early or several years after the onset of AS; they are usually heralded by clusters of AS or absence status and may be infrequent. The syndrome is lifelong and often resistant to medication. A family history of epilepsy is common. Lips and chin myoclonia are by themselves insufficient to justify a syndromic individualization, because of a possible moderate myoclonic component in CAE and JAE [8].

However, there is still a debate on classification and concepts of absence epilepsies: discrete syndromes or biological continuum? [16]. In 2001, the ILAE Task Force [17] proposed to individualize three syndromes with absence seizures in idiopathic generalized epilepsies: Childhood absence epilepsy, Epilepsy with myoclonic absences, Idiopathic generalized epilepsies with variable phenotypes (Juvenile absence epilepsy, Juvenile myoclonic epilepsy). Absence epilepsy of early childhood, Eyelid myoclonia with absences (Jeavons' syndrome), Perioral myoclonia with absences were not recognized as new epileptic syndrome. The Task Force views the development of specific classification as a continuing work in progress, so new epileptic syndrome recognized as specific entity could emerge in the future.

Prognosis

Outcome of epilepsy may be expressed as remission of seizures, with or with out medication; evolution to one seizure type to another; or as intellectual, social, or vocational outcome. A number of patients become seizure free during treatment with antiepileptic drugs and remain so after their discontinuation. A meta-analysis of studies on absence was performed in 1996 [18] to ascertain whether the outcome of abence epilepsies can be stated unequivocally. 23 study cohorts with a total of 2 303 patients were included. Remission rates range from 0,21 to 0,89. The authors concluded that the remission rated differed substantially due to heterogeneity between the studies in inclusion criteria, methods, follow up length, and outcome definitions. One half of the patients developed generalized tonic-clonic seizures in the course of the disease. The proportion seizure free was 0,78 for patients with absence seizures only, and 0,35 for those who developed tonic-clonic seizures. The authors concluded as well that early prediction of outcome in patients who presents with absence seizures cannot be provided with certainty.

The evidence present in the literature is inconclusive concerning evolution and prognosis of CAE. A first reason is poor case classification. Heterogenous conditions have been encompassed within "petit mal" and AS belong to several epileptic syndromes. Thus prognosis has been based on a symptom rather than a syndromic diagnosis. Generally speaking, retrospective studies in adults do not allow a reliable outcome estimate of childhood epilepsies because of lack of accurate initial data. As all AS beginning in childhood do not belong to CAE, their persistence in adulthood must be considered with reservations. For instance, in 26 adults with onset of typical AS when aged 2-10 years AS persisted in adulthood, and they had also GTCS; retrospectively, only one patient would have been classified as having CAE if strict syndrome criteria had been applied [19]. However some of the published data are detailed enough to allow an identification of CAE cases and to select these cases. Another difficulty arises from too short a follow up period. Patients must be followed beyond eighteen or twenty years of age. In series in which 20 years is given as mean age at follow up, some patients are still adolescents at risk for later GTCS or myoclonic seizures. In a personal series, some patients were aged 23-30 years when their first GTCS occurred. The literature and hence the text of the international classification of epileptic syndromes are likely to be too pessimistic. Too arguments may be proposed. In 1924, at a time when no anti-absence drug existed, Adie was thinking that even if AS persist for a long time, they ultimately cease, never to return (Adie, 1924). In a Swedish population-based study, a 91 per cent remission rate was found when patients with absence epilepsy had only absences [20]. Hence a statement: "CAE, if properly defined, may have an excellent prognosis with complete remission of absences and only a slighter higher risk than of normals of infrequent GTCS in adult life" [13]. However, as to date this optimism is not based on indisputable data, some older studies will be quoted, in spite of their selection bias. The included patients had received anti-absence medication, diones since 1945; then ethosuximide since 1951, and later sodium valproate.

Prognosis of absence seizures

AS persist for a mean time of 6.6 years [21], disappear between age 3-19 years, mean age 10.5 [22] or 14 years [21]. "The tendency for petit mal to cease is present at all ages and not just at puberty". In about a quarter of patients the attacks cease before the age of 15 and by the age of 30 years petit mal had ceased in about three quarters of the patients [23]. In this study, with a follow up of about 5 years, only 3 per cent of patients experienced AS beyond 50 years of age. In another study [24], of the 92 uncontrolled patients, 89 were aged 20 or younger at the time of cessation of AS. Thus, AS persistence is a rare occurrence which is reported in about 6 per cent of patients [25]. Attacks become less frequent and are most apt to occur when patients are tired, excited, sleep-deprived or during a menstrual period [21]. AS tend to be very short, and not very troublesome to the patient [26].

Two favorable prognostic signs are age at onset of AS and medication efficacy. In patients early diagnosed and followed beyond 20 years of age, AS had disappeared in 95 and 90 per cent of cases according to an age at onset of 8 or 10 years [27, 28]. Their cessation soon after prescription of a convenient antiepileptic drug is considered as a favorable sign [21, 29].

Prognosis of generalized tonic-clonic seizures

Cessation of AS does not mean recovery. Generalized tonic-clonic seizures may appear, whether AS persist or have disappeared for several years. Most often, GTCS occur 5 to 10 years after onset of AS, i.e. mainly between 8 and 15 years of age [24, 30, 31], and sometimes beyond 20 and even 30 years of age [25, 26]. They have been considered as infrequent and easily controlled [21, 25, 30, 32]. Some authors proposed to distinguish two groups of patients; in one of them, GTCS begin usually beyond 16 years of age, are rare, and even a unique seizure, and a precipitating factor (sleep deprivation, stress) is constant; in the other group, they usually begin between 8 and 15 years of age and recur without provocative factor other than irregular therapy [31].

It has been estimated that GTCS occurred in 36-60 per cent of patients with onset of AS in childhood [21, 24, 25, 30, 32]. These figures are of dubious significance: childhood AS are not necessarily CAE.

Different risk factors were have been suggested, as follows:
- *age at onset of AS*. The later the onset, the higher the risk of convulsive seizures [25, 30, 32, 33, 34, present study]. Onset between 4-6 years of age and 8-10 were compared [34]. Fifty-two patients followed beyond 20 years of age had an early diagnosed strictly defined CAE; according to an onset before 9 years of age or between 9 and 10 years, 16 and 44 per cent of them, respectively, developed GTCS [27];
- *absence status*, especially when they occur late in the course of epilepsy [31];
- *sex*: although AS are more frequent in girls, AS + GTCS are more frequent in boys [25];
- *EEG*. Usually, clinical/EEG correlation is fair. However, the predictive value of the EEG is not absolute; SW discharges may persist after clinical recovery and conversely GTCS may occur in spite of a normalized EEG [20]. When initial tracings show a posterior delta rhythm, GTCS rarely occur [20, 25, 32, 35]. An abnormal background activity, multiple spikes, focal abnormalities were considered as unfavorable signs, but are likely to correspond to erroneous diagnoses;
- *therapy*. With an early institution of effective therapy, GTCS occurred in 30 per cent of cases, and 68 per cent after incorrect therapy [34]. GTCS manifested in 85 per cent of incorrectly treated patients [31].

Many other symptoms and clinical signs were examined as predictors of outcome without conclusive result [38].

A change of CAE into epilepsy with complex partial seizures has been reported. It corresponds to erroneous diagnosis: either AS with automatisms [21, 31, 36], or absence epilepsy other than CAE.

Complete remission

A wide range of remission rates has been given: 33 to 78 per cent. Reasons are as follows: (1) patients with absence epilepsies other than CAE were included; (2) patient's age at last clinic visit, with for instance control in 82 per cent of patients when beyond 18 years of age but only 65 per cent in those beyond 20 [31]; (3) follow up duration, with relapse in 19 per cent of patients who had been seizure-free 2 years or more [31]; and (4) therapy: with an early and adequate therapy, 70 per cent of patients were controlled and only 18 per cent with an incorrect therapy [34].

Social prognosis

Social adaptation of patients having had CAE is often poor, even if they are in remission [10, 22, 31, 37]. One-third of patients appear to have such troubles [32]. Young adults in whom typical absence has been diagnosed in childhood, particularly those without remission of their seizures have greater psychosocial difficulties than those with a non neurologic chronic disease [38]. A psychomotor slowing beginning late in follow up has been found in some patients with AS persisting after the age of 30 to 61 years [26]. It was supposed to be multifactorial in origin.

Personal Data

Further studies on cohort of well defined patients with absence epilepsy are needed. In 1994 we published a cohort of 43 patients (a total of 570 absences were recorded) (Hirsch *et al.*, 1994). From this study with short term follow up, the only reliable clinical criteria about the course of the disease appears to be the early onset of generalized tonic-clonic seizures and the nature of the precipitating factors (hyperventilation or intermittent light stimulation). The terms "childhood absence epilepsy", "juvenile absence epilepsy" and "eyelid myoclonia with absences" can be misleading and we proposed to individualize three categories: (i) "pure" absence epilepsy, (ii) generalized epilepsy with absences and tonic-clonic seizures, (iii) generalized epilepsy with photosensitive absences and tonic-clonic seizures. To confirm or invalidate this proposal we decided in 2001 to review the long term prognosis of this cohort. The objective of the study was to have a long term evolution (remission of absences, occurrence of late onset GTCS, continuation of AED's treatment, social adjustment).

Patients and methods

Data were collected from the initial 43 patients who have been followed now at least eight years. The only criterion for including a patient in the study was the video-EEG recording of typical absences defined by complete, or almost complete, loss of responsiveness, concomitant with bilateral and synchronous spike and wave discharges with a rhythmicity of 2-4 Hz. The only criterion for excluding a patient from this study was the existence of cerebral lesions. Video-EEG recordings were carried out for about 2 h: they included several hyperventilation and one intermittent light stimulation (ILS). Interictal EEG abnormalities, precipitating factors, type of absence seizures were analyzed. The patient history indicated the sex, the age of onset, the possible association with other types seizures. Several EEG recordings performed allowed us to evaluate the course of the disease under treatment.

A standardized interview of patient and family, focused on social adjustment was performed in 2001.

Results

Among 43 patients in the initial study, 40 were included, 3 patients were lost at follow up. Analysis was performed on 40 patients. Median age at onset for absence seizures was 6,5 years (2-32), Mean age at onset was 8,0 ± 5,0 years. Median follow up duration was 12 years, Mean follow up duration was 9 years. At the time of EEG-video recording, 17 patients (42%) showed simple absence seizures and 23 (58%) complex absence seizures. 47,5% showed generalized tonic-clonic seizures during the course of the epilepsy. Photosensitivity were observed in 8 patients (20%). Absence were induced by hyperventilation in 23 patients (58%). A complete remission for absence epilepsies could be estimated in the present study for 47,5% patients. At time of follow up patients were divided in three groups. Main results are summarized in *table I*.

Group 1 (n = 19) were formed of patients *untreated* at time of follow up showing *no absence seizure and generalized tonic-clonic seizure.*

This group of patients was formed of 9 males and 10 females. The mean 6,9 years and median 6 years (2-15) age at onset was during childhood. However, an early age 2 years, or a late age at onset 15 years was not always synonymous with poor prognosis. Absences were frequent (several to many per day), the main provocative factor was hyperpnea. Beside the loss of responsiveness, ictal symptoms varied in a given patient from one absence to another. The symptoms were associated with not stereotyped automatisms, moderated clonic and/or clonic components of the limbs and different types of eyelid and eye movement (rhythmic blnking, myoclonias, tonic deviation of the eyeballs, vertical nystagmus) in 69% of patients. Mild perioral myoclonias were observed in three patients and marked

Table I. Main characteristics in three group of patients. (Group 1: patients untreated complete seizures remission, Group 2: patients treated with seizures remission, Group 3: patients treated with no seizures remission)

	Group 1 (n = 19)	Group 2 (n = 4)	Group 3 (n = 17)
Age at onset (Years)	6,9 ± 3,1	7,7 ± 2,1	10,3 ± 6,6
Follow up (Years)	12,5 ± 3,9	8,2 ± 1,3	21,2 ± 5,7
Type of absence	Complex 68% Simple 32%	Complex 50% Simple 50%	Complex 53% Simple 47%
Provocative factors	Photosensitivity 5% Hyperpnea 63%	Photosensitivity 25% Hyperpnea 50%	Photosensitivity 35% Hyperpnea 64%
Ictal EEG	2-4 c/s SW 100% Poly-spikes 10%	2-4 c/s SW 100% Poly-spikes 20%	2-4 c/s SW 100% Poly-spikes 50%
Interictal EEG	Posterior Delta 15%	Posterior Delta 25%	Posterior Delta 11%
Occurrence of GTCS	5%	0%	100%
Age at GTCS (Years)	15	NR	13,5 ± 4,2
Effective AED's	VPA 75% ESM 10% LTG 15%	VPA 25% VPA + LTG 50% LTG 25%	VPA 47% VPA + LTG 41% others 12%
Time since effectiveness (Months)	14,5 ± 11,0	21,7 ± 15	NR
Treatment Duration (Years)	6,5 ± 4,7	Ongoing	Ongoing

myoclonias of the limbs and body axis in two. Ictal EEG was uniform with bilateral synchronous spike-and-wave discharges (2,5-4 Hz). Interictal EEG revealed a mild not-significant asymmetry in three patients and posterior delta activity which disappeared upon opening of the eyes in three. VPA monotherapy was effective in 75% of patients, two patients were treated with ethosuximide (ESM) and three lamotrigine (LTG) monotherapy. Two patients were initially incorrectly treated (carabamazepine and/or phenytoine, and/or phenoberbital). In one patient, even after more of 15 years of ineffective treatments, LTG monotherapy achieved a complete seizures control and could be stopped with out relapse of seizure or EEG abnormalities. 30% of patients achieved baccalaureate, 70% stopped in junior high school. 61% of patients reported schooling problems. However, 100% of patients considered that their social adjustment was satisfactory.

Group 2 (n = 4) were formed of patients still *treated* at time of follow up showing *no absence seizure and generalized tonic-clonic seizure.*

This group of patients was formed of 1 male and 3 females. Patients in Group 2 have similar characteristics than those in Group 1. However, they were individualized until it was not possible to assert a complete clinical and EEG remission without stopping treatment.

Group 3 (n = 17) were formed of patients still *treated* at time of follow up showing *absence seizures and/or generalized tonic-clonic seizures.*

This group of patients was formed of 8 males and 9 females The mean 10,3 years and median 9 years (3-32) age at onset was during late childhood or adolescence. Absences were less frequent, the main provocative factor was hyperpnea. Beside the loss of responsiveness, ictal symptoms varied in a given patient from one absence to another. Simple absence were as frequent that complex absence. Sustained perioral myoclonias were observed in one patient, marked myoclonias of the limbs and body axis in one and, systematic eyelid myoclonia in one. During the follow up period all patients had at least one generalized tonic-clonic seizures with a median delay of occurence of 13 months (7-20). Ictal EEG was uniform with bilateral synchronous spike-and-wave discharges (2,5-4 Hz), however 50% of patients showed polyspikes associated within 2,5-4 Hz absences. Interictal EEG reveal posterior delta activity which disappeared upon opening of the eyes in two. VPA monotherapy was effective in 43% of patients, a combination of more than one AEDs was needed in 57% of patients. 20% of patients achieved baccalaureate, 80% stopped in junior high school. All patients reported schooling problems. 80% of patients considered that their social adjustment was satisfactory.

Conclusion

Complete remission of absence seizures varied in the literature from 33 to 78% and is 47% in the present study. Generalized tonic-clonic seizures may appear, whether absence seizures persist or have disappeared for several years. It has been estimated that GTCS occurred in 36-60 per cent of patients with onset of absence seizures in childhood. These figures are of dubious significance: childhood onset absence seizures are not necessarily "pure absence epilepsy". In the present study, 47,5% of patients showed generalized tonic-clonic seizures during the course of the epilepsy. Most often, GTCS occur 5 to 10 years after onset of absence seizures, mainly between 8 and 15 years of age and sometimes beyond 20 and even 30 years of age. They have been considered as infrequent and easily controlled. Even with a complete remission of seizures the social adaptation of patients is often poor. Age at onset and medication efficacy are favorable prognostic signs. Photosensitivity, early occurrence of generalized tonic-clonic seizures, poly-spikes as an ictal pattern of absences are unfavorable prognostic signs.

References

1. Commission on Classification and Terminology of the International League Against Epilepsy. Proposal for revised classification of epilepsies and epileptic syndromes. *Epilepsia* 1989; 30: 389-99.
2. Adie WJ. Pyknolepsy: a form of epilepsy occurring in children, with a good prognosis. *Brain* 1924; 47: 96-102.
3. Janz D, Beck-Mannagetta G, Spröder B, Spröder J, Waltz S. Childhood absence epilepsy (pyknolepsy) and juvenile absence epilepsy: one or two syndromes? In: Wolf P, ed. *Epileptic seizures and syndromes*. London: John Libbey & Company, 1994: 115-26.
4. Wirrell EC, Camfield CS, Camfield PR, Gordon KE, Dooley JM. Long-term prognosis of typical childhood epilepsy: remission or progression to juvenile myoclonic epilepsy. *Neurology* 1996; 47: 912-8.
5. Panayiotopoulos CP, Obeid T, Waheed G. Absences in juvenile myoclonic epilepsy: a clinical and video-electroencephalographic study. *Ann Neurol* 1989a; 25: 391-7.
6. Panayiotopoulos CP, Obeid T, Waheed G. Differenciation of typical absence seizures in epileptic syndromes. A video EEG study of 224 seizures in 20 patients. *Brain* 1989b; 112: 1039-56.
7. Panayiotopoulos CP. The clinical spectrum of typical absence seizures and absence epilepsies. In: Malafosse A, Genton P, Hirsch E, Marescaux C, Broglin D, Bernasconi R, eds. *Idiopathic generalized epilepsies: clinical, experimental and genetic aspects*. London: John Libbey & Company Ltd, 1994: 75-85.
8. Hirsch E, Blanc-Platier A, Marescaux C. What are the relevant criteria for a better classification of epileptic syndromes with typical absences? In: Malafosse A, Genton P, Hirsch E, Marescaux C, Broglin D, Bernasconi R, eds. *Idiopathic generalized epilepsies: clinical, experimental and genetic aspects*. London: John Libbey & Company Ltd, 1994: 87-93.
9. Doose H. Absence epilepsy of early childhood. *Eur J Pediatr* 1994; 153: 372-7.
10. Lugaresi E, Pazzaglia P, Franck L, Roger J, Bureau-Paillas M, Ambrosetto G, Tassinari CA. Evolution and prognosis of primary generalized epilepsy of the petit mal type. In: Lugaresi E, Pazzaglia P, Tassinari CA, eds. *Evolution and prognosis of epilepsy*. Bologna: Aulo Gaggi, 1973: 2-22.

11. Jeavons PM. Nosological problems of myoclonic epilepsies in childhood and adolescence. *Dev Med Child Neurol* 1977; 19: 3-8.
12. Appleton RE, Panayiotopoulos CP, Acomb BA, Beirne M. Eyelid myoclonia with typical absences: an epilepsy syndrome. *J Neurol Neurosurg Psychiatry* 1993; 56: 1312-6.
13. Panayiotopoulos CP. Absence epilepsies. In: Engel J, Pedley TA, eds. *Epilepsy: a comprehensive textbook*. Philadelphia: Lippincott-Raven, 1997: 2327-46.
14. Giannakodimos S, Panayiotopoulos CP. Eyelid myoclonia with absences in adults: a clinical and video-EEG study. *Epilepsia* 1996a; 37: 36-44.
15. Panayiotopoulos CP, Ferrie CD, Giannakodimos S, Robinson RO. Perioral myoclonia with absences. In: Duncan JS, Panayiotopoulos CP, eds. *Typical absences and related epileptic syndromes*. London: Churchill Livingstone, 1995: 221-30.
16. Berkovic SF, Andermann F, Andermann E, Gloor P. Concepts of absence epilepsies: discrete syndromes or biological continuum? *Neurology* 1987; 37: 993-1000.
17. Engel J. A proposed diagnostic scheme for people with epileptic seizures and with epilepsy: Report of the ILAE Task Force on classification and terminology. *Epilepsia* 2001; 42: 1-8.
18. Bouma PAD, Westendorp JG, van Dijk JG, Peters ACB, Brouver OF. The outcome of absence epilepsy: A meta-analysis. *Neurology* 1996; 47: 802-8.
19. Giannakodimos S, Panayiotopoulos CP. Idiopathic generalized epilepsies in adults with onset of absences in childhood. *Epilepsia* 1996b; 37 (Suppl 4): 87.
20. Hedström A, Olsson I. Epidemiology of absence epilepsy: EEG findings and their predictive value. *Pediatr Neurol* 1991; 7: 100-4.
21. Currier RD, Kooi KA, Saidman LJ. Prognosis of pure petit mal. *Neurology* 1963; 13: 959-67.
22. Hertoft P. The clinical, electroencephalographic and social prognosis in petit mal epilepsy. *Epilepsia* 1963; 4: 298-314.
23. Gibberd FB. The prognosis of petit mal. *Brain* 1966; 89: 531-8.
24. Livingston S, Torres I, Pauli LL, Rider RV. Petit Mal epilepsy. Results of a prolonged follow up study of 117 patients. *JAMA* 1965; 194: 227-32.
25. Oller-Daurella L, Sanchez ME. Evolucion de las ausencias tipicas. *Rev Neurol (Barcelona)* 1981; 9: 81-102.
26. Gastaut H, Zifkin BG, Mariani E, Salas Puig J. The long-term course of primary generalized epilepsy with persisting absences. *Neurology* 1986; 36: 1021-8.
27. Loiseau P, Duché B, Pedespan JM. Absence epilepsies. *Epilepsia* 1995a; 36: 1182-6.
28. Loiseau P, Duché B, Pedespan JM. Splitting or lumping absence epilepsies. *Epilepsia* 1995b; 36: 116.
29. Loiseau P, Cohadon F, Cohadon S. Le petit mal qui guérit, guérit rapidement. *J Med Lyon* 1966; 1108: 1557-65.
30. Charlton MH, Yahr MD. Long-term follow up of patients with petit mal. *Arch Neurol* 1967; 16: 595-8.
31. Dieterich E, Baier WK, Doose H, Tuxhorn I. Long-term follow up of childhood epilepsy with absences at onset. *Neuropediatrics* 1985; 16: 149-54.
32. Loiseau P, Pestre M, Dartigues JF, Commenges D, Barberger-Gateau C, Cohadon S. Long-term prognosis in two forms of childhood epilepsy: typical absence seizures and epilepsy with rolandic (centrotemporal) EEG foci. *Ann Neurol* 1983; 13: 642-8.
33. Lennox WG, Lennox MA. *Epilepsy and related disorders*. Boston: Little, Brown and Co, 1960: 546-74.
34. Bergamini L, Bram S, Broglia S, Riccio A. L'insorgenza tardiva di crisi Grande Male nel Piccolo Male puro. Studio catamnestico di 78 casi. *Archives Suisses de Neurologie, Neurochirurgie et de Psychiatrie* 1965; 96: 306-17.
35. Cobb WA, Gordon N, Matthews SC, Nieman EA. The occipital delta rhythm in petit mal. *Electroencephalogr Clin Neurophysiol* 1961; 13: 142-3.
36. Sato S, Dreifuss FE, Penry JK. The effect of sleep on spike-wave discharges in absence seizures. *Neurology* 1973; 23: 1335-45.
37. Mirsky AF, Duncan CC, Levav ML. Neuropsychological and psychophysiological aspects of absence epilepsy. In: Duncan JS, Panayiotopoulos CP, eds. *Typical absences and related epileptic syndromes*. Edinburgh: Churchill Livingstone, 1995: 112-21.
38. Wirrell EC, Camfield CS, Camfield PR, Dooley JM, Gordon KE, Smith B. Long-term psychosocial outcome in typical absence epilepsy. *Arch Pediatr Adolesc* 1997; 151: 152-8.

Prognosis of idiopathic myoclonic epilepsies

Pierre Genton, Philippe Gelisse, Pierre Thomas, Charlotte Dravet

Prognosis of epileptic syndromes may be particularly difficult to establish when the natural course of such epilepsies stretches over many years, especially when patients have to move from the hands of a child neurologist or pediatrician into those of an adult neurologist – and are consequently often "lost sight of". Fortunately, the epileptic syndromes implied in the (however artificial) category of idiopathic myoclonic epilepsies are few, and their extension is limited to relatively homogenous age classes. Moreover, our work in a specialized epilepsy centre has allowed us to bridge the gaps between age classes, and many data on the long-term evolution of such epilepsies have been gathered over the years here and elsewhere.

Epilepsies that are "myoclonic" and "idiopathic"

Myoclonic seizures, or myoclonic jerks, can be found in various forms of focal and generalized epilepsies, and do not constitute a very specific clinical trait. However, their occurrence in idiopathic epilepsies is limited, in practice, to two main, clearly differentiated entities and to their clinical variants or related syndromes. According to the 1989 international classification of epilepsies [1], only two forms of idiopathic myoclonic epilepsies can be listed, both belonging to the category of idiopathic generalized epilepsies (IGE). One is benign myoclonic epilepsy in infancy (BMEI), and concerns infants and young children, and the other is juvenile myoclonic epilepsy (JME), which concerns adolescents and adults. The former is fairly infrequent, while the latter is probably the most common type of recognizable epileptic syndrome. However, other less commonly recognized syndromes can also be discussed in this context.

BMEI was first described by Dravet and Bureau [2] and a recent review of this entity [3] has confirmed the existence of this uncommon, yet easily identifiable syndrome. BMEI occurs in normal infants, and is characterized by the onset, typically between the ages of 6 months and 3 years, of bilateral, massive myoclonic jerks that do not occur in cluster but rather at random, sometimes at awakening, and that are always associated with diffuse spike-wave (SW) discharges on the EEG [4]. Mental development and neuroimaging are normal. Clinical variants have been described:

– A form characterized by the occurrence of reflex myoclonic seizures, that shares all the other features of the syndrome [5]: in such patients, all or most of the sudden, massive jerks are triggered by an unexpected stimulation, mostly by sudden contact; in the usual, classical form, jerks can also be elicited by ILS in 10% of the cases [4], and this reflex component is not considered to constitute a significant prognostic marker of BMEI.

– Some patients have a somewhat later onset, in early childhood (ages 3 to 7) rather than in infancy [6, 7].

These clinical variants appear as comparatively frequent, and might account for a sizeable proportion of the total cases of BMEI, which remains an uncommon condition. BMEI is thus probably more than a syndrome confined to "infancy", as its name would indicate. But BMEI is probably also the purest of idiopathic myoclonic epilepsies, since no other seizure type is found during the typical clinical course in infancy and early childhood.

In contrast, JME appears as a very common, though still somewhat underdiagnosed condition. The description of JME was made progressively over the years (references in [8]), but the first comprehensive account of this common and easily recognizable form of epilepsy was published by Janz and Christian in 1957 [9]. The ICE gives the following description of JME:

Juvenile myoclonic epilepsy appears around puberty and is characterized by seizures with bilateral, single or repetitive, arrhythmic, irregular myoclonic jerks, predominantly in the arms. Jerks may cause some patients to fall suddenly. No disturbance of consciousness is noticeable. The disorder may be inherited, and sex distribution is equal. Often, there are generalized tonic-clonic seizures and, less often, infrequent absences. The seizures usually occur shortly after awakening and are often precipitated by sleep deprivation. Interictal an ictal EEGs have rapid, generalized, often irregular spike-waves and polyspike-waves; there is no close phase correlation between EEG spikes and jerks. Frequently, the patients are photosensitive. Response to appropriate drugs is good.

A review of the clinical and EEG characteristics of this syndrome have been published recently [8, 10]. None of the clinical and EEG traits of JME is highly specific. It is not easy, in many cases and according to several authors, to draw distinct lines between JME and other syndromes of IGE that have onset or high prevalence in adolescents, i.e. juvenile absence epilepsy (JAE) [11], epilepsy with generalized tonic-clonic seizures on awakening (or awakening Grand Mal, AwGM) [12], or even the most benign forms of IGE with rare GTCS [13]. Some authors have linked these syndromes into a broader category of IGE of adolescence with variable phenotypes, which has been included as a recommendation for an update on the ICE by the ad hoc commission of the International League Against Epilepsy [14]. The fact is that a sizeable proportion of patients with JAE experience, besides typical absences, GTCS and myoclonic jerks, and that up to 29% of patients with AwGM experience myoclonic jerks. It will thus be necessary to discuss briefly the prognosis of these forms of IGE, only to see whether it differs significantly from the prognosis of JME.

Other epileptic syndromes or diseases could be discussed in this chapter:

– Myoclonic seizures (as well as typical absences or GTCS) may also occur in the context of reflex epilepsies: the concept of praxis-induced seizures was indeed established recently [15] and refers in part to the group of "noogenic" epilepsies outlined some years earlier [16]. Some of these patients have a typical form of primary reading epilepsy and/or praxis-induced seizures [17]. It appears now clearly indeed that such reflex epilepsies, including primary reading epilepsy, are actually either related with JME or common in patients with JME when properly sought [18]. All these forms of reflex epilepsies in which seizures are triggered by mental, cognitive or and association of mental activity and specific movements (praxis) are commonly associated with myoclonus, which may appear clinically as generalized or focal.

– Among the reflex epilepsies, seizures associated with photosensitivity especially inthe context of JME or of IGE, are often characterized by marked myoclonic components; the myoclonias are massive and bilateral as in JME, or sometimes limited to eyelids or to the cephalic segment.

– A recently recognized syndrome of adult-onset idiopathic generalized myoclonic epilepsy, resembling JME in many ways, was recently reported from the US and Germany [19]: these were adult patients of either sex, with onset in adulthood of GTCS and myoclonus, some of whom had a family history of late-onset IGE. Some patients with a JME-like grouping of clinical and EEG symptoms had been described in unexpected age classes some years earlier [20].

– The concept of idiopathicity would be stretched by the inclusion, in this chapter, of patients with late-onset myoclonias in the context of Alzheimer's disease or of dementia in elderly Down syndrome patients [21], or of patients with Unverricht-Lundborg disease (ULD), a type of progressive myoclonus epilepsy that is not associated with mental deterioration and that stabilizes, with a remission from seizures in most patients, in middle adulthood [22]. Nor will we discuss here the adult-onset benign myoclonic epilepsy reported from Japan and characterized mostly by slowly progressive but invalidating myoclonus [23] although this condition, much like ULD, is "idiopathic" as epilepsy and myoclonus are its only clinical symptoms.

– There is another well-recognized epileptic syndrome of childhood that is characterized by idiopathicity and the association of myoclonic seizures with other seizure types, especially with myoclonic-astatic seizures: the Doose syndrome, or myoclonic-astatic epilepsy.

However, these epilepsies will either be discussed elsewhere (the Doose syndrome), or belong to other clinical groupings (of symptomatic epilepsies), or are too rare to warrant a study on prognosis. We shall limit our study to BMEI and JME and their clinical variants.

Prognosis of benign myoclonic epilepsy in infancy and related syndromes

In all patients with BMEI reported in the literature, the spontaneous evolution of the epilepsy was benign. Untreated patients do not develop other seizure types, like GTCS or typical absences. Some interictal myoclonus may be found in a minority of cases [6]. Full seizure control is obtained using valproate monotherapy in a large majority of patients (review in 3), although some may require high doses of VPA or cotherapy. The reflex type of BMEI may remit spontaneously without treatment. Photosensitivity on the EEG, which is far from present in all patients at diagnosis, may appear after diagnosis and even after remission from seizures [6, 24, 25]. There is however no report on clinical seizures triggererd by light in such patients. Myoclonic jerks usually disappear under treatment, and the active period of epilepsy lasts less than 1 year in a majority of cases. Longer evolutions with active epilepsy (lasting 4 to 6 years) were noted in the first publications, before the condition had been recognized and treated. Treatment may be withdrawn after (or even before) the age of 6 in case of longlasting seizure control. Patients with persisting photosensitivity are usually treated during several more years.

However, there are two problems that dominate the long-term outcome of this typically very benign condition:

– The first is the possible occurrence of GTCS, usually after age 10 and usually during drug withdrawal. Most of these patients can be taken off medication somewhat later, and in all the cases reported GTCS were easily controlled by VPA, which was successfully withdrawn later in a majority of the cases with adequate documentation [3]. Thus this long-term complication is still amenable to simple monotherapy, and is probably also an age-dependent clinical phenomenon.

– The second is represented by concerns on the neuropsychological development of patients with BMEI. According to Dravet *et al.* [3], 83% of patients retain a normal development. Among the patients who experience developmental problems, some may have an independent co-pathology (in the Marseille series, one had Down syndrome, and another one developed a psychosis after age 10 years but had had myoclonic jerks until age 5 and had persisting photosensitivity). In the other cases, the presence of developmental problems may be related to a delayed diagnosis with a long period (usually several years) with persisting seizures. Some of these patients can improve over time [26], and all the other ones had mild intellectual deficits, attended specialized schools but none was institutionalized.

Overall, BMEI remains a very benign condition. The reflex form may have an even better than average prognosis. Little is known about the long-term evolution in patients with later onset, but they respond very well to valproate and the clinical manifestations apparently stop before adolescence [7]. BMEI appears as an age-related idiopathic myoclonic epilepsy, with a clinical expression that does not extend beyond childhood, and, although photosensitivity in the EEG lab may persist after the cessation of the clinical attacks, most authors have stressed that treatment can be withdrawn safely during childhood and that there are no transitional forms with JME, which concerns a very distinct age class. Although there are no data on the long-term prognosis of BMEI in terms of schooling and professional activity – which is not unexpected, given the very pediatric nature of this condition which is rarely followed up into adulthood – all markers point to a good prognosis in this respect.

Prognosis of juvenile myoclonic epilepsies and related syndromes

As most forms of IGE, JME has a reputation of benignity and was first considered as a minor form of epilepsy with a good prognosis, and described as such [27]. However, the word "benign" was withdrawn from the denomination of this syndrome following the early recognition of the long duration and pharmacodependency of this syndrome [28]. Recent data have further contributed to give a "mixed" picture of the outcome of this condition, which may indeed be severe in some cases: given the high prevalence of JME, this less than benign evolution may thus concern many patients.

About 85% of patients with JME experience total seizure control [29, 30], most of them on VPA monotherapy. In an age where one of the golden rules of clinical epileptology was to withdraw medication after two years of total seizure control, clinicians quickly became aware of the fact that patients with JME had a very high rate of relapse, with reapparance of myoclonic jerks and of GTCS in more than 90% of the cases within 1-2 years [28]: clinicians were thus taught at the same time that JME was a specific and recognizable epileptic syndrome, and that treatment was probably given for a lifetime. Thus JME stands out as a pharmacodependent form of epilepsy. However, withdrawal was usually attempted in young or middle-aged adults, and there are no reliable data on the natural course of JME in older age classes. Indirect data point to a slow decrease of seizure risk. This may be due to changes in lifestyle, with less risk of sleep deprivation and excessive, acute consumation of alcohol, and this results in the possibility to maintain JME patients who have reached both full seizure control and adulthood or middle age on low-dose valproate [31].

Thus about 15% of all JME patients are drug-resistant. This proportion should theoretically exclude lifestyle issues: patients with irregular sleep-wake schedules and excessive intake of alcohol are at risk of persisting seizures in spite of adequate treatment. Low compliance may also be a factor or co-factor of drug resistance in JME. It should be kept in mind that patients with JME are particularly exposed to paradoxical aggravation due to the choice of inadequate drugs, such as carbamazepine or phenytoin [32]. If all such confounding factors are eliminated, truly resistant patients remain, and little is known about the factors of severity of JME in such cases. Our recent findings have shown that the presence of brain lesions,that may be considered as coincidental findings, on neuroimaging do not influence the clinical expression and prognosis (i.e. response to treatment) in JME [33]. Only clinical markers may predict (to some degree) resistance to treatment [34]: while gender, early age at onset, presence of photosensitivity and even delay in diagnosis are not associated with drug resistance, there are two independent factors of severity, i.e. the association of three seizure types (myoclonic jerks, GTCS and typical absences) on one hand, and the presence of psychiatric problems on the other hand. Conversely, the association of typical absences and myoclonic jerks appears to define a more benign subtype of JME. It has also been stressed that numerous patients, who exhibit only myoclonic jerks, have a very benign condition, to the point that they often may escape medical attention [35].

Compared with other form of IGE, JME is characterized by a high prevalence of psychological and psychiatric problems. It had already been noted by Janz and Christian in 1957 [9] that many patients had a lighthearted, hedonistic approach to life and were highly unreliable, especially in matters of compliance to lifestyle recommendations and drug therapy. This particular psychological profile was confirmed by later studies [36, 37]. Recent surveys have stressed the high prevalence of subtle frontal lobe dysfunctions [38], or the existence of psychiatric problems in up to 26.5% of patients with JME [39]. Such problems, which are significantly associated with drug resistance, may cause difficulties in social integration [36].

Another point was recently made when it was shown that JME may be associated with sudden unexpected death (SUDEP). Isolated cases of SUDEP in idiopathic generalized epilepsy had been reported before, and we showed that 2 such cases had occurred in the follow up of our cohort of 170 cases [40]: besides one patient who died due to complications of anorexia nervosa, two female patients were found dead in the morning after a probable, unwitnessed seizure, and both had severe psychiatric comorbidity.

Other forms that resemble JME but occur in other age classes [19, 20] have been described as benign and easily treatable: not much is known about the actual prognosis of these uncommon observations.

In JME, the overall prognosis thus remains good: JME is and remains a frequent, treatable form of epilepsy that should be easily recognized and managed with a rational approach to choice of drug (avoiding potentially aggravating agents), lifestyle issues, and a long-term perspective that takes into account the pharmacodependency of this condition. Patients with uncontrolled seizures are at risk of SUDEP, however uncommon this complication may appear in the context of this idiopathic epilepsy. A poorer prognosis is present when patients have multiple seizure types, and especially when significant psychiatric problems are present. Thus JME is and remains a benign condition in most patients, but may present as a severe disorder in some.

Conclusions

Any epileptologist will agree that neither the concept of idiopathicity nor the word "myoclonic" mean much in terms of outcome and overall prognosis. However, when put together, they delineate a few epileptic syndromes or diseases among which BMEI and JME stand out. The former has a very good prognosis, the latter is characterized by pharmacodependency and – however few patients may be concerned – by the risk of complications, including SUDEP, and poor social adjustment. In other forms of myoclonic and idiopathic epilepsies, the prognosis spans a wide spectrum. In the present state of our knowledge, it is clear that the elements and factors of prognosis that have been gathered are mainly clinical and reflect the spontaneous evolution of the conditions. With new insights into the basic mechanisms of these elepsies, the prognosis will probably be based on a more rational approach to diagnosis and therapy. We can only hope that this will occur soon.

References

1. Commission on classification and terminology of the international league against epilepsy: proposal for revised classification of epilepsies and epileptic syndromes. *Epilepsia* 1989; 30: 389-99.
2. Dravet C, Bureau M. L'épilepsie myoclonique bénigne du nourrisson. *Rev Electroenceph Neurophysiol Clin* 1981; 11: 438-44.
3. Dravet C, Bureau M. Benign Myoclonic epilepsy in infancy. In: Roger J, Bureau M, Genton P, Dravet C, Tassinari CA, Wolf P, eds. *Epileptic syndromes in infancy, childhood and adolescence (third edition)*. London-Paris: John Libbey (in press).
4. Dravet C, Bureau M, Roger J. Benign myoclonic epilepsy in infants. In: Roger J, Bureau M, Dravet C, Dreifuss FE, Perret A, Wolf P, eds. *Epileptic syndromes in infancy, childhood and adolescence, 2nd ed*. London, Paris: John Libbey Eurotext Ltd, 1992: 67-74.
5. Ricci S, Cusmai R, Fusco L, Vigevano F. Reflex myoclonic epilepsy: a new age-dependent idiopathic epileptic syndrome related to startle reaction. *Epilepsia* 1995; 36: 342-8.
6. Giovanardi Rossi P, Parmeggiani A, Posar A, Santi A, Santucci M. Benign myoclonic epilepsy: long-term follow up of 11 new cases. *Brain Dev* 1997; 19: 473-9.
7. Guerrini R, Dravet C, Gobbi G, Ricci S, Dulac O. Idiopathic generalized epilepsies with myoclonus in infancy and childhood. In: Malafosse A, Genton P, Hirsch E, Marescaux C, Broglin D, Bernasconi R, eds. *Idiopathic generalized epilepsies. Clinical, experimental and genetic aspects*. London: John Libbey, 1994: 267-80.
8. Genton P, Gélisse P, Thomas P. Juvenile myoclonic epilepsy today: current definitions and limits. In: Schmitz B, Sander T, eds. *Juvenile myoclonic epilepsy. The Janz syndrome*. Petersfield, UK, and Philadelphia, USA: Wrightson Medical Publishing, 2000: 11-32.
9. Janz D, Christian W. Impulsiv Petit-Mal. *Dtsch Z Nervenheilk* 2000; 176: 346-86.
10. Waltz S. The EEG in juvenile myoclonic epilepsy. In: Schmitz B, Sander T, eds. *Juvenile myoclonic epilepsy. The Janz syndrome*. Petersfield, UK, and Philadelphia, USA: Wrightson Medical Publishing, 2000: 41-56.
11. Wolf P. Juvenile Absence Epilepsy. In: Roger J, Bureau M, Dravet Ch, Dreifuss FE, Perret A, Wolf P, eds. *Epileptic syndromes in infancy, childhood and adolescence (2nd edition)*. London: John Libbey, 1992: 307-12.
12. Wolf P. Epilepsy with grand mal on awakening. In: Roger J, Bureau M, Dravet Ch, Dreifuss FE, Perret A, Wolf P, eds. *Epileptic syndromes in infancy, childhood and adolescence (2nd edition)*. London: John Libbey, 1992: 329-41.
13. Oller-Daurella L, Sorel L. L'épilepsie Grand Mal bénigne de l'adulte. *Acta Neurol Belg* 1989; 89: 38-45.
14. Engel J Jr. A proposed diagnostic scheme for people with epileptic seizures and with epilepsy: report of the ILAE task force on classification and terminology. *Epilepsia* 2001; 42: 1-8.
15. Inoue Y, Seino M, Kubota H, Yamakaku K, Tanaka M, Yagi K. Epilepsy with praxis-induced seizures. In: Wolf P, ed. *Epileptic seizures and syndromes*. London: John Libbey, 1994: 81-92.
16. Gastaut H. Synopsis and conclusion of the international colloquium on reflex seizures and epilepsies. In:

Beaumanoir A, Gastaut H, Naquet R, eds. *Reflex seizures and reflex epilepsies.* Genève: Éditions Médecine et Hygiène, 1988: 497-507.

17. Wolf P, Mayer T. Juvenile myoclonic epilepsy: a syndrome challenging syndromic concepts? In: Schmitz B, Sander Th, eds. *Juvenile myoclonic epilepsy. The Janz Syndrome.* Petersfield: Wrightson Biomedical, 2000: 33-9.

18. Matsuoka H, Takahashi T, Sasaki M, Matsumoto K, Yoshida S, Numachi Y, Saito H, Ueno T, Sato M. Neuropsychological EEG activation in patients with epilepsy. *Brain* 2000; 123: 318-30.

19. Gilliam F, Steinhoff BJ, Bittermann HJ, Kuzniecky R, Faught E, Abou-Khalil R. Adult myoclonic epilepsy: a distinct syndrome of idiopathic generalized epilepsy. *Neurology* 2000; 55: 1030-3.

20. Gram L, Alving J, Sagild JC, Dam M. Juvenile myoclonic epilepsy in unexpected age groups. *Epilepsy Res* 1988; 2: 137-40.

21. Genton P, Paglia G. Epilepsie myoclonique sénile? Myoclonies épileptiques d'apparition tardive dans le syndrome de Down. *Epilepsies* 1994; 6: 5-11.

22. Roger J, Genton P, Bureau M, Dravet C. Progressive myoclonus epilepsies in childhood and adolescence. In: Roger J, Bureau M, Dravet C, Dreifuss FE, Wolf P, Perret A, eds. *Epileptic syndromes in infancy, childhood and adolescence, second edition.* London-Paris: John Libbey Eurotext, 1992: 381-400.

23. Okino S. Familial benign myoclonus epilepsy of adult onset: a previously unrecognized myoclonic disorder. *J Neurol Sci* 1997; 145: 113-8.

24. Ribacoba Montero R, Salas Puig J. Benign myoclonic epilepsy in childhood. A case report (in Spanish). *Rev Neurol* 1997; 25: 1210-2.

25. Lin YP, Itomi K, Takada H, Kuboda T, Okumura A, Aso K, Negoro T, Watanabe K. Benign myoclonic epilepsy in infants: video-EEG features and long-term follow up. *Neuropediatrics* 1998; 29: 268-71.

26. Cassé-Perrot C, Dravet C, Genton P. Épilepsie myoclonique sévère, épilepsie myoclonique bénigne, épilepsie myoclono-astatique (Doose) : étude neuropsychologique (résultats préliminaires). *Epilepsies* 1997; 9: 191-4.

27. Asconapé J, Penry JK. Some clinical and EEG aspects of benign juvenile myoclonic epilepsy. *Epilepsia* 1984; 25: 108-14.

28. Delgado-Escueta AV, Enrile-Bacsal F. Juvenile myoclonic epilepsy of Janz. *Neurology* 1984; 34: 285-94.

29. Wolf P. Juvenile myoclonic epilepsy. In: Roger J, Bureau M, Dravet Ch, Dreifuss FE, Perret A, Wolf P, eds. *Epileptic syndromes in infancy, childhood and adolescence (2nd edition).* London: John Libbey, 1992: 313-27.

30. Genton P, Salas Puig J, Tunon A, Lahoz C, Gonzalez Sanchez M. Juvenile myoclonic epilepsy and related syndromes: clinical and neurophysiological aspects. In: Malafosse A, Genton P, Hirsch E, Marescaux C, Broglin D, Bernasconi R, eds. *Idiopathic generalized epilepsies: clinical, experimental and genetic aspects.* London: John Libbey, 1994: 253-65.

31. De Toffol B, Autret A. Treatment of juvenile myoclonic epilepsy with low-dose sodium valproate. *Rev Neurol* 1996; 152: 708-10.

32. Genton P, Gélisse P, Thomas P, Dravet C. Do carbamazepine and phenytoin aggravate juvenile myoclonic epilepsy? *Neurology* 2000; 55: 1106-9.

33. Gelisse P, Genton P, Raybaud Ch, Thomas P, Dravet C. Structural brain lesions influence do not influence the prognosis of juvenile myoclonic epilepsy. *Acta Neurol Scan* 2000; 102: 188-91.

34. Gelisse P, Genton P, Thomas P, Rey M, Samuelian JC, Dravet C. Clinical factors of drug resistance in juvenile myoclonic epilepsy. *J Neurol Neurosurg Psychiatry* 2001; 70: 240-3.

35. Jain S, Padma MV, Maheshwari MC. Occurrence of only myoclonic jerks in juvenile myoclonic epilepsy. *Acta Neurol Scand* 1997; 95: 263-7.

36. Lund M, Reintoft M, Simonsen N. Eine kontrollierte soziologische und psychologische Untersuchung von Patienten mit juveniler myoklonischer Epilepsie. *Nervenarzt* 1976; 47: 708-12.

37. Tsuboi T. Primary generalized epilepsy with sporadic myoclonias of myoclonic petit mal type. Stuttgart: Thieme, 1977.

38. Devinsky O, Gershengorn J, Brown E, Perrine K, Vazquez B, Luciano D. Frontal functions in juvenile myoclonic epilepsy. *Neurol Neuropsychol Behav Neurol* 1997; 10: 243-6.

39. Gelisse P, Genton P, Samuelian JC, Thomas P, Bureau M. Troubles psychiatriques dans l'épilepsie myoclonique juvénile. *Rev Neurol* 2001b; 157: 297-302.

40. Genton P, Gélisse P. Unexpected mortality in juvenile myoclonic epilepsy. *Acta Neurol Scand* 2001; 104: 125-9.

Prognosis of idiopathic localisation-related epilepsies

Christine Brasselet, Jacques Motte

In the literature, there is an obvious confusion between the two concepts of idiopathic epilepsy and benign epilepsy: they can sometimes both be used for the same epileptic syndrome but they cannot be considered as synonyms. The concept of benign epilepsy is related to the evolution of the disease with time and a spontaneous remission before the child becomes an adult. The notion of idiopathic epilepsy is an etiologic consideration; an epileptic syndrome may be idiopathic and still not have a spontaneous remission or a great response to antiepileptic drugs. Moreover, the International Classification of Epilepsies [1] talks about idiopathic epilepsies (*i.e.* without any underlying neurologic lesion) in opposition with cryptogenic and symptomatic syndromes (lesional epilepsies). Nevertheless, all idiopathic localisation-related epileptic syndromes are not mentioned in the international classification. Genton and Guerrini [2] summarised the non-rolandic types in *table I*. Thus, we think that the term "benign epilepsy" should not be used, and our purpose here is to talk about the idiopathic, or age-related, localisation-related epilepsies which are known to have a benign evolution, that is mainly benign childhood epilepsy with centro-temporal spikes (BECTS). We will have only a few words about some other syndromes: benign childhood epilepsy with occipital paroxysms (BCEOP), atypical benign partial epilepsy, idiopathic childhood epilepsy with frontal paroxysms and idiopathic partial epilepsy in infancy.

Benign childhood epilepsy with centro-temporal spikes

Definition – Epidemiology

Typical BECTS

BECTS was described for the first time by Nayrac and Beaussart [3]. It has an incidence rate of 5-21/100 000 in the age group of 0-15 years and a prevalence rate in all epilepsies

Table I.

Denomination of syndromes	Authors	Year
Primary reading epilepsy	Bickford	1956
Landau-Kleffner syndrome	Landau and Kleffner	1956
Epilepsy with continuous spike-waves during slow sleep	Patry	1971
Benign partial seizures of adolescence	Loiseau	1978
Benign psychomotor epilepsy	Dalla Bernadina	1980
Benign partial epilepsy with extreme somatosensory evoked potentials	De Marco	1981
Idiopathic epilepsy of childhood with occipital paroxysms	Gastaut	1982
Atypical benign partial epilepsy	Aicardi	1982
Benign frontal lobe epilepsy	Beaumanoir	1983
Idiopathic partial epilepsy in infants	Watanabe	1987
Familial infantile convulsions	Vigevano	1992
Continuous localised EEG discharges during sleep	Galetti	1992
Familial frontal lobe epilepsy	Scheffer	1993
Idiopathic partial epilepsy with photic-induced occipital seizures	Guerrini	1994

of 8-23% [4]. It has its onset between 3 and 13 years, with a peak at 7-8 years and resolves by the age of 16 years. The sex ratio is approximately 3 boys for 2 girls [5]. The children suffering from BECTS have a normal psychomotor development at the age of the first seizure.

Partial (lateralised), oro (hemi)facial and/or oropharyngeal tonic and/or tonic-clonic and/or clonic muscle contractions with speech arrest and hypersalivation are the main motor and vegetative symptoms, which manifest at the tongue, mouth, chin and cheek [4]. The involvement of the glottis and pharynx (> 50%) produces guttural sounds. Post-ictal Todd paralysis occurs in 10% of the cases. Somatosensory symptoms may consist in paresthesia in parts of and/or in the whole oropharyngeal region (tongue, cheek, gum, teeth, lips).

The ictal symptoms may spread to the ipsilateral upper extremity and to the leg, and then generalise secondarily. Secondarily generalised tonic-clonic seizures (GTCS) are a frequent seizure type: they are present in one to two thirds of children. There are no reports on primary GTCS. Duration of seizures is from a few seconds to a few minutes.

Seizures occur in 51-80% of cases while the child is asleep. In 15%, they occur both during sleep and awakening and in 10-20% only when the child is awake. In the case of diurnal seizures, video recording is unusual and has been recently reported [6].

Frequency of seizures is low; in 10-20% of cases only one seizure is described, 60-70% may have 2 to 10 seizures and in 10-20% of cases, seizures may be more frequent and difficult to treat. Clusters of seizures may occur in one night or within a short period of time [7].

A typical EEG pattern is described as follows: rolandic paroxysms defined as spikes or spike-waves simultaneously recorded over the posterior frontal, central, mid-temporal and occasionally the parietal regions with a maximum amplitude over the centro-temporal region [1]. The classical EEG picture shows high voltage, usually diphasic spikes or sharp waves with prominent aftercoming slow waves. Blom *et al.* [8] noted that 30% of cases show spikes only during sleep, and approximately 60% of cases show a unilateral spike focus. The EEG background is usually normal.

In the presence of a typical clinical history, normal neurologic exam and typical EEG findings, no further investigations are required to make the diagnosis of BECTS. The treatment criteria vary from one author to the other but it seems reasonable to withhold any treatment if the child and family are comfortable with this approach [5]. Treatment is usually started if the seizures occur daily, if they are recurrent, secondarily generalised or disturbing the child or family.

Atypical semiology of BECTS

Cases presenting similarities with BECTS but with different, non-characteristic seizure type have been recognised, although their precise relationship with BECTS is not clearly established [9]. Such atypical seizures are often part of syndromes with various other manifestations such as language or cognitive deficits that clearly separate them from BECTS (Atypical benign partial epilepsy, continuous spike wave during sleep, Landau-Kleffner syndrome, syndrome of status of rolandic seizures).

These syndromes share several but not all of the main characteristics of BECTS. Most are marked by partial motor seizures, usually nocturnal and affecting principally the face and oropharyngeal muscles. All feature the typical blunted sharp waves highly suggestive of rolandic epilepsy and a significant increase of paroxysmal activity during sleep.

However, they also clearly differ from BECTS by the greater intensity of the EEG paroxysms, the characteristics of seizures, which often become bilateral and often present inhibitory characteristics, which are not obvious in BECTS.

Scheffer *et al.* [10] described a three-generation family with autosomal dominant inheritance of an epileptic syndrome resembling BECTS. In addition, affected patients have speech dyspraxia and cognitive impairment. This disorder is related to BECTS but also shares some features with two rare, more severe childhood syndromes with partial epilepsy: focal epileptiform discharges and speech dysfunction, which are Landau-Kleffner syndrome (LKS) [11] and the syndrome of epilepsy with continuous spike and wave during slow-wave sleep (CSWS) [12].

A French team of Strasbourg has recently described a new family presenting this syndrome [13]. They reported 10 members on 3 generations with a resembling syndrome: an association of BECTS, mental retardation predominating with language and oro-motor dysfunction.

Controversy exists as to whether LKS or CSWS are separate entities or variations of the same disorder. Fejerman [14] and Doose [15, 16] have proposed that the various atypical syndromes could form a continuum, with a common underlying mechanism, and modulated by the duration, predominant location and diffusion of the epileptic activity. BECTS would then be only part of a spectrum of disorders of hereditary brain maturation with BECTS forming the benign common end and LKS and CSWS the severe, uncommon end of the spectrum.

BECTS prognosis

Epileptic prognosis

Long-term prognosis in BECTS is excellent, except for a few rare exceptions, with almost all patients achieving long-term remission by mid-adolescence [5]. De Romanis *et al.* [17]

followed 150 children with BECTS for 16 years. All children were treated for 2 years and after this time more than 80% remained seizure-free when treatment was stopped.

Beaussart [18] studied 85 cases after withdrawal of treatment and showed that all patients except one were seizure-free.

Loiseau et al. [19] followed 168 patients past the age of 20 years, and in his population, 98% remained seizure-free as adults and 2% developed rare generalised seizures.

Bouma et al. [20] performed a meta analysis of studies on BECTS and found that 50% of patients were in remission at 6 years of age, 92% at 12 years of age and 99.8% at 18 years of age.

Nevertheless, some factors might interfere with this good prognosis.

Loiseau et al. [19] found that age at onset was a good predictive factor for duration of the active period of the epilepsy: the earlier the onset, the longer the active period. Also, patients with multiple seizures at onset have significantly longer active disease periods than patients who have isolated ones [20].

Although seizure duration is usually brief, *status epilepticus* may be seen, and a few cases have been reported. The prevalence varies from 7 to 11% [7, 21]. A few cases of status epilepticus manifesting as anterior operculum syndrome have also been described [22, 23] with patients presenting prolonged speech and oromotor dysfunction with intermittent facial twitching and very frequent, sometimes continuous, bilateral spikes on the EEGs, which increased in sleep and sometimes evolved into CSWs. All patients recovered completely between 6 months and 8 years.

As far as EEG is concerned, as BECTS is an age-related syndrome, EEG manifestations tend to disappear with the disease at a certain age and regardless of the age at onset. With recovery spikes disappear first from the waking record and later from the sleeping one [24]. Sigfrid and Heijbel [25] reinvestigated a group of 26 patients with BECTS reported 10 years before. The EEGs were taken during wakefulness or drowsiness. 24 patients' recordings were normal and two showed slight, episodic bilateral abnormalities of a non-specific nature. No rolandic spikes were found.

In all cases, EEG recordings normalised within 6 months to 6 years [26]. There is no known relation between the intensity of the EEG manifestations and the frequency or length of seizures or the duration of the active period of the disease.

As we said before, therapy in BECTS mainly consists in reassuring the child and his family and avoiding overprotection. Drug therapy is necessary in only a minority of patients.

Carbamazepine and phenobarbital have been reported to cause electroclinical aggravation in some cases but the incidence of drug-induced aggravation in BECTS has never been established. Corda et al. [27] retrospectively studied 98 cases of BECTS; 82 had received one or more treatments, often successively and in association. They concluded that aggravation of BECTS caused by antiepileptic drugs happens only rarely. For these authors the only drugs that could be implicated were carbamazepine and phenobarbital, and the risk of aggravation is minor. It may occur only during certain periods coinciding with spontaneous worsening of the disease. The pharmacodynamic effect of the drug may then appear deleterious, although no aggravation is apparent in other patients. According to Corda, no antiepileptic drug provokes a systematic aggravation in patients with BECTS.

Neuropsychological prognosis

Normal neurological and cognitive findings have been considered a prerequisite for the diagnosis of BECTS. Neuropsychological problems have been described in the acute phase of the disease, but the long-term outcome has not been fully evaluated.

Many early studies [11, 26, 28] noted frequent behavioural problems, hyperactivity, inattention and learning disorders in children with BECTS, but these difficulties were attributed to the social stigma of epilepsy or to side effects of antiepileptic treatment [5].

Recently, Massa *et al.* [29] tried to demonstrate EEG or clinical markers predictive of neuropsychological complications in BECTS. According to their study, clinical deterioration was not linked with seizure characteristics but was significantly correlated with the persistence of three of those EEG patterns for more than three months: a slow wave focus, multiple asynchronous spike and wave (SW) foci, long rhythmic SW clusters, generalised SW discharges and an abundance of interictal abnormalities during wakefulness and sleep.

In a further study [6], the same team showed a significant correlation between the persistence of SW-related symptoms (*i.e.* brief neurological or neuropsychological phenomena having a strict temporal relation with individual components of isolated focal or generalised spike and waves) and a worsening of the epilepsy. They concluded that, during the evolution of the syndrome, a combination of at least three of the criteria mentioned above for a period of at least three months is predictive of cognitive complications in BECTS.

Recent studies have more carefully addressed the question of neuropsychological impairment in BECTS. D'Allessandro *et al.* [30] performed an extended battery of neuropsychological tests on 44 patients with BECTS and normal controls. All patients had been off treatment and seizure-free for a minimum of 6 months before testing. There was no significant difference in IQ scores between "rolandics" and controls, but BECTS performed significantly poorer on tests of attention, visuomotor performances and semantic fluency. Those with bilateral discharges scored the lowest whereas those with only right-sided discharges scored the highest. A follow-up assessment on 13 patients free of seizures and EEG abnormalities for at least 4 years showed that the neuropsychological abnormalities had disappeared, demonstrating the normalisation of neuropsychological problems after remission of the epilepsy.

Transient cognitive impairment (TCI) is a well-identified phenomenon resulting in discrete neuropsychological deficits during the period of infraclinical epileptic discharges, which are responsible for impaired psychosocial functioning in daily life [31]. Binnie's results [32, 33] in studying children with rolandic spikes with or without the clinical pattern of BECTS suggest a direct link between epileptic activity and cognitive functions.

The direct role of the epileptic discharges in causing this TCI in rolandic epilepsy could be confirmed if it could be shown that effectively suppressing them with antiepileptic drugs improves the cognitive function concerned [34]. Until now, only Sulthiame appears to be able both to control seizures and suppress EEG discharges in some cases of rolandic epilepsy, but precise data are very limited [34]. Anyway, this TCI can be subtle, but sometimes persistent or recurrent, and thus sufficient to interfere with school progress.

Other authors have tried to demonstrate the existence of neuropsychological disorders in BECTS in studying the relation between lateralised hemispheric function such as language and the topography of paroxysmal abnormalities [31]. The nature of the deficit found on neuropsychological testing has been shown to correlate with the side of centrotemporal discharge in children with BECTS. Piccirilli *et al.* [35] studied language lateralisation in 22 right-handed children who had a left or right rolandic focus and a group of normal right-handed controls, using a dual task procedure. All controls and patients with right centro-temporal discharge showed left lateralisation of language as expected, whereas those with a left focus demonstrated a different pattern, implying a bilateral representation of language functions. These results raised the possibility that focal epileptic activity may alter cerebral mechanisms underlying cognitive activity.

Hommet *et al.* [31] evaluated the long-term neuropsychological consequences of BECTS and particularly studied the relation between paroxysmal abnormalities and cerebral language lateralisation. They compared the performances of a group of patients in remission from BECTS who had an initial right or left focus, to a control group of adults with complete recovery from childhood absence epilepsy and to thirty-three patients without any significant past neurological history. No difference was found in the three populations concerning the overall cognitive function (memory, language and executive functions). Nevertheless, they demonstrated that BECTS patients in remission following an initial right seizure focus had the same pattern as controls whereas patients with an initial left focus showed a reverse pattern. Their results suggest some reorganisation in language functions according to the initial topography of the focus, as found by Piccirilli *et al.* [35].

In term of psychosocial prognosis, long-term outcome is excellent. Loiseau *et al.* [36] followed 79 patients with BECTS for a mean duration of 15.8 years. No increase in psychiatric problems was noted and almost all patients developed a normal adult personality.

Lerman [24] showed that, if families understood BECTS to be a chronic and disabling disease with probable brain damage, long-term psychosocial outcome was poor. If the benign nature of BECTS was understood and the child was not overprotected, long-term outcome was excellent [5].

Other idiopathic localisation-related epileptic syndromes

Benign childhood epilepsy with occipital paroxysms (BCEOP)

BCEOP was officially identified by Gastaut in 1982 [37]. The prevalence of this syndrome has been overestimated at the time, and many authors now consider it represents about 4% of all epilepsies with onset before 13 years old, and about 19% of benign age – and localisation – related idiopathic epilepsies. It is about one quarter as frequent as BECTS [38]. This syndrome seems to be divided into two entities: the early-onset one, or "Panayiotopoulos-type", is a syndrome of brief or prolonged partial seizures marked by deviation of the eyes and vomiting. The seizures are usually nocturnal and frequently evolve to hemiconvulsions and generalised tonic clonic fits. Onset is between the age of 2 and 8 years, with a peak at 5 years and remission before 12. There is preponderance in girls [39].

The late onset variant, or "Gastaut-type", occurs between 7 and 9 years, with mainly diurnal seizures consisting in visual symptoms, often followed by hemiclonic seizures or automatisms and migraine headache.

The main difficulties come from the fact that the EEG patterns are variable. The typical interictal occipital SW discharges may be found only during short periods in the course of the disease, especially during a few days after a single seizure [40]. They may be absent at the onset of seizures. The morphology of the occipital SW may vary over the time and may change during sleep. The main criterion is that these uni- or bilateral occipital SW attenuate or disappear when eyes are open.

Very few studies have tried to evaluate the prognosis of this syndrome in the past years. In his retrospective work, Panayiotopoulos [38] found an excellent prognosis for 89% of his patients, with no seizure occuring after the age of 12. Nevertheless these results concern the early-onset group of patients, with the peak age around 5 years, which is also the peak age for the appearance of functional occipital spikes in children. Andermann [41] reviewed 63 patients studied by Gastaut and Zifkin ten years before and found no cases where the seizures persisted into middle adulthood, and other types of recurring seizures in adulthood were seen in only 3 patients. The prognosis seems to be poorer in patients whose EEGs show an additional secondary epileptiform disturbance, but are these patients really affected by BCEOP?

Complete seizure control with AEDs was achieved in 38 patients (60%) and seizures persisted in 3 patients followed beyond age 19. The epileptiform EEG may persist for several months or years after the seizures have ceased.

It is considered likely that Panayiotopoulos syndrome represents the early while rolandic epilepsy is the late phenotype of the same syndrome (benign childhood seizure susceptibility syndrome) [38, 39]. Therefore it was expected that a small percentage of children with Panayiotopoulos syndrome could have a similar atypical evolution. Caraballo *et al.* [42] documented this atypical evolution in 2 out of 120 patients. They reported two girls with clinical and electroencephalographic features of BCEOP (Panayiotopoulos type). The first one presented inhibitory seizures in the lower limbs associated with behavioural disturbances and aphasia. EEG showed bilateral SW while awake and CSWS. Control of seizures, improvement of behaviour and partial restoration of cognitive functions were achieved with benzodiazepines. Five years later, EEG recording showed only isolated right occipital spikes, and she presented moderate mental retardation and dysphasia.

The other girl was diagnosed with BCEOP at age 4. Three years later, repeated inhibitory seizures and absences appeared. EEG recording was similar to the first girl's. Ethosuximide was added to valproate and clobazam and the seizures disappeared. The EEG showed less frequent bilateral occipital spikes. Eighteen months later, she has been seizure-free for more than a year and her neuropsychological profile showed mild mental retardation.

More recently, Ferrie *et al.* [43] presented a girl who initially had a prolonged autonomic status epilepticus typical of Panayiotopoulos syndrome, followed by seizures with concurrent symptoms of rolandic epilepsy. She then had an atypical evolution with atypical absences, absence status epilepticus, atonic seizures and mild impairment of scholastic performance. This represents an atypical evolution of intermediate severity compared to the cases reported by Caraballo *et al.* She did not have any behavioural problems, and the EEG during sleep was well organised without CSWS. Her scholastic performance was only mildly affected, probably as a result of frequent atypical absences. A significant improvement followed when lamotrigine was added to valproate and clonazepam, and her school results improved. A further video-EEG was almost normal.

That is the reason why clinicians, whilst rightly stressing the benign nature of Panayiotopoulos syndrome, should be aware that occasional patients with atypical evolution could be encountered. Further, these cases illustrate the links between this syndrome and rolandic epilepsy, which can both be considered as part of the benign childhood susceptibility syndrome [38, 39].

Atypical benign partial epilepsy (ABPE)

This particular form of BECTS was first described in 1982 by Aicardi and Chevrie [44]. They reported seven normally developed children who fulfilled the main criteria for rolandic epilepsy. They additionally suffered from generalised minor seizures (*i.e* atonic-astatic, myoclonic seizures and atypical absences) and showed a marked activation of epileptic discharges up to a discontinuous asymmetrical slow spike wave activity during sleep [45]. They demonstrate an excellent prognosis for epilepsy (with remission at age 9-12) and mental development. In 1989, Doose [46] analysed the clinical symptomatology of children with focal sharp slow waves and spikes of genetic origin and reported four patients closely resembling those described by Aicardi and Chevrie. Because of semiologic features common with Lennox-Gastaut syndrome and a much less benign course in all cases with frequent mental deficit, Doose proposed the term pseudo-Lennox syndrome (PLS) [46]. The author observed broad overlaps between ABPE and rolandic epilepsy, and also emphasised features common to CSWS and LKS.

In recent years, very few studies have focused on ABPE, and the existence of this syndrome has not been generally recognised.

Hahn *et al.* [45] recently investigated the clinical spectrum of ABPE to evaluate its long-term prognosis and investigate its relationship with rolandic epilepsy, CSWS and LKS.

They conclude that ABPE represents an electroclinical entity with a broad spectrum of focal generalising seizures. The EEG is characterised by generalising predominantly multifocal sharp slow-waves and spikes. There are definitely symptomatologic features common with BECTS but also with CSWS and LKS. The aetiology of ABPE or PLS is multifactorial. In a unifying pathogenic concept of idiopathic partial epilepsies by Doose and Baier [22], the responsible basic mechanism has been hypothetically termed hereditary impairment of brain maturation. That is the reason why we think the term age – and localisation – related epilepsies is the most appropriate for these epileptic syndromes.

Anyway, further investigations are needed to elucidate the clinical and electroencephalographic features of PLS as well as the cognitive outcome of this syndrome.

Idiopathic partial epilepsy with frontal paroxysms

This syndrome has been described for the first time by Beaumanoir and Nahory [47]. They presented 11 children with frontal lobe epilepsy of good prognosis, who all had been seizure-free for at least 5 years. According to Loiseau *et al.* [48] this type of epilepsy accounts for approximately 11% of all cases of idiopathic focal epilepsies.

Raffo [49] reported 5 cases of this idiopathic partial frontal epilepsy and synthesised the electroclinical characteristics of the two series. The age at onset ranges from 2 to 8 years, seizure frequency from one seizure per month to several per week and duration of the active period from 1 to 6 years.

The seizures are of several types, diurnal (complex partial seizures, motor automatisms, sometimes absence-like seizures) and nocturnal (hemifacial motor seizures, versive, with sometimes a post-crisis deficit and/or secondarily generalised seizures).

As for BCEOP, the EEG findings are heterogeneous and no defined pattern has been demonstrated: some patients show patterns compatible with the diagnosis of BECTS, others have only focal slow activity; the ictal patterns are shifting frontal discharges. During sleep, activation and diffusion of the anomalies is observed. This leads to be very careful before making a diagnosis of idiopathic partial epilepsy with frontal paroxysms.

The epileptic outcome is spontaneously favourable.

In terms of neuropsychological outcome, TCI have been observed [49], particularly in short-term memory and executive functions, during the active period of the epilepsy with a normalisation after the remission of the disease.

To our knowledge, no other studies have focused on this syndrome and further investigations are therefore needed especially concerning the neuropsychological outcome of these children.

Idiopathic partial epilepsy in infancy

This syndrome was described for the first time by Watanabe [50]. He reported nine infants with complex partial seizures beginning between the age of 3 and 20 months. They all presented with clusters of seizures, with motion arrest, decreased responsiveness, staring or blank eyes, mostly with automatisms and mild convulsive movements. The prognosis was excellent at follow-up. Four of the nine children had a familial history of benign seizures in infancy.

The same authors [51] later reported another group of seven children with secondarily generalised seizures in clusters, and with the same age at onset. The initial ictal symptoms were motion arrest or staring during a few seconds followed by tonic-clonic generalisation. All patients were seizure-free with follow-ups between 3 and 12 years.

A French multicenter study [52] described 34 patients with constant clinical and EEG characteristics: age at onset around 6 months, brief partial seizures, sometimes secondarily generalised, happening in clusters with 2 to 12 episodes per day during a few days (mean 2.5). The ictal EEG showed focal discharges and a slow aspect or focal spikes were observed on the inter-ictal recording, whereas EEG at distance from seizures was normal. Twelve out of the thirty-four cases were familial. Various antiepileptic drugs can be administrated and are efficacious within a few hours. They are stopped after 1 to 3 years and no recurrence is observed. Excellent outcome is the rule in terms of epilepsy as well as neuropsychological prognosis.

Nevertheless, paroxysmal choreo-athetosic episodes, occurring a few years after the initial seizures, have recently been reported by various authors [53-55]. These episodes could correspond to frontal seizures but Koch *et al.* did not observe any EEG abnormalities on the critical video-EEG recording. Low doses of carbamazepine were effective with complete disappearance of the dyskinetic attacks. The neuropsychological profile of the girl was normal, with a global IQ at 117 and a discrepancy between verbal IQ (123) and performance IQ (105). Her school performances were normal.

It may be hypothesised that epileptic infantile seizures and the later choreo-athetosic attacks are two different manifestations, at two different stages of development, of the same neuronal membrane dysfunction, their respective occurrences depending on brain maturation.

Conclusion

Among the localisation-related epilepsies in children, there are some age-related syndromes. This term is, according to us, better than "idiopathic" or "benign".

These syndromes usually have an excellent epileptic prognosis. Concerning the neuropsychological outcome of these syndromes, we have shown that, particularly in BECTS with left focal focus, there is a reorganisation of the hemispheric specialisation concerning the language function, due to the localisation of the epileptic manifestations. Further studies on the subject are certainly needed.

The main interest of knowing the outcome of an epileptic syndrome is to be able to predict this prognosis at the beginning of the manifestations. That is the reason why the initial diagnosis of the syndrome has to be extremely precise and be based upon indisputable criteria. Unfortunately, it does not seem to be the case for the syndromes we have described except for BECTS. We must then wonder whether the cases with atypical evolution really belong to the right syndrome or whether they correspond to diagnosis errors.

References

1. Commission on Classification and Terminology of the International League against Epilepsy. Proposal for classification of epilepsies and epileptic syndromes. *Epilepsia* 1989; 30: 389-99.
2. Genton P, Guerrini R. Idiopathic localisation-related epilepsies: the non-rolandic types. In: Wolf P, eds. *Epileptic seizures and syndromes*. London: John Libbey, 1994: 241-56.
3. Nayrac P, Beaussart M. Les pointes ondes prérolandiques : expression EEG très particulière. *Rev Neurol* 1958; 99: 201-6.
4. Stephani U. Typical semiology of benign childhood epilepsy with centrotemporal spikes. *Epileptic Disord* 2000; 2 (Suppl 1): S3-S4.
5. Wirrell EC. Benign epilepsy of childhood with centrotemporal spikes. *Epilepsia* 1998; 39 (Suppl 4): S32-S41.
6. De Saint-Martin A, Carcangiu R, Arzimanoglou A, *et al*. Semiology of typical and atypical rolandic epilepsy: a video-EEG analysis. *Epileptic Disord* 2001; 3: 173-81.
7. Wirrell EC, Camfield PR, Gordon KE, Dooley JM, Camfield CS. Benign partial epilepsy: atypical features are very common. *J Child Neurol* 1995; 10: 455-8.
8. Blom S, Heijbel J. Benign epilepsy of children with centrotemporal foci. Discharge rate during sleep. *Epilepsia* 1975; 16: 133-40.
9. Aicardi J. Atypical semiology of rolandic epilepsy in some related syndromes. *Epileptic Disord* 2000; 2 (Suppl 1): S5-S9.
10. Scheffer IE, Jones L, Pozzebon M, Howell RA, Saling MM, Berkovic SF. Autosomal dominant rolandic epilepsy and speech dyspraxia: a new syndrome with anticipation. *Ann Neurol* 1995; 38: 633-42.
11. Landau WM, Kleffner FR. Syndrome of acquired aphasia with convulsive disorder in children. *Neurology* 1957; 7: 523-30.
12. Tassinari CA, Bureau M, Dravet C, *et al*. Epilepsy with continuous spikes and waves during slow sleep. In: Roger J, Bureau M, Dravet C, Dreifuss FE, Perret A, Wolf P, eds. *Epileptic syndromes in infancy, childhood and adolescence*. London: John Libbey, 1992: 245-56.
13. Finck S. Épilepsie à paroxysmes rolandiques, dyspraxie bucco-linguale, déficience mentale de transmission autosomique dominante : une nouvelle famille. Mémoire du Diplôme inter-universitaire de Neuropédiatrie 2001.
14. Fejerman N. Atypical evolutions of benign partial epilepsies in children. *Internat Pediatr* 1996; 11: 351-6.
15. Doose H, Baier WK. Benign partial epilepsy and related conditions: multifactorial pathogenesis with hereditary impairment of brain maturation. *Eur J Pediatr* 1989; 149: 152-8.
16. Doose H, Neubauer B, Carlsson G. Children with benign focal sharp waves in the EEG. Developmental disorders and epilepsy. *Neuropediatrics* 1996; 27: 227-41.
17. De Romanis F, Feliciani M, Ruggieri S. Rolandic paroxysmal epilepsy: a long-term study in 150 children. *Ital J Neurol Sci* 1986; 7: 77-80.
18. Beaussart M. Benign epilepsy of children with rolandic (centrotemporal) paroxysmal foci: a clinical entity. Study of 221 cases. *Epilepsia* 1972; 13: 795-811.
19. Loiseau P, Duche B, Cordova S, Dartigues JF, Cohadon S. Prognosis of benign childhood epilepsy with centrotemporal spikes: a follow up study of 168 patients. *Epilepsia* 1988; 29: 229-35.
20. Bouma PAD, Bovenkerk AC, Westendorp RGJ, Bronwer OF. The course of benign partial epilepsy of childhood with centrotemporal spikes: a meta-analysis. *Neurology* 1997; 48: 430-7.
21. Deonna T, Ziegler AL, Despland PA, van Melle G. Partial epilepsy in neurologically normal children: clinical syndromes and prognosis. *Epilepsia* 1986; 27: 241-7.
22. Colamaria V, Sgro V, Carabello R, Simeone M, Zullini E, Fontana E, *et al*. Status epilepticus in benign rolandic epilepsy manifesting as anterior operculum syndrome. *Epilepsia* 1991; 32: 329-34.
23. Deonna T, Roulet E, Fontan D, Marcoz JP. Speech and oromotor deficits of epileptic origin in benign partial epilepsy of childhood with rolandic spikes. *Neuropediatrics* 1993; 24: 83-7.
24. Lerman P. Benign partial epilepsy with centrotemporal spikes. In: Roger J, Bureau M, Dravet C, Dreifuss FE, Perret A, Wolf P, eds. *Epileptic syndromes in infancy, childhood and adolescence*. London: John Libbey Eurotext, 1992: 189-200.
25. Blom S, Heijbel J. Benign epilepsy of children with centrotemporal EEG foci: a follow-up study in adulthood of patients initially studied as children. *Epilepsia* 1982; 23: 629-32.

26. Lerman P, Kivity S. Benign focal epilepsy of childhood: a follow up of 100 recovered patients. *Arch Neurol* 1975; 32: 261-4.
27. Corda D, Gelisse P, Genton P, Dravet C, Baldy Moulinier M. Incidence of drug induced aggravation in benign epilepsy with centrotemporal spikes. *Epilepsia* 2001; 42: 754-9.
28. Heijbel J, Bohman M. Benign epilepsy of children with centrotemporal foci: intelligence, behavior and school adjustment. *Epilepsia* 1975; 16: 679-87.
29. Massa R, de Saint-Martin A, Carcangiu R, *et al*. EEG criteria predictive of cognitive complications in idiopathic focal epilepsy with rolandic spikes. *Neurology* 2001; 57: 1071-9.
30. D'Allessandro P, Piccirilli M, Tiacci C, *et al*. Neuropsychological features of benign partial epilepsy in children. *Ital J Neurol Sci* 1990; 11: 265-9.
31. Hommet C, Billard C, Motte J, *et al*. Cognitive function in adolescents and young adults in complete remission from benign childhood epilepsy with centro-temporal spikes. *Epileptic Disord* 2001; 3: 207-16.
32. Binnie CD. Significance and management of TCI due to subclinical EEG discharges in children. *Brain Dev* 1993; 15: 23-30.
33. Binnie CD, de Silva N, Hurst A. Rolandic spikes and cognitive functions. In: Benign localised and generalised epilepsies of early childhood. *Epilepsy Res* 1992; (Suppl 6): 71-4.
34. Deonna T. Rolandic epilepsy: neuropsychology of the active epilepsy phase. *Epileptic Disord* 2000; 2 (Suppl 1): S59-61.
35. Piccirilli M, d'Allessandro P, Tiacci C, Ferroni A. Language lateralization in children with benign partial epilepsy. *Epilepsia* 1988; 29: 19-25.
36. Loiseau P, Pestre M, Dartigues JF, *et al*. Long term prognosis in two forms of childhood epilepsy: typical absence seizures and epilepsy with rolandic EEG foci. *Ann Neurol* 1983; 13: 642-8.
37. Gastaut H. A new type of epilepsy: benign partial epilepsy of childhood with occipital spike waves. *Clin Electroencephalogr* 1982; 13: 13-22.
38. Panayiotopoulos CP. Benign childhood epilepsy with occipital paroxysms: a 15 year prospective study. *Ann Neurol* 1989; 26: 51-6.
39. Panayiotopoulos CP. Early onset benign childhood occipital seizure susceptibility syndrome: a syndrome to recognize. *Epilepsia* 1999; 40: 621-30.
40. Guerrini R, Dravet C, Vigliano P, *et al*. Childhood idiopathic occipital epilepsy. *Epilepsia* 1993; 34 (Suppl 2): 178.
41. Andermann F, Zifkin B. The benign occipital epilepsies of childhood: an overview of the idiopathic syndromes and of the relationship to migraine. *Epilepsia* 1998; 39 (Suppl 4): S9-S23.
42. Caraballo RH, Astorino F, Cersosimo R, Soprano A.M, Fejerman N. Atypical evolution in childhood epilepsy with occipital paroxysms (Panayiotopoulos type). *Epileptic Disord* 2001; 3: 157-62.
43. Ferrie CD, Koutroumanidis M, Rowlinson S, Sanders S, Panayiotopoulos CP. Atypical evolution of Panayiotopoulos syndrome: a case report. *Epileptic Disord* 2002; 4: 35-41.
44. Aicardi J, Chevrie JJ. Atypical benign partial epilepsy of childhood. *Dev Med Child Neurol* 1982; 24: 281-92.
45. Hahn A, Pisthol J, Neubauer BA, Stephani U. Atypical benign partial epilepsy/pseudo-Lennox syndrome. Part I: Symptomatology and long-term prognosis. *Neuropediatrics* 2001; 32: 1-8.
46. Doose H. Symptomatology in children with focal sharp waves of genetic origin. *Eur J Ped* 1989; 149: 210-5.
47. Beaumanoir A, Nahory A. Les épilepsies bénignes partielles : 11 cas d'épilepsies partielle frontale à évolution favorable. *Rev Electroencéphalogr Neurophysiol Clin* 1983; 13: 207-11.
48. Loiseau P, Duche B, Loiseau J. Classification of epilepsies and epileptic syndromes in two different samples of patients. *Epilepsia* 1991; 32: 303-9.
49. Raffo E. Épilepsie idiopathique à paroxysmes frontaux : à propos de 5 observations. Mémoire de diplôme inter-universitaire de Neurologie Pédiatrique. 2000.
50. Watanabe K, Yamamoto N, Negoro T, *et al*. Benign complex partial epilepies in infancy. *Pediatr Neurol* 1987; 3: 208-11.
51. Watanabe K, Negoro T, Aso K. Benign partial epilepsy with secondarily generalised seizures in infancy. *Epilepsia* 1993; 34: 635-8.
52. Gautier A, Pouplard F, Bednarek N, *et al*. Convulsions bénignes du nourrisson. Étude collaboratrice française. *Arch Pediatr* 1999; 6: 32-9.

53. Koch C, Bednarek N, Motte J. Benign epileptic seizures in infancy followed by paroxysmal choreo-athetosis during adolescence. *Epileptic Disord* 1999; 1: 141-2.
54. Echenne B, Rivier F, Humbert CV, Roubertie A, Cheminal R, Malafosse A. Les convulsions familiales bénignes du nourrisson. *Arch Pediatr* 1999; 6: 54-8.
55. Sceptetowski P, Rochette J, Berquin P, *et al.* Familial infantile convulsions and paroxysmal choreo-athetosis: a new neurological syndrome linked to the pericentrometric region of human chromosome 16. *Am J Hum Genet* 1997; 61: 889-98.

Prognosis of Lennox-Gastaut syndrome

Alexis Arzimanoglou

Lennox-Gastaut syndrome (LGS), along with West and Dravet syndromes, is one of the most malignant epilepsy syndromes of childhood. The characteristic clinical and EEG features have been extensively reported [1-5]; however, there is considerable confusion surrounding the concept of the Lennox-Gastaut syndrome, and its definition remains a subject of dispute. As a result, studies on long-term outcome are very difficult to interpret, as they do not necessarily discuss prognosis of the same types of patients. In particular, when discussing prognosis and long-term evolution, issues related whether the definition is based on the presence of diffuse slow spike-wave complexes only or bursts of rapid rhythms during sleep may be of primary importance. The presence or absence of atonic or tonic seizures may be of similar importance. Finally age at onset of each type of seizure within this syndrome and, even more important, timing of the appearance of the different EEG abnormalities are almost never taken into account when defining the syndrome and even less when discussing its long-term outcome.

The most widely accepted *definition* for Lennox-Gastaut syndrome is that of a disorder characterized by a combination of multiple, brief seizures, the most characteristic of which are tonic, atonic, and atypical absence seizures as well as episodes of nonconvulsive and tonic status epilepticus. From the EEG standpoint, slow (< 2.5 Hz) spike-wave complexes and bursts of rapid (10-Hz) rhythms during slow sleep often corresponding to minimal or subclinical seizures are most important for diagnosis. Other types of focal or generalized seizures often occur, simultaneously with, preceding or following the typical attacks. Psychomotor retardation is present in almost all cases. The syndrome may be cryptogenic in children with a previously normal development or symptomatic of congenital or acquired brain anomalies.

There are no definitive estimates of the *incidence* of Lennox-Gastaut syndrome. Published figures indicate that it may represent between 3% and 10.7% of the epilepsies of childhood [6], but the true incidence is impossible to determine because of the various definitions of the syndrome. Boys are more often affected than girls. The onset of LGS is age-dependent [7] with a peak incidence between one and seven years, although cases with a later onset, in adolescence or adulthood, are occasionally reported [8]. Prevalence was estimated at about 2.6 per 10 000 children in the general population at 10 years of age [9].

The *short-term mortality* has been estimated at 4.2 to 7% of those affected, in part secondary to tonic status [10]. Up to 10% of children with LGS die prior to reaching 11 years of age [11, 12].

Estimates of the frequency of a family history of epilepsy among patients with the Lennox-Gastaut syndrome are highly variable. Discrepancies are, once again, probably due to variability in the types of epilepsy included in the different published reports. A family history of febrile seizures or of epilepsy has been reported in 48% of patients in one series [13]. The familial influence seems greater in patients with the cryptogenic rather than the symptomatic form. Other types of seizure disorders, especially West syndrome, often precede the Lennox-Gastaut syndrome.

Several studies are available on the electro-clinical characteristics and reactivity to AEDs of patients with LGS. However, the long-term evolution and prognosis has not been carefully investigated, and reports involving large series of patients are relatively few [5, 14-17].

Many authors suggest that Lennox-Gastaut syndrome is a nonspecific response of the one to seven-year-old brain to diffuse or occasionally localized damage [10, 18]. Blume [19] recently discussed the pathogenesis of LGS and suggested that the occurrence of factors enhancing excitability during a vulnerable period of cortical and thalamic development, as when the child's nervous system is still immature, may permanently establish a bilateral diffuse epileptogenic system in the brain. Frontal lesions may be particularly apt to produce the picture of Lennox-Gastaut syndrome [20]. Elucidation of the long-term evolution would contribute to understanding the underlying pathophysiology.

Methodological issues

A comprehensive debate on the prognosis of a given syndrome should imply that we are dealing with a well-defined clinical entity and that we have at our disposal prospectively collected data on the natural evolution of the disease for a substantial number of patients, who have been rigorously evaluated according to pre-defined criteria. Unfortunately, as far as LGS is concerned, the only point that all authors agree on is that there is still considerable confusion surrounding its definition.

Thus, it is almost impossible to discuss, for example, *the significance of bursts of rapid rhythms during sleep* without examining them within the context of a representative series of patients and comparing those patients who do to those who do not have this feature at various points during the course of their disorder. If we all agree that maturational processes within the nervous system influences and may be influenced by a given type of EEG abnormality or type of discharges, how can we seriously discuss the influence of these electrographic findings on long-term outcome when we do not precisely know the age at which they first appeared?

Other methodological difficulties are the direct result of a *number of other variables to be considered*, particularly when discussing complex syndromes such as LGS. These include the various underlying etiologies, presence of various types of seizures, use of specific drug therapies and combinations of drugs that are often indicated for different types of seizures (for example one patient with LGS may have received a given drug because of intractable myoclonic seizures while another may have received the same drug for the persistence of tonic seizures), duration of treatment; initial treatments used; and other factors as well.

Another bias stems from the fact that most of the published data on the prognosis of LGS come from *retrospective series*. The inherent problem with such studies is that they include patients not on the basis of the presumed or suspected diagnosis at onset but on the diagnosis made after some years of observation. Such retrospective diagnoses are usually influenced by what is generally thought to be the typical evolution and outcome for the syndrome. We do not currently have sufficient data on the mechanisms involved to allow a similar consideration of prognosis in several clinical scenarios such as: a) patients who do not present with all of the key features of LGS at onset but who go on to develop classic LGS during the course of their epilepsy; b) patients who initially present with a partial epilepsy and then evolve into a typical LGS; and c) patients who have a typical LGS picture at onset but who then evolve towards a non-typical form.

We strongly believe that *"prognosis" can only be part of the description of a given epilepsy syndrome and that it should never be part of the criteria for making a diagnosis.* We are aware of the fact that, for many epilepsy syndromes, all symptoms are not always present at onset and that epilepsies change with age. However, in order to discuss prognosis, we should first agree on the critical period by the end of which one should be able to confirm or discard the diagnosis of LGS.

Under certain circumstances, one of the more challenging aspects of LGS is the distinction from other childhood epilepsies that might mimic either its EEG or clinical pattern. Comparison between the evolution of LGS patients and the evolution of entities presenting with only part of the symptoms is almost impossible with the existing available data. For example, when trying to compare LGS to myoclonic-astatic epilepsy [21], several problems are introduced by the simple fact that the ILAE classification of the epilepsies did not define the two syndromes on the basis of the same criteria. LGS was defined primarily based upon its electroclinical features, while, as Doose emphasizes, myoclonic-astatic epilepsy was defined mainly on etiological criteria and a genetic predisposition.

The above mentioned and other methodological difficulties explain why evidence from the literature is particularly difficult to use in this field. Different studies produce different answers to most questions. In the present review we will discuss available data on prognosis of LGS. Whenever reported, the diagnostic criteria used in each published series will be presented.

Prognosis of seizures in Lennox-Gastaut syndrome

The persistence of seizures is of primary importance because the unpredictable occurrence of attacks influences the quality of all aspects of everyday life. This is particularly true in LGS as seizures are a common cause of injury. The seizures that occur in Lennox-Gastaut syndrome are of several types [3, 5, 14, 22, 23]. Brief tonic, atonic, myoclonic, and myoatonic attacks, atypical absences, and absence status or mixed tonic and absence or purely tonic status represent the primary ictal manifestations. They are frequently associated with other less characteristic types of seizures.

Seizure types in LGS

Tonic seizures are probably the most common and most characteristic type, although they are estimated to occur in anywhere from 17% [3] to 55% [5] and even up to 95% of cases [14]. The higher incidence is observed when sleep tracings are systematically obtained. Tonic attacks are typically activated by sleep. They are much more frequent during non-REM sleep than during wakefulness and do not occur during REM sleep. Tonic seizures that occur in series may be reminiscent of infantile spasms although the duration of the individual contractions tends to be longer, especially when Lennox-Gastaut syndrome follows infantile spasms. The autonomic phenomena (flushing or pallor, rarely cyanosis; hypersalivation) may be prominent.

Atonic seizures are frequent and occur in 26% to 56% of patients. Most such seizures are quite brief, lasting one to four seconds [4, 24, 25]. In the briefest attacks, patients may show only head nodding or sagging at the knees. If a fall occurs, the patient usually picks himself up immediately and resumes what he was doing. There is no detectable alteration of consciousness or postictal confusion, but severe injuries to the nose or teeth may result. Atonic attacks are often initiated by a myoclonic jerk [4, 22, 26] that also may supervene at the same time as the atonic fit, e.g., a myoclonic jerk of the arms with an atonic fall. The incidence of *myoclonic seizures* in Lennox-Gastaut syndrome is variably estimated at 11% to 28% of patients [5, 6, 27]. *Atypical absences* occur in 17% to 60% of patients with LGS.

Nonconvulsive status is common in Lennox-Gastaut syndrome [11, 28, 29]. It is marked by obtundation, apathy, stupor, or a slight blurring of consciousness, interspersed with atonic or myoclonic head nods, fluttering of eyelids, or slight erratic myoclonus of the face or segments of the limbs. Facial expression is slack, there is drooling of saliva, and speech is slurred or disappears altogether. Episodes of absence status may be so subtle as to be hardly noticeable or sufficiently intense to confine the patient to bed. The episodes often occur on awakening [30]. In some patients, the myoclonic component is prominent (myoclonic status). The episodes of status, when subtle, may be difficult to distinguish from the interictal state [6, 29, 31]. Duration is variable, from hours to days and occasionally weeks. Tonic status may appear suddenly, at times following intravenous administration of benzodiazepines [32-34] *or progressively*. Mixed tonic and absence status is one of the most common types of status in this syndrome. It consists of an uninterrupted series of short tonic seizures alternating with atypical absences.

Any combination of seizures can be encountered, and, in virtually all patients, good periods alternate with bad ones. During bad periods there is often an apparent deterioration of mental performance and an increase in the frequency of EEG abnormalities.

Prognosis of seizures in typical cases

As they progress to adulthood, patients with tonic seizures, nonconvulsive or tonic status epilepticus, and rapid discharges during sleep are most likely to continue manifesting the same seizure types. Beaumanoir [35] studied a group of 103 patients followed for a mean of 19.7 years and divided it into two subgroups: (a) patients with a typical presentation from onset including tonic fits, nonconvulsive or tonic status and 10-Hz discharges during slow sleep 75% of whom continued to exhibit an unchanged pattern at the end of follow-up; and (b) patients with less typical features, often following the occurrence of initial partial seizures, who mainly evolved to what appeared to be a partial epilepsy with complex partial or multifocal seizures. In this group, the patients tended to loose the characteristics of the Lennox-Gastaut syndrome, and the seizure outcome was better. For these patients, Lennox-Gastaut syndrome seemed to represent an age-related mode of expression of partial epilepsies with temporary diffusion of the paroxysms. Similar results concerning the persistence of tonic seizures in typical patients have been recently reported by Yagi [16]. In typical cases the clinical pattern changes with age. Between 15 and 20 years of age the overall seizure frequency usually diminishes. Atypical absences and drop attacks may become rare but all other types of seizures, including tonic seizures in sleep, persist. In older patients tonic seizures during sleep are probably under-reported.

Prognosis of seizures in atypical cases

Prognosis may also be different in patients who develop atonic or tonic seizures in the course of partial epilepsy [8, 36]. Gastaut and Zifkin [37] came to similar conclusions in their study of 40 patients. In all studies, the occurrence of tonic and atonic attacks was associated with the appearance on the EEG of bilateral fast or slow spike-wave complexes and/or bursts of a 10-Hz recruiting rhythm, especially during sleep. Such secondary spread of initially focal epilepsy may be impossible to distinguish from classic Lennox-Gastaut syndrome. In fact, most such cases fulfill all or most of the criteria for the syndrome. They may even constitute a subgroup of it and thus should not be regarded as representing a different entity. Their practical interest is that they may be due to localized lesions that could conceivably be amenable to surgical treatment. It is indeed possible that many cases of Lennox-Gastaut syndrome are due to undetectable focal lesions or areas of dysfunction. Studies with PET have given variable results [38-40] but 5 of the 15 cases studied by Chugani and collaborators [41] had focal areas of hypometabolism. Likewise, other investigators [40] also recorded focal pathological areas.

Prognosis is difficult to establish for patients who, at onset, present exclusively with myoclonic-astatic seizures. Most of them will have a long-term evolution that differs from the evolution of LGS. However, some patients will later also develop tonic seizures and/or bursts of rapid rhythms during sleep, thus fulfilling the criteria for LGS [70].

Treatment strategies and prognosis

Effects of treatment with AEDs have been published based upon numerous open-label studies, but only a few placebo-controlled studies have been done in this area (for a detailed review see Aicardi and Arzimanoglou 1996 [42]; Crumrine PK 2001 [43]; Trevathan E. 2002 [44]). In a few publications a significant reduction of seizures has been reported, particularly with new AEDs. *Sodium valproate* has been the mainstay of therapy for the past 20 years. The *benzodiazepines* have also been extensively used, sedation and development of tolerance representing their main limits. Among the new AEDs, *felbamate* was the first drug shown to be effective in LGS [45]. Experience has remained limited because a few months following its commercialization, concerns were raised over the risk of hepatotoxicity and aplastic anemia. Recent data suggests that the risk is not as high as was initially thought, and therefore the use of the drug may be justified in severe cases [46]. *Lamotrigine* [47], probably because of its wide spectrum of effectiveness, has also provided promising results in open [48-51] and controlled studies [52]. In the double-blind, placebo-controlled study, 33% of the lamotrigine group and 16% of the placebo group experienced more than a 50% reduction in the frequency of all major seizure types, including drop attacks. Global evaluations of patient's functioning in terms of speech, language, and attention were significantly improved in the lamotrigine group [52]. A synergistic action between valproic acid and lamotrigine has been reported [53, 54]. In a large open study [55], control of seizures in LGS patients was better with this combination. The efficacy of *topiramate* has also been reported for tonic-clonic seizures, tonic seizures, and drop attacks associated with LGS [56]. Although statistically significant when compared to placebo, reduction of drop attacks occurred in only 14% of the patients taking topiramate. Comparative trials of topiramate, lamotrigine, and felbamate are not currently available.

Favorable results in Lennox-Gastaut syndrome have been reported with the use of ACTH and steroids [6, 57]. However, no controlled study is available and the results may be difficult to assess in patients receiving multiple forms of treatment as well as in syndromes that are known to fluctuate between good and bad periods. The relapse rate seems to be high even with high-dose, prolonged regimens. Some authors [58] recommend the use of such drugs primarily to tide some patients over a particularly difficult period rather than as a long-term, regular therapy. Only palliative surgery can be offered to drug-resistant patients, callosotomy being indicated in selected cases with repeated falls [59]. Few patients experience any benefit from vagus nerve stimulation [60].

Did new treatment strategies modify prognosis?

Overall, the therapeutic options for treatment of Lennox-Gastaut syndrome have expanded during the last fifteen years. According to Papini *et al.* [61], in LGS patients, 31% of seizures that do not occur during slow sleep occur during drowsiness and 54% during inactive wakefulness. Only 8% and 6% of seizures respectively occur during active wakefulness and sleep. The main precipitating factors of seizures in Lennox-Gastaut syndrome are inactivity and drowsiness [62]. It could be assumed that the use of new, less sedating, antiepileptic drugs will result in some indirect benefit.

In terms of overall efficacy, the literature can only confirm that the vast majority of LGS patients remain intractable to treatment, including to the new AEDs. Undoubtedly, a small number of patients experience a reduction in seizure frequency, particularly when appropriately treated from onset with wide spectrum drugs such as valproate or lamotrigine, alone or in combination. For a large proportion of LGS patients, control of drop attacks could positively influence quality of life. Unfortunately, none of the new or old AEDs has led to a meaningful change in the overall prognosis of the syndrome. For the very few patients who rapidly became seizure free there are no available data from controlled trials about the evolution of other components of the syndrome, in particular mental retardation and behavioral problems.

Another issue to consider is the possible harmful effects of the drug treatment itself. Although the overall bad prognosis of the majority of LGS patients seems independent of the various AEDs used during the last twenty years, aggravation due to certain drugs has been reported in individual cases. Controlled or prospective studies are not available. Anecdotal reports, particularly those concerning seizure exacerbation associated with the use of the new drugs, are based on short-term clinical observations that do not take into account the fluctuation between good and bad periods of seizure control that is often seen in LGS. Therefore, apparent worsening of seizures after initiation of a new drug may simply reflect the normal fluctuations seen in LGS and have nothing to do with adverse effects of the new drug itself. The only point that all authors agree on is that prognosis will be worse when a patient is treated with multiple drugs in combination as this can lead to sedation which in turn can cause an exacerbation of seizure occurrence.

Mental retardation, behavioral problems and prognosis

Mental retardation is present before onset of the seizures in 20 to 60% of patients with LGS [5, 6, 14, 63, 64]. As with infantile spasms, such cases are considered secondary or symptomatic. They are often associated with neurological signs, a history of brain injury, and neuroimaging abnormalities. Psychomotor retardation tends to be particularly severe in such patients. In cryptogenic cases, initial mental and neurological development is normal, and mental deterioration is all the more striking when the onset is at several years of age. The proportion of mentally retarded patients increases to 75 to 93% five years after onset [5, 23, 65]. The degree of mental retardation is often severe: Chevrie and Aicardi

[5] found that 55% of their patients had IQs below 50. This was also the case in 48% of Gastaut's patients [14]. Even in the rare patients with normal intelligence, there is extreme slowness in ideation and action. Mental retardation in Lennox-Gastaut syndrome patients is often accompanied by behavioral and personality disturbances. The patients are withdrawn and feel insecure and anxious [14]. Frank psychotic behavior is common [64].

Progressive declines in IQ scores in patients with LGS were initially attributed to lack of new learning rather than loss of previously acquired skills [10, 14]. However, clinical evidence of marked *deterioration* is present in many children, especially in those who have had long periods of previously normal development, and it is difficult to escape the impression of a degenerative CNS disease. There is, however, no other evidence for a neurodegenerative disorder being the basis for LGS, and the process of deterioration is self-limiting with a clear temporal correlation between the presence of intense paroxysmal activity and the deterioration. Indeed, deterioration may well result from the epileptic activity itself. It has been suggested that IQ scores remain constant during remissions and exacerbations of the syndrome, whereas, by contrast, motor reaction time, verbal latencies, and performance on simple cognitive tasks are definitely affected by the patients' current clinical status [66].

In a recent retrospective study Hoffmann-Riem and collaborators [67] reported on the course of the disease, EEG tracings and intellectual function in 101 patients. Tonic seizures and diffuse slow spike-wave complexes on the interictal EEG were necessary for the diagnosis of LGS. Mean age at onset of tonic seizures was 5.2 years (range 2-14 years) and the mean age of the patients at the time of the study was 17 years (range 5-34 years) with an average observation period of 16 years (range 4-31 years). Of note, epilepsy started with tonic seizures allowing the diagnosis of LGS from the onset in only 6% of patients. Overall, only 4% of the patients became seizure-free. Neurological dysfunction was a common feature (24% presented with signs of severe encephalopathy with ataxia and pyramidal signs, inability to walk was noted in 21%, inability to speak in 38%, and impaired motor coordination in 52%). Mental retardation, which legitimately was not one of the inclusion criteria, was evaluated as severe (IQ < 35) in 57 (56%) and mild or moderate (IQ > 35) in 44 (43%) of patients. Multivariate analysis revealed four independent risk factors significantly correlated with severe mental retardation. These were in a decreasing order of importance: nonconvulsive status epilepticus (NCSE) (Odds Ratio (OR) 25.2), a previous diagnosis of West syndrome (OR 11.6), a symptomatic etiology (OR 9.5), and an early age at onset of epilepsy (OR 4.7). The results of this study confirm existing data regarding the role of factors like etiology and age at onset on intellectual deterioration in LGS patients and provide evidence to suggest that, within the setting of this syndrome, NCSE may also play a major role. Similar assumptions about the role of NCSE, were advanced by Doose and Völzke [68] to explain the development of dementia in some patients with "myoclonic-astatic epilepsy".

Episodes of status epilepticus, however, may be only another expression of the severity of an unknown process responsible for both the loss of mental abilities and the epileptic activity. No relation has been found in other studies [28] between cognitive functioning at the end of follow-up and the occurrence of overt episodes of status epilepticus. Moreover a relationship could exist between "bad periods" that may represent minimal status and deterioration. Many patients with the Lennox-Gastaut syndrome develop abnormalities of behavior that include autistic features or hyperkinetic syndrome. Even patients with relatively normal intelligence are usually extremely slow in all their mental processes.

Underlying mechanisms of mental retardation in Lennox-Gastaut syndrome remain to be elucidated and prognosis has not changed despite recent developments in modes of evaluation and treatment.

Available data on long-term prognosis

As already mentioned, Beaumanoir [35] reported on the long-term evolution of LGS patients and underscored the fact that most of the patients with typical symptoms continue to present a similar clinical picture.

According to Ohtahara and Yamatogi [7], three groups can be delineated depending on the clinical course of the disorder and its outcome. Patients in the first group (42 of their 89 patients) continued to display a typical electroclinical picture of Lennox-Gastaut syndrome; those in the second group (19 patients) developed other types of EEG discharges, mainly focal ones; those in the third group (28 patients) presented multiple independent spike foci after first having the typical EEG features. Patients in the second group fared better than those in the other groups, and only 40.5% of them were mentally retarded. Of patients who developed multiple independent spike foci, 47.4% were retarded, and 60% continued to have "minor" seizures. Compared to patients in the other two groups, patients in the first group more often belonged to the symptomatic type of Lennox-Gastaut syndrome and had more frequently evolved from infantile spasms.

Oguni *et al.* [15] studied long-term prognosis of LGS in 72 patients followed for more than 10 years. Patients were included if they had more than two types of seizures (including generalized tonic seizures) as well as diffuse EEG slow spike-and-wave complexes with or without rapid rhythms during sleep. Mean age at epilepsy onset was two years four months (range, one month to 14 years). The diagnosis was first made in the age range from two to 15 years with peak occurrence at five years. Cryptogenic LGS was diagnosed in 21 patients and symptomatic in 51, of whom 24 had previously had West syndrome (West plus group). At last examination, the mean age was 21 + 5 years in the cryptogenic group and 23 + 5 years in the symptomatic group. Follow-up period was 17 + 4 years in the former and 17 + 5 in the latter.

At the end of follow-up, 33% of patients with cryptogenic and 55% with symptomatic LGS no longer displayed the typical characteristics of LGS. In the cryptogenic group, epilepsy was classified as LGS in 14 (67%) patients, as nonspecific symptomatic generalized epilepsy in five (24%) lacking diffuse slow SW complexes or multiple seizure types, as localization related in one, and one patient had no more seizures. In the symptomatic group the diagnosis remained that of LGS in 23 (45%) but was considered as nonspecific symptomatic generalized in 14 (27%), as severe epilepsy with multiple independent spike foci in eight (16%), as localization related in four (8%) and only two patients had no more seizures. More than 60% of the patients had daily or weekly seizures, of which generalized tonic seizures were the most frequent. An IQ score decrease of at least 15 points was demonstrated in nine of the 11 patients with cryptogenic LGS who were able to retake the test and in seven of the nine patients with symptomatic LGS. Deterioration of gait over several years was a prominent feature in 12 patients and, according to the authors, seemed to be due largely to progression of the epileptic encephalopathy caused by repeated seizures.

Ohtsuka *et al.* [69] reported the clinical and EEG features of 89 patients with LGS who were followed for more than 5 years and found that only 31 (34.8%) still had the characteristic LGS features at the time of last observation. Of those, 28 had progressed to severe epilepsy with multiple independent spike foci. Similar results, confirming that the characteristic LGS features disappear with age in 30 to 50% of the cases are also reported by Beaumanoir [35] and Oller-Daurella [64]. Cryptogenic LGS appears to have a more homogeneous clinical picture since evolution to other syndromes is seen less often [15].

Yagi [16] also reported on evolution of LGS in 102 patients observed for an average of 16 years (range 10-20). Mean age at epilepsy onset was 4.3 years (range, 2 months to

18 years). All patients had more than one type of seizure but, this being a retrospective study, the authors did not state whether all had tonic seizures during the early stages of the disorder. Twenty-two patients had evolved from West syndrome to LGS, 36 began as unspecific epilepsies, either generalized or localization-related, and 44 began primarily with the electroclinical characteristics of LGS. At the end of the study, eight had been completely seizure free for more than a year, and the remaining 94 patients still had seizures. Nearly all of the 94 had tonic seizures (52 as the only type of seizures, 17 of whom had them in sleep). The characteristic clinical symptoms and EEG discharges continued in one third of the subjects. At the end of the survey, 5 patients were students at a special school for the handicapped, twelve had regular jobs, one was a housewife, seven were working part-time, 19 were under custodial care at home, 29 were working either at work centers or industrial training centers, 21 were institutionalized for care, six were hospitalized for treatment of seizures, and two had died.

Aicardi and Levy Gomes [28] studied 10 patients with a *possible mild variant* of the syndrome. All had a normal neurological examination, a relatively late onset (43 months), and a predominance of absence attacks over tonic seizures. They had relatively normal background EEG tracings, a positive response to hyperventilation, and typical 3-Hz absences were sometimes observed early in the course of their disorder. Such cases are reminiscent of the so-called "intermediate petit mal" [68]. However, complete separation of a subgroup was not possible because all patients also fulfilled strict criteria for Lennox-Gastaut syndrome and because several patients with typical Lennox-Gastaut syndrome exhibited similar features.

Concluding remarks

Lennox-Gastaut syndrome is one of the most severe forms of childhood epilepsy. Because of mental retardation and other neurological deficits, only a very few patients are ultimately able to live independent lives. Approximately 80% of patients will continue to have seizures. The repetition of absences and episodes of status epilepticus as well as the use of high-dosage drug therapy probably play important roles in augmenting the effects of mental deficiency by interfering with education and secondary to latent anticonvulsant toxicity.

Despite discrepancies and methodological biases, it becomes clear that the clinical picture of the syndrome is characterized by the presence of all known general predictors for a bad prognosis: presence of neurological and mental abnormalities; presence of several types of seizures; presence of particularly intractable types of seizures, including tonic and atonic; a relatively early age of onset; prolonged episodes of nonconvulsive status; and a progressive course, which apparently is not significantly affected by existing therapeutic strategies.

The syndrome is probably heterogeneous, and this heterogeneity is reflected in the outcome. The proportion of severely retarded patients is estimated to be as high as 72% for secondary cases and 22% for cryptogenic cases. Lennox-Gastaut syndrome that occurs after infantile spasms is significantly more severe although patients in whom myoclonic seizures and atypical absences are prominent may do substantially better. Although the overall prognosis of Lennox-Gastaut syndrome is extremely severe, rare patients fare relatively well and do not have mental retardation or psychiatric disturbances. Apparently, the development of new AEDs and new treatment strategies during the last decade has not radically affected the overall prognosis.

The evidence that the clinical manifestations of LGS often change with age raises the question of whether the fundamental pathophysiology differs in patients in whom the underlying LGS evolves into other epilepsy syndromes compared with those patients who retain all of the characteristics of LGS. Oguni speculated that diffuse as well as multifocal cortical epileptogenesis could produce both diffuse slow spike-wave abnormalities and LGS features during childhood. Later, as a result of changes brought about during normal maturational processes, multifocal epileptogenesis would no longer be able to generate diffuse slow spike-waves. In addition, there may be a biologic continuum between true LGS that retains all of its characteristic features and LGS that ultimately evolves into various other epilepsy syndromes in adolescence and adulthood.

References

1. Dravet C. *Encéphalopathie épileptique de l'enfant avec pointe-onde lente diffuse.* Thèse. Marseille, 1965.
2. Gastaut H, Roger J, Soulayrol R, *et al.* Childhood epileptic encephalopathy with diffuse slow spike-waves (otherwise known as "petit mal variant") or Lennox syndrome. *Epilepsia* 1966; 7: 139-79.
3. Niedermeyer E. The Lennox-Gastaut syndrome, a severe type of chilhood epilepsy. *Dtsch Z Nervenheilk* 1969; 195: 263-82.
4. Schneider H, Vassella F, Karbowski K. The Lennox syndrome: a clinical study of 40 children. *Eur Neurol* 1970; 4: 289-300.
5. Chevrie JJ, Aicardi J. Childhood epileptic encephalopathy with slow-spike wave: a statistical study of 80 cases. *Epilepsia* 1972; 13: 259-71.
6. Beaumanoir A, Dravet C. The Lennox-Gastaut syndrome. In: Roger J, Bureau M, Dravet C, Dreifuss FE, Perret A, Wolf P, eds. *Epileptic Syndromes in infancy, childhood and adolescence*, 2nd ed. London: John Libbey, 1992: 115-32.
7. Ohtahara S, Yamatogi Y. Evolution of seizures and EEG abnormalities in childhood onset epilepsy. In: Wada JA, Ellingson RJ, *Clinical Neurophysiology of Epilepsy. EEG Handbook* (revised series, vol. 4). Amsterdam: Elsevier, 1990: 457-77.
8. Roger J, Rémy C, Bureau M, Oller-Daurella L, Beaumanoir A, Favel A, Dravet C. Le syndrome de Lennox-Gastaut chez l'adulte. *Rev Neurol (Paris)* 1987; 143: 401-5.
9. Trevathan E, Murphy CC, Yeagrin-Allsopp M. Prevalence and descriptive epidemiology of Lennox-Gastaut syndrome among Atlanta children. *Epilepsia* 1997; 38: 1283-8.
10. Erba G, Browne TR. Atypical absence myoclonic, atonic, and tonic seizures and the "Lennox-Gastaut syndrome". In: Browne TR, Feldman RG, eds. *Epilepsy, Diagnosis and Management.* Boston: Little Brown, 1983: 75-94.
11. Beaumanoir A, Foletti G, Magistris M, Volansche D. Status epilepticus in the Lennox-Gastaut syndrome. In: Niedermeyer E, Degen R, *The Lennox-Gastaut Syndrome*, New York: Alan R. Liss, 1988: 283-99.
12. Rai PV, Fulop T, Ercal S Clinical course of Lennox-Gastaut syndrome in institutionalized adult patients, In: Niedermeyer E, Degen R, eds. *The Lennox-Gastaut syndrome.* New York: Alan R. Liss, 988: 409-18.
13. Boniver C, Dravet C, Bureau M, Roger J. Idiopathic Lennox-Gastaut syndrome. In: Wolf P, Dam M, Janz D, Dreifuss F, *Advances in Epileptology, 16th Epilepsy International Symposium.* New York: Raven Press, 1987: 195-200.
14. Gastaut H, Dravet C, Loubier D, Giove C, Viani F, Gastaut JA, Gastaut JL Evolution clinique et pronostic du syndrome de Lennox-Gastaut. In: Lugaresi E, Pazzaglia P, Tassinari CA, eds. *Evolution and Prognosis of Epilepsies*, Bologna: Aulo Goggi, 1973: 133-54.
15. Oguni H, Hayashi K, Osawa M. Long-term prognosis of Lennox-Gastaut syndrome. *Epilepsia* 1996; 37 (Suppl 3): 44-7.
16. Yagi K. Evolution of Lennox-Gastaut syndrome: a long-term longitudinal study. *Epilepsia* 1996; 37 (Suppl 3): 48-51.
17. Heiskala H. Community-based study of Lennox-Gastaut syndrome. *Epilepsia* 1997; 38: 526-31.
18. Aicardi J. The problem of the Lennox syndrome. *Dev Med Child Neurol* 1973; 15: 77-81.
19. Blume WT. Pathogenesis of Lennox-Gastaut syndrome: considerations and hypotheses *Epileptic Disord* 2001; 3: 183-96.
20. Bancaud J, Talairach J. Semiology of frontal lobe epilepsy seizures in man. In: Chauvel P, Delgado-Escueta AV, Halgren E, Bancaud J, eds. *Frontal lobe seizures and epilepsies*, New York: Raven Press, 1992: 3-58.

21. Dravet C. Le syndrome de Lennox-Gastaut et ses frontières. *Epilepsies* 1996; 8: 73-88.
22. Gastaut H, Tassinari CA. Ictal discharges in different types of seizures. In: *Epilepsies: Handbook of Electroencephalography and Clinical Neurophysiology, Vol. 13, Part A*, Amsterdam: Elsevier, 1975: 13A-45.
23. Livingston JH. The Lennox-Gastaut syndrome. *Dev Med Child Neurol* 1988; 30: 536-40.
24. Chayasirisobhon S, Rodin EA. Atonic-akinetic seizures. *Electroencephalogr Clin Neurophysiol* 1981; 50: 225.
25. Gastaut H, Regis H. On the subject of Lennox's akinetic petit mal. *Epilepsia* 1961; 2: 298-305.
26. Gastaut H, Broughton R, Roger J, Tassinari CA. Generalized convulsive seizures without local onset. In: Vinken PJ, Bruyn GW, *Handbook of Clinical Neurology, Vol. 15: The Epilepsies*. Amsterdam: Elsevier, 1974: 107-29.
27. Dravet C, Roger J, Bureau M, Dalla Bernardina B. Myoclonic epilepsies in childhood. In: Akimoto H, Kazamatsuri H, Seino M, Ward A, *Advances in Epileptology: XIIIth Epilepsy International Symposium*. New York: Raven Press, 1982: 135-40.
28. Aicardi J, Levy Gomes A. The Lennox-Gastaut syndrome: clinical and electroencephalographic features. In: Niedermeyer E, Degen D. *The Lennox-Gastaut Syndrome*. New York: Allan Liss, 1988: 25-46.
29. Dravet C, Natale O, Magaudda A, Larrieu JL, Bureau M, Roger J, Tassinari CA. Les états de mal dans le syndrome de Lennox-Gastaut. *Rev EEG Neurophysiol Clin* 1985; 15: 361-8.
30. Doose H. Nonconvulsive status epilepticus in childhood: clinical aspects and classification. In: Delgado-Escueta AV, Wasterlain CG, *Advances in Neurology, Vol. 34: Status Epilepticus*. New York: Raven Press, 1983: 83-92.
31. Porter RJ, Penry JK. Petit mal status. In: Delgado-Escueta AV, Wasterlain CG, Treiman DM, Porter RJ, *Advances in Neurology, Vol. 34: Status Epilepticus*, New York: Raven Press, 1983: 61-7.
32. Tassinari CA, Dravet C, Roger J, Cano JP, Gastaut H. Tonic status epilepticus precipitated by intravenous benzodiazepine in five patients with Lennox-Gastaut syndrome. *Epilepsia* 1972; 13: 431-5.
33. Alvarez N, Hartford E, Douet C. Epileptic seizures induced by clonazepam. *Clin Electroencephalogr* 1981; 12: 57-65.
34. Bittencourt PRM, Richens A. Anticonvulsant-induced status epilepticus in Lennox-Gastaut syndrome. *Epilepsia* 1981; 22: 129-34.
35. Beaumanoir A. Les limites nosologiques du syndrome de Lennox-Gastaut. *Rev EEG Neurophysiol Clin* 1981; 11: 468-73.
36. Pazzaglia P, D'Alessandro R, Ambrosetto G, Lugaresi E. Drop attacks: An ominous change in the evaluation of partial epilepsy. *Neurology* 1985; 35: 1725-30.
37. Gastaut H, Zifkin BG. Secondary bilateral synchrony and Lennox-Gastaut syndrome. In: Niedermeyer E, Degen R. *The Lennox-Gastaut Syndrome*. New York: Alan R. Liss, 1988: 221-42.
38. Gur R, Sussman N, Alavi A, Gur RE, Rosen AD, O'Connor M, Goldberg HI, Greenberg JH, Reivich M. Positron emission tomography in two cases of childhood epileptic encephalopathy (Lennox-Gastaut syndrome). *Neurology* 1982; 32: 1191-4.
39. Iinuma K, Yanai K, Yanagisawa T, Fueki N, Tada K, Ito M, Matsuzawa T, Ido T. Cerebral glucose metabolism in five patients with Lennox-Gastaut syndrome. *Pediatr Neurol* 1987; 3: 12-8.
40. Theodore WH, Rose D, Patronas W, Sato S, Holmes M, Bairamian D, Porter RJ, Di Chiro G, Larson S, Fishbein D. Cerebral glucose metabolism in the Lennox-Gastaut syndrome. *Ann Neurol* 1987; 21: 14-21.
41. Chugani HT, Mazziota JC, Engel J Jr, Phelps ME. The Lennox-Gastaut syndrome: metabolic subtypes determined by 2-Dioxy-2 ^{18}F fluoro-D-glucose positron emission tomography. *Ann Neurol* 1987; 21: 4-13.
42. Aicardi J, Arzimanoglou A. Treatment of the childhood epilepsy syndromes. In: Shorvon SD, *et al.*, eds. *The treatment of Epilepsy*. Blackwell Science, 1996: 199-214.
43. Crumrine PK. Lennox-Gastaut syndrome. *J Child Neurol* 2002; 17: S70-S75.
44. Trevathan E. Infantile Spasms and Lennox-Gastaut syndrome. *J Child Neurol* 2002; 17: 2S9-2S22.
45. The Felbamate Study Group in Lennox-Gastaut Syndrome. Efficacy of Felbamate in childhood epileptic encephalopathy (Lennox-Gastaut Syndrome). *N Engl J Med* 1993; 328: 29-33.
46. Schmidt D, Bourgeois B. A risk-benefit assessment of therapies for Lennox-Gastaut syndrome. *Drug Saf* 2000; 22: 467-77.
47. Dulac O, Kaminska A. Use of lamotrigine in Lennox-Gastaut and related epilepsy syndromes. *J Child Neurol* 1997; 12 (Suppl 1): S23-S28.
48. Timmings PL, Richens A. Lamotrigine as add on drug in the management of Lennox-Gastaut syndrome. *Eur Neurol* 1992; 32: 305-7.

49. Arzimanoglou A, Gérardin V, Moszkowski J, Bidaut-Mazel C. Lamotrigine (Lamictal) in patients with childhood onset intractable epilepsy. *Epilepsia* 1993.
50. Schlumberger E, Chavez F, Palacios E, *et al.* Lamotrigine in treatment of 120 children with epilepsy. *Epilepsia* 1994; 35: 359-67.
51. Donaldson JA, Glauser TA, Olberding LS. Lamotrigine adjunctive therapy in childhood encephalopathy (the Lennox-Gastaut syndrome). *Epilepsia* 1997; 38: 68-73.
52. Motte J, Trevathan E, Arvidsson JFV, *et al.* Lamotrigine for generalized seizures associated with the Lennox-Gastaut syndrome. *N Engl J Med* 1997; 337: 1807-12.
53. Panayiotopoulos CP, Ferrie CD, Knott C, *et al.* Interaction of lamotrigine with sodium valproate. *Lancet* 1993; 341: 445.
54. Brodie MJ, Yuen AW. Lamotrigine substitution study: evidence for synergism with sodium valproate? 105 Study Group. *Epilepsy Res* 1997; 26: 423-32.
55. Arzimanoglou A, Kulak I, Bidaut-Mazel C, Baldy-Moulinier M. Utilisation optimale de la lamotrigine en pratique clinique: résultats d'une étude ouverte multicentrique dans l'épilepsie réfractaire. *Rev Neurol* 2001; 157: 525-36.
56. Sachdeo RC, Glauser TA, Ritter F, Reife R, Lim P, Pledger G. A double-blind, randomized trial of topiramate in Lennox-Gastaut syndrome. Topiramate YL Study Group. *Neurology* 1999; 52: 1882-7.
57. Brett EM. The Lennox-Gastaut syndrome: therapeutic aspects. In: Niedermeyer E, Degen R, eds. *The Lennox-Gastaut syndrome*. New York: Alan R. Liss, 1988: 329-39.
58. Aicardi J. *Epilepsy in children*. New York: Raven Press, 1994.
59. Wilson DH, Reeves A, Gazzaniga M. Cerebral commissurotomy for control of intractable seizures. *Neurology* 1982; 32: 687-97.
60. Valencia I, Holder DL, Helmers SL, Madsen JR, Riviello JJ Jr. Vagus nerve stimulation in pediatric epilepsy: a review. *Pediatr Neurol* 2001; 25: 368-76.
61. Papini M, Pasquinelli A, Armellini M, Orlandi D. Alertness and incidence of seizures in patients with Lennox-Gastaut syndrome. *Epilepsia* 1984; 25: 161-7.
62. Baldy-Moulinier M, Touchon J, Billiard M, Carrière A, Besset A. Nocturnal sleep study in the Lennox-Gastaut syndrome. In: Niedermeyer E, Degen R. *The Lennox-Gastaut Syndrome*, New York: Alan Liss, 1988: 243-60.
63. Markand ON. Slow spike-wave activity in EEG and associated clinical features: often called "Lennox" or "Lennox-Gastaut" syndrome. *Neurology* 1977; 27: 746-57.
64. Oller-Daurella L. Evolution et pronostic du syndrome de Lennox-Gastaut. In: Lugaresi E, Pazzaglia P, Tassinari CA. *Evolution and Prognosis of Epilepsies*. Bologna: Aulo Gaggi, 1973: 155-64.
65. Furune S, Watanabe K, Negoro T, Miyazaki S, Takevchi T, Matsumoto A, Kumagai T, Takahashi I, Maehara M. Long-term prognosis and clinicoelectroencephalographic evolution of Lennox-Gastaut syndrome. *Brain Dysfunct* 1986; 1: 146-53.
66. Erba G, Cavazzuti V. Ictal and interictal response latency in Lennox-Gastaut syndrome. *Electroencephalogr Clin Neurophysiol* 1977; 42: 717.
67. Hoffmann-Riem M, Diener W, Benninger C, *et al.* Nonconvulsive status epilepticus – A possible cause of mental retardation in patients with Lennox-Gastaut syndrome. *Neuropediatrics* 2000; 31: 169-74.
68. Doose H, Völzke E, Petit mal status in early childhood and dementia. *Neuro Pédiatrie* 1989; 10: 10-4.
69. Ohtsuka Y, Amano R, Mizukawa M, Ohtahara S. Long-term prognosis of the Lennox-Gastaut syndrome. *Jpn J Psychiatry Neurol* 1990; 44: 257-68.
70. Kaminska A, Ickowicz A, Plouin P, Bru MF, Dellatolas G, Dulac O. Delineation of cryptogenic Lennox-Gastaut syndrome and myoclonic astatic epilepsy using multiple correspondence analysis. *Epilepsy Res* 1999; 36: 15-29.

Prognosis of Landau Kleffner syndrome and other forms of cognitive epilepsy

Catherine Billard

Acquired Aphasia-Epilepsy syndrome and other forms of cognitive epilepsy (Encephalopathy with electrical status epilepticus during sleep or ESES) are age-dependent and self-limiting syndromes whose distinctive features include characteristic age of onset (with a peak around 4-5 years), heterogeneous seizure types (mostly partial motor unilateral seizures during sleep and absences or falls while awake), a typical EEG pattern (with continuous and diffuse paroxysms during sleep) and variable neuropsychological regression. Despite the long-term favourable outcome of epilepsy and electrical status epilepticus during sleep, the prognosis is guarded because of the persistence of severe neuropsychological and/or motor deficits in approximately half of the patients.

Description of syndromes

Acquired aphasia-epilepsy syndrome

Acquired aphasia-epilepsy syndrome (often called Landau Kleffner syndrome) is characterized by particular childhood aphasia, usually receptive, paroxymal EEG abnormalities Clinically manifest seizures may not occur or occur infrequently. Two hundred forty-eight publications were reported by Panayiotopoulos in 1999 [1]. First described by Landau [2] in an institution for deaf children, until the 1980s the proposed pathogenesis of Landau Kleffner syndrome ranged from an epilepsy-related syndrome to a particular encephalitic condition. After this date, several publications (for review [3]), emphasized the possibility of that symptoms were a direct consequence of the epileptic disorder. The Venice symposium later summarized the main clinical, neuropsychological and neurophysiologic characteristics:

1. Clinical features: the acquired aphasia occurs in previously normal children between 2 and 8 years of age, with a peak between 5 and 7 years. The type of aphasia typically seen is verbal agnosia but all types of aphasia can occur. Hyperkinesia, impairment of affective development and personality disorders have been described, with different degrees of severity.

2. Epileptic seizures are mentioned in 80% of cases but are usually rare, nocturnal and clinically heterogeneous (generalised tonic-clonic, simple partial motor, atypical absences, unilateral seizures).

3. Neurophysiological characteristics: epileptic activities are represented by multiple foci of high amplitude repetitive spikes and spikes and waves. Sleep, particularly sleep onset, has a marked activating effect on EEG abnormalities. The sleep EEG presents a pattern of continuous, bilateral spikes and waves, consistent with the occurrence of Continuous Spike Wave during Slow Wave Sleep (CSWS), and suggesting a partial or complete overlap between aphasia-epilepsy and Encephalopathy with ESES.

Encephalopathy with ESES other than aphasia-epilepsy (AE)

The first description of Epileptic Status induced by Slow Wave Sleep (ESES) in children was published by Patry [4], describing 6 children with an unusual EEG pattern occurring almost continuously during sleep, for variable lengths of time (months to years). Five children were mentally retarded and two of these failed to acquire language. Later the Commission on Classification and Terminology of the International League against Epilepsy adopted the term of Continuous Spikes during Slow Wave Sleep (CSWS) [5]. However, over the years evidence has been reported demonstrating that neuropsychological and/or motor impairments are prominent features of the condition and determine the usually poor prognosis. Tassinari [6] therefore recently proposed the term of Encephalopathy with ESES, defined as an age-related and self time limited disorder of unknown aetiology characterized by the following features:

1. Epilepsy is characterized by constantly present seizures, occurring between 2 months and 12 years of age, frequently nocturnal and of unilateral type, but also partial motor seizures, absences, "generalized" tonic-clonic or complex partial seizures. The severity and frequency of seizures frequently change during ESES and three groups have been proposed:
– Group 1 with rare nocturnal motor seizures,
– Group 2 with unilateral partial motor seizures or generalized tonic-clonic seizures, mainly occurring during sleep, and absences during wakefulness,
– Group 3 with rare nocturnal seizures and atypical absences with atonic or tonic components leading to sudden falls.

Negative myoclonus is frequent during wakefulness and contributes to motor impairment.

2. Neuropsychological impairment during ESES has the appearance of a further decrease in performance, marked impairment of IQ, deterioration of language, temporo-spatial disorientation, behavioural changes and occasionally psychotic states. The pattern of cognitive deterioration presumably depends on the prevalent localization of the discharges: both temporal paroxysmal abnormalities are associated with language disorders, mental and behavioural deterioration evoking a frontal syndrome has been described with interictal frontal foci, dystonia, dyspraxia, unilateral deficit or acquired opercular syndrome are the most disabling motor disorders. The association of ESES with dysphasia is not well documented. Finally ESES without behavioural disorders has been described in several reports [7].

3. The Neurophysiological pattern is characterized by continuous bilateral and diffuse slow waves occurring as soon as patients fall asleep and persisting through all the slow sleep stages. A SW index ranging from 86 to 100% is considered an essential feature for the diagnosis of Encephalopathy with ESES, but variations in paroxysmal activity night by night have not been studied and it is possible that the same clinical conditions (seizures and cognitive deterioration) may occur with less frequent paroxysmal activity.

Signs of brain lesions are seen in 30 to 60% of ESES cases not classed as Landau Kleffner syndrome and 3% of Landau Kleffner aphasia epilepsy, characterizing the symptomatic forms.

The criteria of diagnosis of Encephalopathy with ESES are not as clear as those of aphasia-epilepsy. In typical aphasia-epilepsy the development of the child is normal until the deterioration of language and the deterioration is clear. In most cases the symptoms are limited to language deterioration. In Encephalopathy with ESES the deterioration is often not so clear: probably because the onset of the symptoms (behaviour disorders) is not so evident as loss of language.

Prognosis of syndromes

All these features demonstrate that Encephalopathy with ESES is a more heterogeneous syndrome than Landau Kleffner aphasia. They also explain the heterogeneity of prognosis according to the symptoms, age of onset, duration of epilepsy, kind of antiepileptic treatment and of quality of rehabilitation. These features are similar to those of West Syndrome.

However prognosis can be predicted in terms of the epilepsy and, more importantly, in terms of the cognitive outcome.

Prognosis in terms of epilepsy

Montovani and Landau [8] reported the first long term follow-up of patients with Landau Kleffner syndrome and none of their patients continued to have seizures. Rossi [9] reported that seizures disappeared in all patients and mean age at disappearance was 7 years 10 months. Paquier [10] described the follow-up of 6 patients and reported that seizures ceased in 5 and persisted in the form of Grand Mal in one case. The EEG abnormalities disappeared in most of the cases. In the follow-up of the 7 cases described by Deonna [11], all but one were seizure free and had normal EEG. The last had monthly grand mal seizures and non-specific focal EEG abnormalities.

In the follow-up of 25 patients with encephalopathy with ESES who were seizure free [12], the mean duration was 8 years and 6 months. The mean age at the last consultation was 18 years. The treatment regimes varied: At last follow-up, 15 patients were without treatment, 5 patients were on very low dose monotherapy, and 5 patients were still receiving a combination of 2 drugs. Seizures disappeared in all cases, whether symptomatic or cryptogenic, and whether epilepsy had been severe or not. Mean duration of epilepsy was about 12 years, ranging from 4 years 4 months to 14 years 11 months. In 31%, the disappearance of seizures coincided with the onset of ESES. In 44% of cases, seizures disappeared before the end of ESES, and in 25% of cases they persisted after the end of ESES, becoming rare and consisting of absences without falls, and generalized clonic or clonic-tonic seizures. EEG was normal during wakefulness and sleep in 8 cases, with progressive normalization occurring at a mean of 3 months after the end of ESES. Repeated awake and sleep EEG recordings showed that normalization may continue for an average of 15 years. In 5 cases, it was normal when awake, while showing focal abnormalities during sleep. In 12 cases, focal abnormalities existed during awake and sleep recordings. In all cases, cyclic organization of sleep was normal: all stages of sleep were present at normal percentages, with normal sleep pattern in all cases. No diffuse abnormalities were recorded.

One case was reported in a mentally retarded patient aged 21 years, still persisting at the age of 25 years. Thus encephalopathy with ESES is not a strictly age-related disorder [13].

Prognosis in terms of neuropsychological outcome

This is probably the most difficult point to summarize. In fact, there are some reports of long term outcome but the children did not have similar cognitive deficits during the acute phases (complete chronic agnosia, fluctuating aphasia or mild language disorders for AE, severe frontal syndrome or mild right hemisphere function disorders in Encephalopathy with ESES). The age of onset is not the same, and thus nor is the level of cognitive or language development at the beginning of ESES. The duration of ESES is not the same and varies from several months to many years. The outcome was spontaneous in the first publications and depended on the effect of treatment in later reports. Since the 1990s, the need for active treatment of EEG abnormalities in AE and Encephalopathy with ESES has been recognized, but there are few recommended treatments [14]: Ethosuccimide, Benzodiazepine (particularly Clobazam), Corticotherapy, and more recently subpial resection. The rehabilitation programmes in AE, and principally in Encephalopathy with ESES, vary. Further longitudinal studies will clarify the prognosis of Landau Kleffner syndrome with early diagnosis, good therapeutic recommendations and evaluated rehabilitation.

Several reports of long term follow-up of Landau Kleffner syndrome have described an improvement, although complete recovery is not always achieved.

Mantovani [8] evaluated 9 patients 10 to 28 years after the onset of aphasia. Four patients recovered, one had mild language dysfunction and 4 had moderate language disability. Four of the five patients with the best language outcome had decreased visuo-perceptive function as measured by the Benton Revised Visual retention test (RBVRT), whereas the three adults with moderate language disorders had normal RBVRT scores. The outcome in Mantovani's patients was similar to that in the other 11 cases reported in his publication and followed-up for longer than 10 years (3 normal, 5 with intermediate language difficulty and 2 severely aphasic). He concluded that: "The variability of outcome of similarly affected children remains one of the most puzzling feature of this disorder". In Paquier's long term follow-up of 6 cases [10], 2 patients remained severely impaired in comprehension and production of language, 3 patients had slight language deficit 19 and 8 years after the onset of aphasia, without interference with professional or school life, and one patient recovered totally. In Deonna's report [11], 7 cases of LK syndrome were re-evaluated 10 years later. One man recovered completely, one had a normal oral language but is severely dyslexic, four had no language comprehension and no expressive speech, and only one learned and is using sign language with some efficiency. In this study, as in others performed before the current treatment recommendations, there was no progressive deterioration in cognitive function and no psychotic disorder despite the severe communication handicap. The long term outcome showed that the clinical picture varied at onset, as well as during the course of the illness. The long term outcome of aphasia was quite unpredictable, despite the fact that epilepsy and EEG abnormalities regressed or disappeared with the years. Rossi's [9] reported similar results in 11 patients with long term follow-up. Perhaps earlier active antiepileptic treatment with EEG normalization will change the difficulty of predicting neuropsychological outcome. However, the disorder tends to stabilize with time without personality disorder.

The evolution of aphasia was related to the scores of a dichotic listening task [15]. Recovery from aphasia went together with the evolution of the dichotic listening pattern, progressing from a bilateral low score (associated with severe aphasia) to unilateral channel extinction (aphasia of moderate severity) and then a normal pattern (total recovery). Although channel extinction tended to involve mainly the dominant channel (3 cases), in 2 patients it affected the non-dominant channel. This long lasting dichotic extinction revealed a permanent dysfunction in the temporal auditory system that may be the consequence of the presence of an active epileptogenic focus during the critical period of functional differentiation of the temporal cortex.

Precise studies of long term perception disabilities [16] have revealed that there is a dissociation between the discrimination of environmental sounds and phonological auditory discrimination, the latter being more impaired than the former. This suggests that the primary deficit of receptive aphasia is an impairment of auditory phonological discrimination, rather than generalized auditory agnosia.

A report of a 27-year-old woman with chronic agnosia following Landau Kleffner syndrome diagnosed at 4 years, growing up in a hearing/speaking community with some exposure to manually coded sign language [17], showed that Signed English is her preferred mode of communication. Comprehension and production of spoken language remained severely compromised and disruptions in auditory processing could be observed. Linguistic analysis of spoken and sign language indicated that the sign language phonology was normal and spoken language phonology was impaired because of deprivation of auditory input during a period critical for the development of phonology. Other reports on long term evolution of severe cases confirmed the normality of the linguistic system in sign language but not in oral language [18, 19].

In summary, the outcome is different from one case to another, auditory processing deficits remain in cases without complete recovery, suggesting a temporal lobe dysfunction.

The description of neuropsychological outcome of Encephalopathy with ESES is still more difficult to summarize. Psychomotor development prior to ESES may be normal or retarded, the onset of cognitive regression is often not as clear as in AE, and the rehabilitation method is still unknown. A longitudinal study of a previously normal boy with partial seizures and continuous spike waves during sleep [20] revealed prolonged insidious reversible stagnation of learning and slight language disability. In Tassinari's series, 16 out of the 25 cases were normal prior to ESES. In all these cases (as in AE), improvement in performance and/or behaviour, albeit always slow and often only partial, was noted after the end of ESES. The impairment of specific temporo-spatial orientation and memory and in language skills disappeared in all subjects. However, compared to LKS, IQ remained low in 50% of cases, and behaviour disorders persisted in 50% of cases. The same poor cognitive and behaviour prognosis was demonstrated by Morikawa [21]. Only 50% of patients had normal lives, but none were able to receive further education, and 50% had to live in sheltered living situations. The poor prognosis is not attributed to the age of discovery of ESES, in contrast to LKS where prognosis depends on age of onset of aphasia. Prognosis is not attributed to the severity of epilepsy or to the severity of associated disorders, and the presence or absence of brain lesions were not involved. It may, however, be related to the duration of ESES. It may also be related to the type of rehabilitation. The quality of rehabilitation is known to be essential in LK syndrome, and probably appropriate rehabilitation is also important in Encephalopathy with ESES, but the rehabilitation of non-verbal disabilities is unknown and unpractised in Europe.

The long term prognosis of Landau Kleffner syndrome and encephalopathy with ESES is not dependent on the prognosis of the epilepsy: in all cases, in spite of a good evolution of seizure frequency and EEG paroxysmal activity, most often with complete recovery, the neuropsychological and psychosocial outcome is often poor whatever the severity of the epilepsy. The prognosis depends on the neuropsychological disorders. The neuropsychological outcome varies according to the severity of disorders in the acute phase, the age of onset, the duration of ESES, and the types of rehabilitation and education programmes...

Early diagnosis (before a long period of cognitive disorders), an active antiepileptic drug (directed against EEG abnormalities), and active and evaluated neuropsychological rehabilitation are the best guarantee of less significant neuropsychological sequelae.

References

1. Panayiotopoulos CP. Severe syndromes of mainly linguistic and neuropsychological deficits, seizures or both and marked EEG abnormalities from the rolandic and neighbouring regions. In: Panayiotopoulos CP, ed. *Benign childhood partial seizures and related epileptic syndromes*. London: John Libbey, 1999: 337-60.
2. Landau WM, Kleffner FR. Syndrome of acquired aphasia with convulsive disorder in children. *Neurology* 1957; 7: 523-30.
3. Billard C, Autret, Lucas B, De Giovanni E, Gillet P, Santini JJS, De Toffol B. Are frequent SW during Non-REM sleep in relation with an acquired neuropsychological deficit. *Neurophysiol Clin* 1990; 20: 439-53.
4. Patry G, Lyagoubi S, Tassinari CA. Subclinical electrical status induced by sleep in children. *Arch Neurol* 1971; 24: 242-52.
5. Commission on classification and terminology of the international league against epilepsy. Proposal for revised classification of epilepsies and epileptic syndromes. *Epilepsia* 1989; 30: 389-99.
6. Tassinari CA, Rubboli G, Volpi L, Meletti S, d'Orsi G, Franca M, Sabetta AR, Riguzzi P, Gardella E, Zaniboni A, Michelucci R. Encephalopathy with electrical status epilepticus during slow sleep or ESES syndrome including the acquired aphasia. *Child Neurophysiology* 2000; 111 (Suppl 2): S94-S102.
7. Gökyit A, Caliskan A. Diffuse spike-wave status of 9 years duration without behavioural change or intellectual decline. *Epilepsia* 1995; 34: 210-3.
8. Mantovani JF, Landau WM. Acquired aphasia with convulsive disorder: course and prognosis. *Neurology* 1980; 30: 524-9.
9. Rossi PG, Parmeggiani A, Posar A, Scaduto MC, Chiodo S, Vatti G. Landau-Kleffner syndrome: long-term follow-up and links with electrical status epilepticus during sleep (ESES). *Brain Dev* 1999; 21: 90-8.
10. Paquier PF, Ran Dongen HR, Loonen CB. The Landau-Kleffner syndrome or acquired aphasia with convulsive disorder. Long-term follow-up of six children and a review of the recent literature. *Arch Neurol* 1992; 49: 354-9.
11. Deonna T, Peter C, Ziegler AL. Adult follow-up of the acquired aphasia-epilepsy syndrome in childhood. Report of 7 cases. *Neuropediatrics* 1989; 20: 132-8.
12. Bureau M, Cordova S, Dravet C, Roger J, Tassinari CA. Épilepsie avec pointes-ondes continues pendant le sommeil lent (POCS). Évolution à moyen et long terme (à propos de 15 cas). *Epilepsies* 1990; 2: 86-94.
13. Mariotti P, Della Marca G, Iuvone L, Mennuni GF, Guazelli M, Marchette S, Mazza S. Is ESES/CSWS a strictly age-related disorder? *Clin Neurophysiol* 2000; 111: 452-6.
14. Marescaux C, Hirsch E, Fink S, *et al*. Landau-Kleffner syndrome. A pharmacologic study of five cases. *Epilepsia* 1990; 31: 768-77.
15. Metz-Lutz MN, Hirsch E, Maquet P, de Saint Martin A, Rudolf G, Wioland N, Marescaux. Dichotic listening performances in the follow-up of Landau and Kleffner syndrome. *Child Neuropsychology* 1997; 3: 47-60.
16. Korkman M, Granstrom ML, Appelquist K, Liukkonen E. Neuropsychological characteristics of five children with Landau-Kleffner syndrome: dissociation of auditory and phonological discrimination. *Journal of International Neuropsychological Society* 1998; 4: 566-75.
17. Roulet E, Davidoff V, Prelaz AC, Morel B, Rickli F, Metz-Lutz MN, Boyes Braem P, Deonna T. Sign language in childhood epileptic aphasia (Landau-Kleffner syndrome). *Dev Med Child Neurol* 2001; 43: 733-44.
18. Baynes K, Kleg JA, Brentari D, Kussmaul C, Poizner H. Chronic auditory agnosia following Landau-Kleffner syndrome: a 23 year outcome study. *Brain Lang* 1998; 63: 381-425.
19. Sieratzki JS, Calvert GA, Brammer M, David A, Woll B. Accessibility of spoken, written and sign language in Landau Kleffner syndrome: a linguistic and functional MRI study. *Epileptic Disord* 2001; 3: 79-89.
20. Deonna T, Davidoff V, Maeder-Ingvar M, Zesiger P, Marcoz JP. *Eur J Paediatr Neurol* 1997; 1: 19-29.
21. Morikawa T, Seini M, Watanabe M. Long-term outcome of ESES syndrome. In: Beaumanoir A, Bureau M, Deonna T, Mira L, Tassinari CA, eds. *Continuous spikes and waves during slow waves sleep. Electrical Status Epilepticus during Slow Sleep*. London: John Libbey, 1995: 27-36.

Prognosis of epileptic encephalopathy with electric status epilepticus during sleep

Christine Bulteau

Although strict criteria of abnormal electroencephalogram (EEG) activity were described thirty years ago, electric status epileptic during slow sleep (ESES) remains a rare and poorly understood epileptic syndrome.

ESES must be considered as an epileptic encephalopathy age-dependant syndrome [1] since the neurological deterioration mainly results from epileptic activity as in severe myoclonic epilepsy in infancy or Lennox-Gastaut syndrome during childhood. The unusual fact is that the prognosis of this epileptic syndrome concerns neuropsychological deterioration but is not due to the seizures.

Patry *et al.* [2] first reported continuous spike-and-wave activity during slow sleep (CSWS) as "the subclinical electrical status epilepticus induced by sleep in children" in a group of 6 epileptic children at Centre Saint-Paul in Marseille, France. The presence of continuous EEG abnormalities affecting 85% of slow wave sleep was the main criterion for diagnosing this condition. Tassinari *et al.* [3] completed the description with some non-specific neuropsychological characteristics and introduced the term ESES. The International League Against Epilepsy [4] classified ESES as a syndrome with both focal and generalized electro-clinical features. Nevertheless the distinction between an EEG pattern and a true epileptic syndrome has not yet been completely resolved and many terms are used: ESES, Epileptic encephalopathy with CSWS, and the syndrome with CSWS. The literature reports many groups of patients with the CSWS EEG pattern but with various types of seizures, different cognitive disturbances, and a wide range of outcomes [5]. Strict criteria from a clinical point of view (age of onset, seizure type, duration and type of cognitive impairment) are notably missing. Such criteria are essential to making an early diagnosis and instituting appropriate treatment.

Description of the syndrome

Age of onset

Onset is during childhood, generally between two and ten years. There is a male preponderance.

Seizure

Seizures are rare and usually occur during sleep. They may initially go unnoticed at the onset of the disorder. The seizures include simple or complex partial as well as various kinds of generalized seizures, particularly atypical absences and drop attacks. No tonic seizures are observed. Epilepsy in the ESES syndrome is more severe than in the Landau-Kleffner syndrome as, in the latter group, patients may have no seizures during the time they are experiencing disruption of cognitive functions. When CSWS is present, around 70% of the children have seizures.

Neuropsychological features

Before the diagnosis of ESES there may be a history of normal or mildly delayed development. The crucial clinical symptom of ESES syndrome is the regression of intellectual abilities which is variable in terms of characteristics and severity. This regression develops at the onset of the disorder and lasts until the CSWS disappears. The acquired neuropsychological deficit is not the same in all patients and various clinical patterns are seen. All cognitive functions seem to be disrupted during the period when CSWS is evident on the EEG. The specific cognitive impairments already reported in the literature are described below.

Some patients with verbal agnosia appear as though they were deaf. Within a few months, they lose the ability to speak. By contrast, there is spared praxis and visuo-motor abilities. This condition is well known as the acquired-epileptic-aphasia or Landau-Kleffner syndrome [6]. Other types of language dysfunction are possible with severe expressive language impairment [7].

Acquired frontal syndrome with behavioral changes has been described [8]. Attention deficit as the initial change is followed by hyperactivity, disinhibition, impulsiveness and aggressiveness. At the worst phase, loss of the sense of danger, echopraxia, ritualistic behaviors, and mimic psychosis may occur. The cognitive profile corresponds to a deficit in verbal and non-verbal reasoning, temporal disorientation, and a disorder of judgment. Sometimes, neuropsychological testing is impossible because of the global deterioration.

Praxia dysfunction with oro-bucco-facial apraxia [9] has been reported. Patients become unable to perform voluntary movements of their mouth, including kissing, oral expression and eating. Drooling may also occur.

Temporal-spatial disorder with Gerstmann syndrome has been described only rarely [10].

In many patients, the cognitive regression occurs in children who were previously normal in terms of their psychomotor development. The regression is typically identified by the family; however, it is frequently not clearly evident to the clinician when the child is first brought to medical attention for signs of psychomotor stagnation or psychomotor delay. Only the emergence of subsequent cognitive and behavioral abnormalities may be noticed in the medical history. Frequently the diagnosis is overlooked until children have seizures and therefore undergo an EEG.

EEG

The EEG tracing during wakefulness exhibits mainly focal diphasic spike-wave activity. In the patients with language or executive function impairment, the EEG shows respectively temporal or frontal lobe activity. When there are drop attacks, the epileptiform abnormalities mainly involve the rolandic region. Motor dysfunction with loss of ability to walk is due to brief and repeated episodes of loss of tone, so-called negative myoclonus [11]. Sometimes generalized spike-wave during a few seconds is characteristic of atypical absences. But some patients exhibit a more severe EEG pattern with a "continuous spike-wave discharges during awakening" with no clinical manifestation other than substantial attentional difficulties.

During slow sleep, bilateral, continuous, high frequency spike-wave activity (1.5-5 Hz) is always present. A quantitative measure of the EEG abnormalities is the spike-wave index (SWI), which is the sum of all spike and slow wave minutes multiplied by 100 and divided by the total Non-REM minutes. The proportion of the EEG tracing with spikes should be > 85% during slow wave sleep although, for some children (for example within the Landau-Kleffner group) the spike-wave index may be around 50% [12]. Much remains to be done to validate this index and determine which specific epileptiform patterns should be included in it. For example, some children may have continuous diphasic spike-wave during slow sleep but also bursts of polyspike-waves [13] which may be interspersed with focal slow wave or generalized discharges.

One must bear in mind that an asleep EEG recording may be difficult to obtain in children and is therefore not routinely requested in children older than four years even if seizures appear. This is particularly true in retarded children with behavioral problem. In our experience, we use very rarely the chlorhydrate for sedation; it doesn't seem to modify the CSW EEG pattern. But we need futher study to confirm this feeling.

Etiology

The etiologies associated with ESES can be either cryptogenic or symptomatic, the later largely resulting from pre- or perinatal vascular insults, including ulegyria and leukomalacia. Among the migration disorders, polymicrogyria is most often associated with CSWS, whereas other cortical developmental disorders are not [12]. Guerrini *et al.* hypothesized that the preservation of horizontal neuronal connections seen in polymicrogyric cortices may allow the propagation and spreading of the spike and wave discharges [14].

Treatment

The relationship between the neuropsychological disorder and the ESES phenomenon is not clearly understood but several studies demonstrated varying degrees of improvement in language and social behavior with EEG normalization. It is generally agreed that ESES does not respond to conventional antiepileptic drugs (AEDs) such as phenobarbital and phenytoin. Carbamazepine must be avoided because it could precipitate the occurrence of CSWS and could play a role in prolonging it [15]. The response to sodium valproate is uncertain and inconsistant. Benzodiazepines (BZ) are effective particularly in some cryptogenic cases. Steroids appear to have a favorable and lasting effect and are justified when benzodiazepines are ineffective (most often in symptomatic patients). Corticosteroids should be administered for about 18 months in order to assure suppression of the epileptic process associated with CSWS during the age-dependant period of development when the syndrome is expressed. In a retrospective study of 33 children treated with benzodiazepines in monotherapy, CSWS disappeared in 33% of cryptogenic and 12.5% of symptomatic cases. Hydrocortisone was used in 27 children with a normalization of the EEG in all cryptogenic cases but in only 35% of the symptomatic group [12]. Many studies indicate that the early reversal of clinical and EEG abnormalities may improve the overall outcome of children with ESES.

Prognosis

Descriptions of the long-term outcome of ESES are not well documented. Complete reversibility of cognitive disorders has been described in this syndrome [3].

There are some factors which may influence prognosis. These include age of onset, duration and severity of cognitive impairment, response to antiepileptic treatment and effect of psychological and specific educational therapies [16].

The data from the literature confirm the favorable outcome of this syndrome with respect to seizures.

The outcome of the EEG abnormalities is difficult to evaluate due to the considerable variability in the AEDs used and the duration of their use. The longer the duration of CSWS, the more damage it causes. Monotherapy with benzodiazepine or use of corticosteroids appears to have favorable and lasting effects. CSWS is now considered a disorder that occurs during a vulnerable period in brain development and is due to rapid secondary generalization (e.g. a secondary bilateral synchrony) from one or several cortical foci. The cerebral metabolic pattern observed in epilepsy with the CSWS pattern suggests focal or multifocal dysfunction of associative cortical areas which may impede normal formation of synapses [17]. The early resolution of the electrical status by stopping this hypersynchrony may prevent cognitive decline. During the recovery period, the CSWS becomes fragmented or fluctuates, and the spike-wave discharges diminish and eventually disappear completely. This improvement in the EEG is accompanied by progressive clinical improvement.

Regardless of the duration of the active epileptic process, one must consider that possible reorganization of cortical functions has to take place in the brain after the end of the ESES period. This period may have been quite prolonged. This expected reorganization may not occur very effectively in symptomatic patient with cerebral damage or in retarded children. More generally, we can expect that if a focal epileptic dysfunction arises in a cerebral area mediating the emergence of a specific cognitive function, the disorder will be more severe than if it appears after the stabilization of this function. These various areas affected and the outcome of the disorder can involve different skills in different patients, depending on the maturational stage of the functions involved at disease onset. For example, in the case of the Landau-Kleffner syndrome with verbal auditory agnosia, the earlier the onset, the more severe the consequences [18]. The later outcome of this syndrome is extensively described in the chapter devoted to it by C. Billard.

Descriptions of the long-term evolution of the acquired epileptic frontal syndrome show that the behavioral disturbances first subside, followed by cognitive and linguistic recovery. The outcome, however, is quite poor. Although patients stabilized, they did not recover fully during the follow-up period. Some patients are even characterized by profound alterations in personality and social conduct.

Prospective studies are needed to improve our understanding of the ESES syndrome. Serial neuropsychological evaluations in correlation with treatment and EEG findings are required. Early diagnosis and rapid initiation of specific treatments are a pre-requisite for recovery.

Aknowledgement

I thank Olivier Dulac for his help in the translation of this article.

References

1. Dulac O. Epileptic encephalopathy. *Epilepsia* 2001; 42 (Suppl 3): 23-6.
2. Patry G, Lyagoubi S, Tassinari CA. Subclinical "electrical status epilepticus" induced by sleep in children. *Arch Neurol* 1971; 24: 242-52.
3. Tassinari CA, Bureau M, Dravet C, Dalla-Bernardina B, Roger J. Epilepsy with continuous spike and waves during slow sleep, otherwise described as ESES (epilepsy with electrical status epilepticus during slow sleep). In: Roger J, Bureau M, Dravet C, Dreifuss FE, Perret A, Wolf P, eds. *Epileptic syndromes in infancy, childhood and adolescence*. London and Paris: John Libbey, 1992: 245-56.
4. Commission on classification and terminology of the international league against epilepsy: proposal for revised classification of epilepsies and epileptic syndromes. *Epilepsia* 1989; 30: 389-99.
5. Galanopoulou AS, Bojko A, Lado F, Moshé SL. The spectrum of neuropsychiatric abnormalities associated with electrical status epilepticus in sleep. *Brain Dev* 2000; 22: 279-95.
6. Billard C, Autret E, Lafon C, *et al*. Aphasie-acquise de l'enfant avec épilepsie. A propos de quatre enfants avec état de mal épileptique infraclinique du sommeil. *Rev Electroencephalogr Neurophysiol Clin* 1981; 11: 457-67.
7. Bulteau C, Jambaqué I, Dulac O, Plouin P. Case reports. Aphasia epilepsy: a clinical and EEG study of six cases with CSWS. In: Beaumanoir A, Bureau M, Deonna T, Mira L, Tasinari CA, eds. *Continuous spike and waves during slow sleep, electrical status epilepticus during slow sleep*. Mariani Foundation Neurology Series:3. London: John Libbey, 1995: 199-201.
8. Roulet-Perez E, Davidoff V, Despland PA, Deonna T. Mental and behavioral deterioration of children with epilepsy and CSWS: acquired epileptic frontal syndrome. *Dev Med Child Neurol* 1993; 35: 661-74.
9. Colamaria V, Sgro V, Carabello R, *et al*. Status epilepticus in benign rolandic epilepsy manifesting as anterior operculum syndrome. *Epilepsia* 1991; 32: 329-34.
10. Badinand N, Bastuji H, De Bellescize J, Cortinovis P, Kocher L, Rousselle C, Revol M. Case reports. Three unpublished new cases of continuous spikes and waves during slow sleep. In: Beaumanoir A, Bureau M, Deonna T, Mira L, Tasinari CA, eds. *Continuous spike and waves during slow sleep, electrical status epilepticus during slow sleep*. Mariani Foundation Neurology Series:3. London: John Libbey, 1995: 186-7.
11. Guerrini R, Dravet C, Genton P, *et al*. Epileptic negative myoclonus. *Neurology* 1993; 43: 1078-83.
12. Bulteau C, Jambaqué I, Dulac O. Aspects neuropsychologiques du syndrome des pointes ondes continues pendant le sommeil lent. *Approche Neuropsychologique des Apprentissages chez l'Enfant* 1997; 41: 5-9.
13. Veggiotti, Beccaria F, Guerrini R, Capovilla G, Lanzi G. Continuous spike and wave activity during slow-wave sleep: syndrome or EEG pattern? *Epilepsia* 1999; 40: 1593-601.
14. Guerrini R, Genton P, Bureau M, Parmegianni A, Salas-Puig X, Santucci M. Multilobar polymicrogyria, intractable drop attack seizures, and sleep-related electrical status epilepticus. *Neurology* 1998; 51: 504-12.
15. Morikawa T, Seino T, Yagi K. Long-term outcome of four children with continuous spikes and waves during slow waves. In: Roger J, Bureau M, Dravet C, Dreifuss FE, Perret A, Wolf P, eds. *Epileptic syndromes in infancy, childhood and adolescence*. London and Paris: John Libbey, 1992: 257-65.
16. Roulet-Perez E. Cognitive Profiles of CSWS Syndrome. In: Jambaqué I, Lassonde M, Dulac O, eds. *Neuropsychology of childhood epilepsy*. New York: Kluwer Academic/Plenum Publishers, 2001: 199-206.
17. Maquet P, Hirsch E, Metz-Lutz MN, Motte J, Dive C, Marescaux C, Franck G. Regional cerebral glucose metabolism in children with deterioration of one or more cognitive functions and continuous spike-wave discharges during sleep. *Brain* 1995; 118: 1497-520.
18. Bishop DVM. Age of onset and outcome in "acquired aphasia with convulsive disorder" (Landau-Kleffner syndrome). *Dev Med Child Neurol* 1985; 27: 705-12.
19. Veggiotti P, Bova S, Granocchio E, Papaglia G, Termine C, Lanzi G. Acquired epileptic frontal syndrome as long-term outcome in two children with CSWS. *Neurophysiol Clin* 2001; 31: 387-97.

Prognosis of convulsive status epilepticus

Hervé Outin, Pierre Thomas

The risk of death associated with convulsive status epilepticus (CSE) was highlighted in the very first descriptions of the phenomenon, which date back to the nineteenth century [1, 2]. Since then, the life-threatening nature of CSE has been emphasized in many review articles [3-7] and consensus conferences [8, 9]. Epidemiological studies [10-18], randomized therapeutic trials [19, 20], and numerous retrospective studies [21-33] of CSE have provided accurate information on mortality in specific populations and have identified various factors that influence the likelihood of death. Conversely, few data are available on the rate and severity of new neurological deficits and cognitive impairments following CSE [22, 33, 34]. A few studies have investigated the risk of recurrent CSE [17, 35, 36] and subsequent epilepsy.

Inadequacies in published data result in uncertainty about the prognosis of convulsive status epilepticus

Methodology of available studies

Considerable methodological variation exists among published studies of survival and functional disability after CSE. Few truly prospective epidemiological studies have been reported [12, 14, 17, 18]. Outcomes data have been derived from randomized therapeutic trials [19, 20] or cohorts such as the Rochester study population [10, 15, 16]. Other studies pooled retrospective and prospective data [33] or used only retrospective data [27, 37]. A meta-analysis of retrospective data is available [1]. The duration of follow up varies widely across studies. Most studies considered outcomes assessed after a follow up of 30 to 60 days [12, 14, 15, 17-20, 22, 32, 33, 38], although a few recorded long-term outcomes (6 months [26] and 12 years [10]).

Difficulties with definitions

The seizure duration required to make a diagnosis of CSE is difficult to define [2, 39, 40]. Based on experimental studies [8, 9, 40-42], CSE is often defined as seizing for at least 30 minutes, either as a continuous seizure or as repeated seizures without recovery of consciousness in the inter-seizure intervals [43]. Although this definition has been widely relied on, particularly in epidemiological studies, it is difficult to use and is often substantially modified [8, 40, 43, 44]. After defining CSE as seizing for at least 30 minutes, the American Consensus Conference recommended that patients seizing for at least ten minutes in the emergency room be treated as cases of CSE [9]. Similarly, the French-Language Society for Critical Care has defined CSE as seizing for five to ten minutes [8]. In a study of out-of-hospital treatment, Alldredge *et al.* [19] defined CSE as seizures lasting 5 minutes or more. In the Veterans Affairs study, patients were included if they had at least two seizures without recovery in the interval or a continuous seizure lasting more than 10 minutes [20]. Claassen *et al.* distinguished continuous seizures lasting more than 10 minutes and repeated seizures for longer than 30 minutes [22]. Others [45] sought to identify the duration beyond which spontaneous termination became unlikely. In a study comparing CSE (seizing for 30 min or longer) to prolonged seizures (10 to 29 minutes), DeLorenzo *et al.* found that 43% of prolonged seizures stopped spontaneously and that in this subgroup none of the patients died [45]. A carefully designed study of characteristics that identify this subset of patients would be useful in that it would help practitioners identify those patients in whom they could defer early initiation of treatments with important side effects, especially anesthetic drugs.

Populations investigated

Some studies of the prognosis of CSE were hospital-based [17], whereas others were population-based [18]. Many studies focused on highly selected populations, such as patients admitted to the intensive care unit [32] or conventional hospital ward [21] or patients older than 60 years [13, 46]. Mortality varied according to the type of healthcare facility, from 1.9% in the study by Scholtes *et al.* conducted in epileptology clinics to 11.9% in teaching hospitals [25]. Data specific to children are sometimes difficult to obtain because many studies included all age groups [10, 14, 15, 17, 18], although others focused on pediatric patients [12, 31, 33, 35, 47, 48]. Among inclusion criteria that require special attention is CSE caused by hypoxia-ischemia, which contributes a larger proportion of patients in recent studies [11]. Hypoxic-ischemic CSE is difficult to differentiate from hypoxic-ischemic encephalopathy, which is often included in published series although it lacks many of the criteria for CSE [18, 49, 50].

Clinical presentation of convulsive status epilepticus

Spontaneously, overt CSE progresses to subtle SE then to purely electrical SE [3, 51]. These three patterns have very different prognoses [20]. In routine practice, the passage from one pattern to another can only be diagnosed electrographically. When EEG criteria are not appropriately incorporated into the definition of status epilepticus, as was the case in some retrospective studies, various diagnostic mistakes can be made. These include failure to recognize subtle SE [50]. The relative proportions of overt and subtle SE are not always specified in study reports. EEG data should be collected more aggressively, as in a study by DeLorenzo *et al.* who performed continuous EEG monitoring for at least 24 hours after clinical control was achieved [45]. Furthermore, difficulties in the interpretation the

EEG can lead to overdiagnosis of CSE, for instance in patients with hypoxic-ischemic encephalopathy, or to underdiagnosis, particularly in patients with periodic epileptiform discharges (PEDs), a pattern whose significance remains debated. Treiman *et al.* believe that PEDs occur at the most advanced stage of subtle SE [51] and, in practice, indicate a very poor prognosis. Other studies excluded patients in whom PEDs were the only EEG abnormality [17]. Another factor that adds to the nosographic confusion is that some authors consider subtle SE as a form of nonconvulsive SE [4, 19, 25, 52].

Mortality in patients with generalized convulsive status epilepticus

Mortality rates

The mortality rate in patients with CSE *(table I)* decreased from the beginning of the twentieth century to the 1970s [41] and since then has shown little change, despite the increasing number of elderly patients and, probably, the inclusion in some studies of patients with hypoxic-ischemic encephalopathy [11]. Mortality is about 20% in adults and 5% in children [1, 6, 8, 9]. From a metaanalysis including 1686 patients, Shorvon concluded that the mortality rate was 18% [1]. The retrospective study by Logroscino *et al.* [15] excluded patients with febrile CSE and found a 30-day mortality rate of 19%. Waterhouse *et al.* [14] prospectively studied 645 children and adults, in whom the two-month mortality rate was 19.6% for intermittent SE and 31.4% for continuous SE. Epileptologists have reported lower rates in patients managed in epilepsy units [25]. When interpreting mortality rates, the distribution of the causes of CSE should be considered. However, very high mortality might be observed in patients with acute brain insults, usually managed in ICUs [44, 50]. In the EPISTAR study conducted in French-speaking Switzerland, mortality was only 7.6%, but the authors carefully excluded patients with hypoxic-ischemic encephalopathy [18]. Alldredge *et al.* reported a 9.4% mortality rate in a study characterized by highly restrictive inclusion criteria [19]. A long-term study of the Rochester cohort [10] found that the ten-year cumulative mortality rate was 43% and that the risk of death was almost three times greater than expected when standardized to the general population.

Prognostic factors

The mortality and morbidity associated with CSE result from many factors, whose respective contributions remain difficult to establish. The cause of the CSE is probably the most important factor, however. In many cases, the cause or causes represent progressive or degenerative disorders that follow their own worsening course. Furthermore, a cause with a particularly poor prognosis, for instance cardiac arrest, may influence the decision to limit treatment. In addition, the systemic repercussions of CSE seem to weigh more heavily on the prognosis than does the seizure activity itself [4, 7]. To date, there is no proof that CSE *per se*, independently from the complications it generates, can directly cause death [1, 50]. Although cardiocirculatory factors have been incriminated, their role remains to be established [53, 54]. In contrast, the adverse effects of the seizures on the brain seem clearly exacerbated by the systemic repercussions of CSE [41, 42]. As early as 1983, Meldrum [55] reported that the main factors of adverse prognostic significance in animals in addition to duration of the CSE were the presence of hypoxia, hypotension, and hyperthermia. Other factors include inadequate or inappropriate management and iatrogenic events related to the aggressive treatments required in CSE.

Table I. Main recently published studies (1996-2002) providing data on the prognosis of convulsive status epilepticus

Author Year	Study design	Sample size	Overall mortality	Comments
Logroscino et al. 2002	Retrospective cohort	145	43% cumulative over 10 years	• Patients with CSE who survived beyond the first month • Duration is a prognostic factor only if the SE is symptomatic and lasts more than 24 h
Claassen et al. 2002	Retrospective cohort	83 SE 74 patients	21% at hospital discharge	• Neurological deterioration in 23% of survivors
Alldredge et al. 2001	Randomised clinical trial	205	9.4% at hospital discharge	• Adults • Selected population • Neurological deterioration in 16.3% of survivors
Shinnar et al. 2001	Prospective cohort	180	0% first month	• Children (1 month-10 years) • Only febrile SE
Coeytaux et al. 2000	Prospective cohort	172	7.6% at hospital discharge	• All age groups • Quality of management • Subtle SE very rare if strict diagnostic criteria are used
Waterhouse et al. 1999	Prospective cohort	646	17.8% first two months (children, 6.2%; adults, 24%)	• Age older than 1 month • Prognosis different between continuous CSE and intermittent CSE
Treiman et al. 1998	Randomised clinical trial	618	36% first month	• Adults • Mortality: 65% if subtle SE 27% if overt CSF
Logroscino et al. 1997	Retrospective cohort	201	19% first month	• Prognosis seems independent from duration
DeLorenzo et al. 1996	Prospective cohort	204 SE 166 patients	22% first month (children, 3%; adults, 26%)	• Patients with CSE who survived beyond the first month • Good analysis of prognosis according to cause

SE: status epilepticus; CSE: convulsive status epilepticus.

Etiological factors

Given the important influence of the cause on the prognosis of CSE, stratification of patients based on this criterion may be desirable in studies of CSE [37]. Shorvon [1] reported that death was clearly related to the cause in more than 90% of cases. Barry and Hauser found that the mortality rate was 54% in CSE related to an acute brain insult as compared to only 16% in patients with a previous history of epilepsy [26]. In a study by Logroscino and Hesdorffer [15], 89% of deaths within the first 30 days occurred among patients with acute symptomatic CSE. In the EPISTAR study, seven of the 13 deaths were clearly related to the cause of the CSE [18]. The long-term study of the Rochester cohort confirmed the excess mortality in the patients with symptomatic CSE and found that ten-year mortality in patients with idiopathic/cryptogenic CSE was similar to that in the population at large [10]. Although this study included only patients who survived for at least 30 days, its results suggest that CSE per se has no marked effect on mortality [56].

Patients with hypoxic-ischemic encephalopathy are too often classified as having subtle SE based on clinical criteria, without careful EEG documentation. The prognosis of hypoxic-ischemic encephalopathy with myoclonus is extremely bleak [57-59]. Consequently, including these patients in studies of CSE biases the results regarding outcomes. For instance, in the EPISTAR study, the mortality rate dropped to 7.6% when patients with hypoxic-ischemic encephalopathy were excluded [18]. In the Richmond cohort, the mortality rate was 22%, but 13% of the patients had hypoxic-ischemic encephalopathy [17]. Similarly, in the Veterans Affairs study, mortality was 36% in the overall population of 518 CSE patients as compared to 65% in the subgroup of 134 patients with subtle SE, 38% of whom had hypoxic-ischemic encephalopathy [20].

Ischemic and hemorrhagic stroke are important causes of CSE, although their contribution has varied across studies. Stroke was the cause of CSE in 17.5% of the adults in the EPISTAR study [18] and in nearly 50% of the adults in the Richmond cohort [17]. Mortality in the Richmond cohort was 32%, i.e., about three times the expected rate for stroke of similar severity without CSE [17]. Waterhouse *et al.* reported that patients with CSE at the acute phase of stroke had an eight-fold increase in mortality as compared to patients with CSE who had a remote history of stroke [60]. In a study by Velioglu *et al.* [61], CSE within one week of stroke occurrence was associated with excess mortality and a higher risk for CSE recurrence. Taken in aggregate, these data are consistent with a direct deleterious effect of CSE on the vascular lesion, perhaps mediated by the acute modifications in brain hemodynamics induced by the multiple seizures.

Conversely, CSE related to anticonvulsant medication withdrawal has a better prognosis, with less than 10% mortality in most studies [6, 8-10, 17, 18, 27, 41]. When no such cause or provocation is apparent (spontaneous CSE), mortality seems to be higher, around 20% [37].

Patient age

Mortality is higher in the youngest and oldest patients. In children, mortality rates range from 3% to 11%. In a short-term study of the very distinctive population of children with febrile CSE, Shinnar *et al.* recorded no deaths [12]. Waterhouse *et al.* reported 38% mortality in patients older than 65 years of age and at least 50% in those older than 80 years of age [13]. Logroscino *et al.* found that the relative risk for death was 67 in the patients aged 65 years or older as compared to those in the 1-19 year age group and that mortality in the patients aged 65 years or older was increased two-fold as compared to the expected mortality rate in the general population of a similar age [10].

Duration of status epilepticus

Data on the duration of CSE are difficult to interpret [29]. Prolonged CSE may simply be a marker for the absence of effective, appropriate treatment. In addition, CSE duration is related to the clinical pattern as, over time, overt CSE gives way to subtle SE. In the Veterans Affairs study, mean SE duration was 2.8 hours in overt CSE (mortality, 27%) and 5.8 hours in subtle SE (mortality, 65%). Regardless of the pattern, mortality is increased two-fold in patients who fail to respond to first-line therapy [20], and earlier administration of second-line therapy is associated with a considerably higher response rate [38].

Overall, longer duration is associated with a worse prognosis [27, 29, 37]. In a retrospective study by Lowenstein *et al.*, CSE duration was shorter in the patients who survived

(2.4 hours) than in those who died (11.2 hours) [27]. In the retrospective study of the Richmond cohort, CSE duration longer than 1 hour showed a highly significant association with death [37]. DeLorenzo *et al.* reported that mortality was 2.6% in patients with CSE durations shorter than 30 minutes and 19% in those with longer durations [62]. Conversely, Logroscino *et al.* found no influence of seizure duration on short-term mortality after adjusting for other risk factors [15]. However, in the long-term study of the same cohort, the relative risk of death in patients with CSE durations longer than 24 hours was 2.3 compared to patients with CSE durations shorter than 2 hours [10], and excess mortality occurred only in those patients with symptomatic CSE. Similar findings have been obtained in children [33].

Pattern of status epilepticus termination

Refractory status epilepticus

Refractory CSE is defined as persistent seizures despite appropriate management. Studies have consistently shown a high mortality rate of about 40% in patients with refractory SE [50]. In the Veterans Affairs study, resistance to two antiepileptic drugs was noted in 38% of patients with overt CSE and in 82% of those with subtle SE. Response rates to administration of a third antiepileptic drug have been extremely low (2% to 5%) [63]. A retrospective study by Mayer *et al.* [38] found that 31% of patients failed to respond within 60 minutes to the successive administration of two antiepileptic drugs and that the mortality rate in this subgroup was 23%. Most deaths were related to intercurrent complications or to the complications of intensive care. Mortality was 61% in a retrospective study of 33 patients with very long duration refractory SE treated ultimately with midazolam [64]. These poor results can probably be ascribed to the fact that, in earlier studies, midazolam was reserved for the least severe cases.

Subtle status epilepticus

Subtle SE was associated with a very poor prognosis in the Veterans Affairs study [20]: the analysis of survival beyond the 30th day showed that 65% of the 134 patients in the subtle SE subgroup died, as compared to 27% of the 384 patients with overt CSE. In this series, the rate of response to drugs was 14.9% among patients with subtle SE and 55.5% among those with overt CSE. However, these results should be interpreted with caution because of the imprecision in the definitions. In the Veterans Affairs study, 24% of the patients had subtle SE, with hypoxic-ischemic encephalopathy as the cause in 38% of cases, whereas in the EPISTAR study, which excluded hypoxic-ischemic encephalopathy, only 1.2% of patients had subtle SE [18]. Many studies lump together subtle SE, myoclonic SE, non-convulsive SE, and EEG patterns suggestive of SE in comatose patients. For instance, Mayer *et al.* included seven patients with "nonconvulsive SE" in "comatose or obtunded patients" [38]. Similarly, among the patients studied by Towne *et al.* [65], 8% had "an EEG pattern suggestive of SE", a pattern whose validity has been challenged by Benbadis *et al.* [66].

Intermittent versus continuous SE

Mortality seems to be lower in patients with intermittent seizures [14]. In adults, SE duration did not differ significantly between these two clinical patterns [14].

Quality of management

Many studies have found evidence that emergency management is often inappropriate. In a study by Celesia, seven of the 27 deaths seemed ascribable either to inadequate monitoring or to errors in the dosage or route of administration of medications [52]. Walker *et al.* reported that only 12% of physicians followed a predefined management protocol [67]. In 1996, the same group conducted an audit of 26 patients admitted to a neurological intensive care unit [68]. Failure to diagnose factitious SE was noted in six patients, four of whom underwent tracheal intubation, and phenytoin therapy was inadequate in nearly half the patients [68]. Among the patients enrolled in the 1964-1985 Rochester cohort who were given appropriate first-line drugs, three in every four received inadequate dosages. Furthermore, when a second antiepileptic drug was given, the dosage was inadequate in 80% of cases [69]. Others [38, 64] have reported poor standardization of therapy and use of inadequate dosages. Scholtes *et al.* found that treatment was suboptimal in 44.7% of patients who died and in 22.7% of those with residual deficits. This contrasts with 10.3% of those with a favorable outcome [25].

Morbidity related to generalized convulsive status epilepticus

There are currently no available published studies specifically designed to evaluate the morbidity related to CSE. An evaluation of morbidity would face considerable methodological difficulties because morbidity directly attributable to SE is difficult to differentiate from morbidity related to the cause and treatment of CSE [1, 5, 22, 41]. A number of experimental and clinical arguments strongly suggest that SE may promote neuronal death, particularly when the seizures are prolonged. For instance, high levels of neuron specific enolase have been found in cerebrospinal fluid from patients with SE [70]. DeGiorgio *et al.* demonstrated neuronal loss in the CA1 and CA3 sectors of the hippocampus in patients who died following CSE, as compared to patients who died from other causes [71]. A few studies have found magnetic resonance imaging evidence of progressive hippocampal atrophy [41]. These data are related to the continuing controversy over whether hippocampal sclerosis can occur as a result of complicated febrile seizures in children [12]. The sequelae of febrile status epilepticus may consist of development or worsening of a neurological deficit, development of mental retardation, subsequent epilepsy, or a combination of these [5].

Neurological and cognitive impairments

Studies in the pediatric age group have yielded conflicting results. Some [31] have found that deficits occurred in 9% to 28% of pediatric patients but were often related to the cause of CSE [33, 48, 72]. On the other hand, a long-term prospective study [73] found favorable cognitive outcomes in children with a history of febrile seizures. Shinnar *et al.* [12] prospectively identified 180 children aged one month to ten years who had febrile CSE over a period of ten years. They were compared to 244 children who had their first febrile seizure, without SE. No deaths were recorded, and there were no cases of new cognitive or motor impairment in the short term. Long-term follow up of this cohort can be expected to provide insight into possible relationships between febrile CSE and the subsequent occurrence of hippocampal sclerosis.

In a 1971 study of adults, Oxbury and Whitty found that 11% of the patients suffered sequelae [30]. Aminoff and Simon reported that the rate of morbidity directly related to CSE was 12.5% [29]. Similar rates were found in another retrospective study [27]. In the recent study by Alldredge *et al.* [19] of 255 selected adults with overt SE, 16.3% of patients had new neurological deficits following the episode. However, the influence of etiological factors complicates the interpretation of overall or individual results. It has been suggested that chronic progressive encephalopathy, sometimes with cerebral atrophy, may occur in 6 to 15% of patients [41]. Claassen *et al.* conducted a retrospective study of 83 episodes of CSE in 74 elderly patients, many of whom had symptomatic CSE. Sixteen (11%) episodes were followed by a one point or greater increase in the Glasgow Outcome Scale (GOS) score [22]. They estimated that the deterioration was probably unrelated to the cause of CSE in seven patients. Mayer *et al.* [38] found a 54% reduction in the GOS score in refractory CSE, although the difference with CSE responsive to first-line therapy was not significant in this small sample sized retrospective study. Very few articles report accurate quantitative data on cognitive sequelae [1, 5, 34].

Epilepsy

The risk of epilepsy is increased after an episode of CSE. Hesdorffer *et al.* reported that the risk of epilepsy in the Rochester cohort was 37% after an episode of CSE and 5% after a single symptomatic seizure [16]. In children with symptomatic seizures, the risk of recurrence may be higher after CSE than after a single seizure [74]. DeLorenzo *et al.* [17] found that 13.3% of their patients experienced recurrent CSE.

Conclusions

Improving the prognosis of CSE requires [1] use of a detailed predefined management protocol [8, 50, 67] involving prompt aggressive treatment and, if in the slightest doubt, continuous EEG recording [43], as well as closer collaboration between neurologists and intensivists [50]. First-line treatment is not consistently successful in terminating the seizures: clearly, there is a need for more effective medications [20], particularly for refractory CSE [38, 43], which will have to be evaluated in randomized therapeutic trials. To gain further insight into the factors that bear on the prognosis of CSE, prospective studies using standardized treatments and patient stratification on age and etiologies are needed.

References

1. Shorvon S. Status Epilepticus. Its clinical features and treatment in children and adults. Cambridge: Cambridge University Press, 1994: 382.
2. Lowenstein DH. Status epilepticus: an overview of the clinical problem. *Epilepsia* 1999; 40: S3-8; discussion S21-2.
3. Treiman DM. Effective treatment for status epilepticus. In: Schmidt D, Schachter SC, eds. *Epilepsy problem solving in clinical practice*. London: Martin Dunitz, 2000: 253-65.
4. Shorvon S. The management of status epilepticus. *J Neurol Neurosurg Psychiatry* 2001; 70 (Suppl 2): II22-7.
5. Loiseau P. Morbidité et mortalité des états de mal épileptiques. *Neurophysiol Clin* 2000; 30: 155-60.
6. Lowenstein DH, Alldredge BK. Status epilepticus. *N Engl J Med* 1998; 338: 970-6.
7. Nouailhat F, Outin HD, Simon N, Merrer J. Status epilepticus and serial seizures. In: Tinker J. ZWM, eds. *Care of the critically ill patient*. London: Springer-Verlag, 1992: 1003-28.
8. Conférence de consensus en réanimation et médecine d'urgence: prise en charge de l'état de mal épileptique (Enfants-Adultes). *Rean Urg* 1995: 387-96.
9. Treatment of convulsive status epilepticus. Recommendations of the Epilepsy Foundation of America's Working Group on Status Epilepticus. *JAMA* 1993; 270: 854-9.
10. Logroscino G, Hesdorffer DC, Cascino GD, Annegers JF, Bagiella E, Hauser WA. Long-term mortality after a first episode of status epilepticus. *Neurology* 2002; 58: 537-41.
11. Logroscino G, Hesdorffer DC, Cascino G, Annegers JF, Hauser WA. Time trends in incidence, mortality, and case-fatality after first episode of status epilepticus. *Epilepsia* 2001; 42: 1031-5.

12. Shinnar S, Pellock JM, Berg AT, O'Dell C, Driscoll SM, Maytal J, Moshe SL, Delorenzo RJ. Short-Term Outcomes of Children with Febrile Status Epilepticus. *Epilepsia* 2001; 42: 47-53.
13. Waterhouse EJ, DeLorenzo RJ. Status epilepticus in older patients: epidemiology and treatment options. *Drugs Aging* 2001; 18: 133-42.
14. Waterhouse EJ, Garnett LK, Towne AR, Morton LD, Barnes T, Ko D, DeLorenzo RJ. Prospective population-based study of intermittent and continuous convulsive status epilepticus in Richmond, Virginia. *Epilepsia* 1999; 40: 752-8.
15. Logroscino G, Hesdorffer DC, Cascino G, Annegers JF, Hauser WA. Short-term mortality after a first episode of status epilepticus. *Epilepsia* 1997; 38: 1344-9.
16. Hesdorffer DC, Logroscino G, Cascino G, Annegers JF, Hauser WA. Incidence of status epilepticus in Rochester, Minnesota, 1965-1984. *Neurology* 1998; 50: 735-41.
17. DeLorenzo RJ, Hauser WA, Towne AR, Boggs JG, Pellock JM, Penberthy L, Garnett L, Fortner CA, Ko D. A prospective, population-based epidemiologic study of status epilepticus in Richmond, Virginia. *Neurology* 1996; 46: 1029-35.
18. Coeytaux A, Jallon P, Galobardes B, Morabia A. Incidence of status epilepticus in French-speaking Switzerland: (EPISTAR). *Neurology* 2000; 55: 693-7.
19. Alldredge BK, Gelb AM, Isaacs SM, Corry MD, Allen F, Ulrich S, Gottwald MD, O'Neil N, Neuhaus JM, Segal MR, Lowenstein DH. A comparison of lorazepam, diazepam, and placebo for the treatment of out-of-hospital status epilepticus. *N Engl J Med* 2001; 345: 631-7.
20. Treiman DM, Meyers PD, Walton NY, Collins JF, Colling C, Rowan AJ, Handforth A, Faught E, Calabrese VP, Uthman BM, Ramsay RE, Mamdani MB. A comparison of four treatments for generalized convulsive status epilepticus. Veterans Affairs Status Epilepticus Cooperative Study Group. *N Engl J Med* 1998; 339: 792-8.
21. Delanty N, French JA, Labar DR, Pedley TA, Rowan AJ. Status epilepticus arising de novo in hospitalized patients: an analysis of 41 patients. *Seizure* 2001; 10: 116-9.
22. Claassen J, Lokin JK, Fitzsimmons BF, Mendelsohn FA, Mayer SA. Predictors of functional disability and mortality after status epilepticus. *Neurology* 2002; 58: 139-42.
23. Krishnamurthy KB, Drislane FW. Relapse and survival after barbiturate anesthetic treatment of refractory status epilepticus. *Epilepsia* 1996; 37: 863-7.
24. Sagduyu A, Tarlaci S, Sirin H. Generalized tonic-clonic status epilepticus: causes, treatment, complications and predictors of case fatality. *J Neurol* 1998; 245: 640-6.
25. Scholtes FB, Renier WO, Meinardi H. Generalized convulsive status epilepticus: causes, therapy, and outcome in 346 patients. *Epilepsia* 1994; 35: 1104-12.
26. Barry E, Hauser WA. Status epilepticus: the interaction of epilepsy and acute brain disease. *Neurology* 1993; 43: 1473-8.
27. Lowenstein DH, Alldredge BK. Status epilepticus at an urban public hospital in the 1980s. *Neurology* 1993; 43: 483-8.
28. Yaffe K, Lowenstein DH. Prognostic factors of pentobarbital therapy for refractory generalized status epilepticus. *Neurology* 1993; 43: 895-900.
29. Aminoff MJ, Simon RP. Status epilepticus. Causes, clinical features and consequences in 98 patients. *Am J Med* 1980; 69: 657-66.
30. Oxbury JM, Whitty CW. Causes and consequences of status epilepticus in adults. A study of 86 cases. *Brain* 1971; 94: 733-44.
31. Aicardi J, Chevrie JJ. Convulsive status epilepticus in infants and children. A study of 239 cases. *Epilepsia* 1970; 11: 187-97.
32. Nouailhat F, Levy-Alcover MA, Goulon M. État de mal épileptique de l'adulte. Étude épidémiologique et clinique en réanimation. *Rev Electroencephalogr Neurophysiol Clin* 1985; 14: 287-92.
33. Maytal J, Shinnar S, Moshe SL, Alvarez LA. Low morbidity and mortality of status epilepticus in children. *Pediatrics* 1989; 83: 323-31.
34. Dodrill CB, Wilensky AJ. Intellectual impairment as an outcome of status epilepticus. *Neurology* 1990; 40: 23-7.
35. Shinnar S, Maytal J, Krasnoff L, Moshe SL. Recurrent status epilepticus in children. *Ann Neurol* 1992; 31: 598-604.
36. Hauser WA, Rich SS, Annegers JF, Anderson VE. Seizure recurrence after a 1st unprovoked seizure: an extended follow up. *Neurology* 1990; 40: 1163-70.

37. Towne AR, Pellock JM, Ko D, DeLorenzo RJ. Determinants of mortality in status epilepticus. *Epilepsia* 1994; 35: 27-34.
38. Mayer SA, Claassen J, Lokin J, Mendelsohn F, Dennis LJ, Fitzsimmons BF. Refractory status epilepticus: frequency, risk factors, and impact on outcome. *Arch Neurol* 2002; 59: 205-10.
39. Coeytaux A, Jallon P. Des difficultés de définir et classer l'état de mal épileptique. *Neurophysiol Clin* 2000; 30: 133-8.
40. Lowenstein DH, Bleck T, Macdonald RL. It's time to revise the definition of status epilepticus. *Epilepsia* 1999; 40: 120-2.
41. Fountain NB. Status epilepticus: risk factors and complications. *Epilepsia* 2000; 41: S23-30.
42. Baldy-Moulinier M, Crespel A. Physiopathologie des crises et des états de mal épileptiques. *Ann Fr Anesth Reanim* 2001; 20: 97-107.
43. Bleck TP. Refractory status epilepticus in 2001. *Arch Neurol* 2002; 59: 188-9.
44. Outin HD, De Jonghe B, Hayon J, Merrer J, Ben M'Barek-Delanoue K, Choquet S, Nouailhat F. Prise en charge des états de mal épileptiques de l'adulte en réanimation. *Rean Urg* 1995: 454-9.
45. DeLorenzo RJ, Waterhouse EJ, Towne AR, Boggs JG, Ko D, DeLorenzo GA, Brown A, Garnett L. Persistent nonconvulsive status epilepticus after the control of convulsive status epilepticus. *Epilepsia* 1998; 39: 833-40.
46. Sung CY, Chu NS. Status epilepticus in the elderly: etiology, seizure type and outcome. *Acta Neurol Scand* 1989; 80: 51-6.
47. Barnard C, Wirrell E. Does status epilepticus in children cause developmental deterioration and exacerbation of epilepsy? *J Child Neurol* 1999; 14: 787-94.
48. Dunn DW. Status epilepticus in children: etiology, clinical features, and outcome. *J Child Neurol* 1988; 3: 167-73.
49. Assal F, Coeytaux A, Jallon P. L'état de mal résistant aux antiépileptiques. *Neurophysiol Clin* 2000; 30: 139-45.
50. Outin H, Liot P, De Jonghe B, Thomas P. Prise en charge des états de mal épileptiques convulsifs réfractaires en milieu de réanimation. *Rev Neurol* (Paris), 2003 (in press).
51. Treiman DM. Electroclinical features of status epilepticus. *J Clin Neurophysiol* 1995; 12: 343-62.
52. Celesia GG. Prognosis in convulsive status epilepticus. *Adv Neurol* 1983; 34: 55-9.
53. Boggs JG, Marmarou A, Agnew JP, Morton LD, Towne AR, Waterhouse EJ, Pellock JM, DeLorenzo RJ. Hemodynamic monitoring prior to and at the time of death in status epilepticus. *Epilepsy Res* 1998; 31: 199-209.
54. Jallon P. Épilepsie et cœur. *Rev Neurol (Paris)* 1997; 153: 173-84.
55. Meldrum BS. Metabolic factors during prolonged seizures and their relation to nerve cell death. *Adv Neurol* 1983; 34: 261-75.
56. Krumholz A, Berg AT. Further evidence that for status epilepticus "one size fits all" doesn't fit. *Neurology* 2002; 58: 515-6.
57. Wijdicks EF, Parisi JE, Sharbrough FW. Prognostic value of myoclonus status in comatose survivors of cardiac arrest. *Ann Neurol* 1994; 35: 239-43.
58. Krumholz A, Stern BJ, Weiss HD. Outcome from coma after cardiopulmonary resuscitation: relation to seizures and myoclonus. *Neurology* 1988; 38: 401-5.
59. Celesia GG, Grigg MM, Ross E. Generalized status myoclonicus in acute anoxic and toxic-metabolic encephalopathies. *Arch Neurol* 1988; 45: 781-4.
60. Waterhouse EJ, Vaughan JK, Barnes TY, Boggs JG, Towne AR, Kopec-Garnett L, DeLorenzo RJ. Synergistic effect of status epilepticus and ischaemic brain injury on mortality. *Epilepsy Res* 1998; 29: 175-83.
61. Velioglu SK, Ozmenoglu M, Boz C, Alioglu Z. Status epilepticus after stroke. *Stroke* 2001; 32: 1169-72.
62. DeLorenzo RJ, Garnett LK, Towne AR, Waterhouse EJ, Boggs JG, Morton L, Choudhry MA, Barnes T, Ko D. Comparison of status epilepticus with prolonged seizure episodes lasting from 10 to 29 minutes. *Epilepsia* 1999; 40: 164-9.
63. Treiman DM, Walton NY, Collins JF, Point P. Treatment of status epilepticus if the first drug fails. *Epilepsia* 1999; 40: 243.
64. Claassen J, Hirsch LJ, Emerson RG, Bates JE, Thompson TB, Mayer SA. Continuous EEG monitoring and midazolam infusion for refractory nonconvulsive status epilepticus. *Neurology* 2001; 57: 1036-42.

65. Towne AR, Waterhouse EJ, Boggs JG, Garnett LK, Brown AJ, Smith JR, Jr., DeLorenzo RJ. Prevalence of nonconvulsive status epilepticus in comatose patients. *Neurology* 2000; 54: 340-5.
66. Benbadis SR, Tatum WO, IV, Towne AR, Waterhouse EJ, Garnett L. Prevalence of nonconvulsive status epilepticus in comatose patients. *Neurology* 2000; 55: 1421-3.
67. Walker MC, Smith SJ, Shorvon SD. The intensive care treatment of convulsive status epilepticus in the UK. Results of a national survey and recommendations. *Anaesthesia* 1995; 50: 130-5.
68. Walker MC, Howard RS, Smith SJ, Miller DH, Shorvon SD, Hirsch NP. Diagnosis and treatment of status epilepticus on a neurological intensive care unit. *Q J Med* 1996; 89: 913-20.
69. Cascino GD, Hesdorffer D, Logroscino G, Hauser WA. Treatment of nonfebrile status epilepticus in Rochester, Minn, from 1965 through 1984. *Mayo Clin Proc* 2001; 76: 39-41.
70. DeGiorgio CM, Heck CN, Rabinowicz AL, Gott PS, Smith T, Correale J. Serum neuron-specific enolase in the major subtypes of status epilepticus. *Neurology* 1999; 52: 746-9.
71. DeGiorgio CM, Tomiyasu U, Gott PS, Treiman DM. Hippocampal pyramidal cell loss in human status epilepticus. *Epilepsia* 1992; 33: 23-7.
72. Yager JY, Cheang M, Seshia SS. Status epilepticus in children. *Can J Neurol Sci* 1988; 15: 402-5.
73. Verity CM, Greenwood R, Golding J. Long-term intellectual and behavioral outcomes of children with febrile convulsions. *N Engl J Med* 1998; 338: 1723-8.
74. Shinnar S, Berg AT, Moshe SL, Petix M, Maytal J, Kang H, Goldensohn ES, Hauser WA. Risk of seizure recurrence following a first unprovoked seizure in childhood: a prospective study. *Pediatrics* 1990; 85: 1076-85.

Prognosis in non-convulsive status epilepticus

Peter W. Kaplan

Introduction

Status epilepticus (SE), the maximum expression of epilepsy [1] is a neurologic emergency, largely recognized for the lasting morbidity and high mortality seen with convulsive status epilepticus (CSE). Prompt diagnosis with rapid control of CSE can improve patient outcomes. Nonconvulsive status epilepticus (NCSE), until recently, was considered a rare form of SE, to a great extent because it was under-recognized and under-diagnosed [2]. Standard texts have included isolated case reports and chapters describing occasional slowly-resolving or permanent cognitive deficits [3-8], but only more recently have larger case series addressed this issue [9-10]. The issue of comatose patients, or ICU patients with multiple organ failure, and electrographic evidence of seizure activity probably represents a definable population [9-13], distinct from the original concept of NCSE [14]. Because NCSE was not believed to cause morbidity or death [9-10, 12, 15-18], rapid intervention and aggressive control was not emphasized in the management of patients with NCSE. There have been few systematic analyses of the prognosis in NCSE.

The problems confronting the determination of prognosis in NCSE

Only more recently has the subject of residual morbidity after status epilepticus been looked at, with its attendant problems of disentangling the consequences of status from those of the condition precipitating status. Even when trying to correlate duration of status with outcome, such confounding features as cause and effect are still present as it is not entirely clear whether particular causes of status result in greater difficulty in controlling status.

At its simplest, the determination of prognosis in NCSE involves defining and identifying the number of patients with NCSE, separating this pleomorphic population into groups of like (absence status epilepticus [ASE] versus complex partial status epilepticus [CPSE]), so as to determine the number of patients in these specific groups who have a given outcome. With respect to determining prognosis for NCSE, each link in this chain has methodologic issues which must be addressed. An outline of these issues is given in *table I*. This paper will examine the different components that need to be defined and then answered to fill in the equation that leads to prognosis. Suggestions regarding definition or guidelines for these components will be provided. Finally, evidence from the literature will be used (clearly retrospectively) to estimate or determine the prognosis for different types of NCSE.

Table I. Determining prognosis in NCSE

- Identification of patients with possible NCSE (suspicion)
- Problems of obtaining an EEG (unavailability of diagnostic tool) after hours and at weekends. Correct interpretation of EEG as NCSE (diagnosis)
- Differentiating insult **causing** NCSE from ictal **consequences** of NCSE (co-morbid confounding factors)
- Lack of data on cognitive or functional status **before** NCSE (lack of premorbid data)
- Differentiating morbid effects of treatment, from the morbidity of the disease itself (cause, disease or cure)
- Correct classification of NCSE type, delineation of comorbidity and stratification by level of consciousness = PROGNOSIS

From Kaplan PW. Behavioral manifestations of non-convulsive status epilepticus. *Epilepsy & Behavior* 2002; 3: 122-39.

The definition of status epilepticus

The definition of status epilepticus given in the WHO Dictionary of Epilepsy [19] has been modified with regard to NCSE by many authors. For the purposes of this paper, I will define NCSE as: A condition of ongoing or intermittent clinical epileptic activity (but not coma) without convulsions associated with electroencephalographic evidence of seizures. In its narrowest sense, this definition represents probable NCSE, since more convincing evidence for NCSE resides not only in its EEG and clinical features, but also in the response to intravenous benzodiazepines since some EEG epileptiform patterns are not status and will not show clinical improvement. However, clinical response to treatment is best avoided in defining a syndrome. In retrospectively estimating prognosis from the literature, however, information to make a determination is usually either inadequate, not provided or is beyond the analytic ability of this presentation. Therefore, I will include the probable group as representing the population of NCSE unless there are compelling reasons to exclude particular cases (e.g. patient deeply obtunded or in coma without EEG or clinical improvement with parenteral AEDs). To be noted later in this paper, are the problems of defining: a) what constitutes ongoing or intermittent clinical epileptic activity (as compared with the patient's often compromised baseline state – with significant psychiatric or mental retardation substrates); b) what constitutes the electroencephalographic evidence of epileptiform activity (let alone seizures) and c) what constitutes proximate clinical and EEG response to AED therapy in assessing prognosis.

Classification/categorization of NCSE

From the foregoing, any type of status epilepticus without convulsions perforce is non-convulsive status epilepticus. From *table II*, it can be seen that this includes simple partial status and possibly electrical status in coma. With such a wide swathe, unless carefully categorized by type, there is the risk of putting together in one cage two very different beasts that share superficially similar descriptions before determining outcome. Imagine, if you will, placing two striped mammalian quadrupeds (zebra and tiger) in one cage and

Table II. A classification of nonconvulsive ictal states

I. **Generalized nonconvulsive status epilepticus (GNSE)**
   A. **Absence status epilepticus (ASE)**
      i. Typical absence status epilepticus (TAS) occurring in idiopathic generalized epilepsies, with 3/sec spike-and-wave
      ii. "De novo" reactive (situation-related) absence status in the elderly usually with neuroleptic medications, or following drug withdrawal
      iii. Absence states with degenerative generalized epilepsies; progressive myoclonic epilepsies
      iv. Secondary generalized NCSE of frontal or temporal lobe origin

   B. **Atypical absence status epilepticus (AASE)**
      i. Seen in childhood with secondary generalized epilepsy, usually with mental retardation (cryptogenic and symptomatic) e.g. with Lennox-Gastaut Syndrome. EEG shows "slow" spike-and-wave at < 2.5 Hz, but other patterns described, e.g. with ring chromosome 20 where high-voltage slow waves predominate, with occasional spikes

IIa. **Simple partial status epilepticus (also see IIb)**
   i. Frontal lobe simple partial NCSE with affective/cognitive features
   ii. Parietal lobe simple partial status with somatosensory features
   iii. Temporal lobe simple partial status with autonomic features
   iv. Occipital lobe simple partial status with visual features, with or without nystagmus

IIb. **Complex partial status epilepticus (CPSE)**
   i. Frontal lobe
   [Fronto polar/fronto-central NCSE, with severe confusion and major behavioral disturbances. [Supplementary motor, cingular, orbito-frontal, dorsolateral frontal lobe epilepsies exist, but localized status is rarely documented]
   ii. Temporal lobe
   iii. Parietal lobe
   Sensory perceptions with formication, numbness, pain and perception of body distortions. Lateral (neocortical) posterior temporal lobe with auditory or visual perceptual hallucinations progressing to disorientation, dysphasia and head movement (nystagmus; staring)
   Opercular/insular with vestibular/autonomic hallucinations (progressing to staring and oral/alimentary automatisms)
   iv. Occipital lobe
   Visual hallucinations, nausea, vomiting, headache, nystagmus, occillopsia

III. **NCSE presentation by age (some overlap with IA and B)**
   i. Neonatal NCSE
   ii. Myoclonic-astatic etiology with AASE
   iii. Electrical status epilepticus during slow sleep (ESES)
   iv. Landau-Kleffner Syndrome (acquired epileptic aphasia)
   v. Minor epileptic status of Brett
   vi. Ring chromosome 20 syndrome
   vii. Rolandic status

IV. **NCSE presentation with learning delay and mental retardation (Some overlap with IA, B, III i-v)**
   i. In children
   ii. In adolescents
   iii. In adults

V. **Electrographic status in coma**
   i. Subtle status usually post convulsive status epilepticus (CSE)
   ii. With major CNS damage, often with multi-organ failure (with facial, perioral and/or limb myoclonias), but without apparent preceding CSE

VI. **Allied ictal states**
   i. Confusion with paroxysmal lateralized epileptiform discharges (PLEDS) or paroxysmal lateralized epileptiform discharges (PLEDS) plus
   ii. Confusion with bilateral independent paroxysmal lateralized epileptiform discharges (BiPLEDs)
   iii. Confusion with bilateral synchronous epileptiform discharges (BiPEDs)
   iv. Epileptic encephalopathies: altered mental status with disorganized diffuse or multifocal epileptiform features (e.g. with hypsarrhythmia; "interictal" severe Lennox-Gastaut syndrome; borderline NCSE vs triphasic wave toxic encephalopathies (e.g. lithium, baclofen)

From Kaplan PW. Behavioral manifestations of non-convulsive status epilepticus. *Epilepsy & Behavior* 2002; 3: 122-39.

drawing peaceful conclusions. For some of the rarer NCSE types, such as simple partial status epilepticus without motor features, there will be a less extensive examination. The greatest attention will be directed at generalized forms of nonconvulsive status epilepticus, principally absence status epilepticus (ASE), and lateralization related CPSE, largely frontal and temporal varieties.

An official classification of SE has not yet been adopted by the International League Against Epilepsy (ILAE), but current classifications usually follow the ILAE classification of seizure types, are based on a combination of pathophysiological, etiological, clinical and EEG features, or are based on age of presentation and/or cognitive status (e.g. neonatal, NCSE in retarded children; particular childhood syndromes [e.g. Landau-Kleffner syndrome; ESES; ring chromosome 20 syndrome]; NCSE in mentally retarded adults; or NCSE arising *de novo* in the elderly [1, 20].

Initially classified into "absence status" and "complex partial status", NCSE has increasingly been seen to represent a heterogeneous group of disorders that includes NCSE with EEG features of both localization-related and generalized epilepsies, encephalopathies with epileptiform activity on EEG, and comatose states with electrographic seizures. By grouping together these widely heterogeneous patient populations, there are (not surprisingly) a wide variety of outcomes [11, 17, 21-27], ranging from no morbidity, to death in about half of affected patients.

Mental status/behavior: change from baseline

Patients at risk for NCSE are often those in whom behavioral changes are the most difficult to identify. For example, patients with significant mental retardation or Lennox-Gastaut syndrome will have a baseline mental and behavioral state that is significantly impaired. For the physician, identifying change in these patients is problematic, and only close observers may be able to identify differences. Patients with psychiatric disorders, psychosis and agitation may also have behavioral changes that are difficult to identify, particularly if ictal behaviors involve these same features. Consequently, awareness of just those behaviors that are seen in these particular populations with NCSE is particularly important for diagnosis [20].

Thus, to define behavioral change from baseline in mental retardation with or without epilepsy, there should be: a) diminished level of consciousness with impaired arousal associated with a worsening in EEG from baseline, including an increase in epileptiform morphologies or, b) the appearance of new behavioral patterns of a type seen in NCSE (such as non-ritualistic automatisms, staring, mutism, facial or body myoclonus); c) regressive behavior, diminished attention span, trance-like states and unexplained vegetative symptoms [20].

EEG evidence of ongoing seizures

Diagnosis of NCSE depends on EEG evidence of seizure activity. Without EEG support, diagnosis is speculative or presumptive and may include a variety of other conditions with altered behavior or cognition not due to seizures (e.g. transient global amnesia, fugue states, psychiatric and psychotic conditions). The clinician often may not think to request an EEG, or EEG cannot be obtained because clinical presentation is after usual working hours, or on weekends. This ascertainment bias will clearly lead to underestimation of the number of patients in NCSE, arguably those with the fewest adverse sequelae. EEG interpretation may be difficult, and extra care is needed to exclude patterns without clinical or epileptic significance, and epileptiform patterns not diagnostic of seizures (such as triphasic waves).

A wide spectrum of EEG morphologies may be seen with NCSE [25, 28-30]. Even if clear seizure patterns are identified, some ambiguous patterns remain, such as PLEDs with lateralized epileptiform discharges, subtle myoclonus with a diminished level of consciousness (whether or not they improve with treatment), and sharply contoured triphasic waves such as those due to intoxications with baclofen or lithium. Even the EEG evidence for seizures may be cryptic. In some patients, seizures may be recorded with implanted electrodes, while simultaneous surface EEG fails to record seizures.

From both the above considerations regarding *behavior and EEG diagnosis*, it can be seen that there is a great potential for underdiagnosis from the behavioral perspective, and either under or over-diagnosis by EEG criteria.

Despite the apparent scarcity of nonconvulsive states, Shorvon suggests that CPSE is a common form of NCSE. By history, it occurs in up to 15% of patients with complex partial seizures and resolves spontaneously [1] [p. 116]. A major problem in determining outcome is assessing morbidity (as the numerator) over the number of cases identified (the denominator). With marked under-recognition, it is very difficult to determine prevalence and morbidity. For example, if a few percent of cases of NCSE are diagnosed by EEG and treated (with the other 98% resolving without sequelae), there is a significant and unwarranted "concentration" of the morbidity of NCSE [31].

The particular issue of coma, and problems of grouping together all patients with EEG status and impaired consciousness

The group of patients with significant obtundation or coma and electrographic seizures represents a particular consideration. This scenario does not conform to the original concept of NCSE which originally denoted the "wandering confused". Also, this population typically exists in intensive care units where there are severely ill patients with multiple organ failure, or with significant concurrent brain damage which may itself determine a poor prognosis. It is important to identify this population according to concurrent medical and neurologic issues as well as level of consciousness and to segregate these patients from other types of NCSE (whether localized or generalized) when establishing prognosis.

Recent literature has included a number of different groups with impaired consciousness and epileptiform activity ranging from those with minimal impairment of vigilance to the comatose, resulting in markedly different outcomes. To better define one of these groups, Treiman coined the term "subtle status" [32], a state often seen as part of the evolution after CSE. Others have described "generalized electrographic status epilepticus" [33], "non tonic-clonic status epilepticus" [12] and "subclinical status" [34]. Although Rohr-le-Floch *et al.* [33], Shorvon [1] and Thomas *et al.* [36] have distinguished frontal from limbic NCSE, many series do not distinguish by extent of obtundation or CNS compromise. Prognosis obtained by "lumping" patient groups together is illustrated by studies showing markedly different outcomes: Patients seen in the emergency room with relative mild obtundation [26] or in the out-patient setting [37] have little morbidity and mortality, whereas those studies in the intensive care setting [11, 27, 33] include comatose patients, (with multiorgan failure, and often-other neurologic insults) and have high morbidity and mortality.

Literature data on outcome in different types of NCSE

Prognosis subsumes morbidity (functional outcome), death, response to therapy and recurrence. The different types of NCSE will be examined along these lines.

With the *caveats* mentioned above, the following represents a compilation of data from the literature, largely using published case series, reviews of the literature on the subject, and some isolated case reports. *Table II* provides a classification of non-convulsive ictal states that can be used as an outline for different NCSE types.

Historically, it was considered rare to die in status epilepticus [1, 38]. Early studies were confined to tonic-clonic status epilepticus, again beset by problems of definition, selection bias and case ascertainment (1). As Shorvon notes, there are no trustworthy population-based data on death rates from status until very recently, and death rates from status in existing data underestimate risks. Case ascertainment may easily miss mild or short-lived cases, those least likely to have significant morbidity. Effective early treatment may also forestall the evolution to status epilepticus, and such cases will be excluded from statistics, thus published figures are maximum estimates [1].

Summary

What follows is a summary of the prognosis in most of the better delineated types of NCSE. Please see *table II* for a more complete classification of NCSE.

I. Generalized nonconvulsive status epilepticus (GNSE)

A) Absence status epilepticus (ASE)

i. Typical absence status epilepticus (TAS)

The term "absence status" has undergone an evolution in the literature from the original understanding that the condition represented children with absence seizures who had status epilepticus characterized by 3 per-second spike-and-wave. Such "typical absence status epilepticus (TAS)" is seen with idiopathic generalized epilepsies, and care must be taken to differentiate this entity from those GNSE cases associated with significant obtundation, or even from bilateral frontal status epilepticus as delineated by Thomas [36]. Misdiagnosis is common and less than 20% of patients may be initially identified [39].

ASE almost invariably rapidly responds to parenteral benzodiazepines. Thomas reported that all his five patients had a prompt response to one injection of benzodiazepines [36]. Granner and Lee in 31 patients, noted improvement in 90% on AEDs [25]. Antecdotally, cases lasting as long as weeks, months or years have had no adverse consequences. One patient had ASE for nine years without sequelae [40]. Nonetheless, serum neuron-specific enolase (NSE), believed to be a marker of acute brain injury has been shown to be raised in ASE [41]. Recurrence is frequent, as noted in the study of Berkovic *et al.*, 1989 in which 23/25 patients [42] had recurrences, on the average over five times per year before treatment; valproate prevented recurrence in 14/18 patients. Others also describe multiple recurrences in six patient [43] (See *table III*). Conversely, Agathonikou found that 86% of the 21 patients with TAS were seizure free at two years [39]. Regarding cognitive outcome, Andermann and Robb concluded that isolated episodes in children and adolescents had no clear significance [44]. Guberman *et al.* studied 13 episodes in 10 patients, and found no adverse consequences [16], a view mirrored by Porter and Penry [45]. Review of these case series and individual case reports reveal no long-term morbidity or death, but no formal follow-up, has been done.

Table IIIa. Outcomes of patients with absence status epilepticus (SE)

Status description	No. Pts.	Consequences
"Spike wave stupor" (1-2 days) (Niedermeyer and Khalifeh, 1965)	6	Several recurrences No long-term sequelae noted
Absence SE (Andermann and Robb, 1972)	38	Few with subsequent amnesia, uncertain duration "No clear prognostic significance"
"De novo" SE in the elderly (Thomas *et al.*, 1992)	11	No recurrences in 5 yr Follow-up No sequelae noted

Table IIIb. Outcomes of patients with complex partial status epilepticus (CPSE)

Status description	No. Pts.	Consequences
CPSE (Mayeux and Lueders, 1978)	1	"Return to normal"
CPSE (Engel *et al.*, 1978)	1	4 episodes of days/3 yrs Severe recent memory loss, lasting at least 3 weeks
Children (McBride *et al.*, 1981)	4	Subsequent normal development
CPSE (Treiman and Delgado-Escuetada, 1983)	2	Short-term memory loss, at least 4 months One with generalized convulsions: "persistent" memory loss
CPSE (Ballenger *et al.*, 1983)	8	Frequently recurrent; "returned to baseline cognitive function"
CPSE (Cockerell *et al.*, 1994)	20	17 with recurrence None with cognitive deterioration (5 with neuropsychologic testing)

Table IIIc. Nonconvulsive status epilepticus of mixed types

Status description	No. Pts.	Consequences
"Late life ictal confusion" (Lee, 1985)	11	"All did well". Followed up to 5 yr
NCSE (Guberman *et al.*, 1986)	10	Often recurrent. 8 pts. With 5 yr follow up: no deterioration
Adults (Dunne *et al.*, 1987)	22	"Did well"; little follow up
Mostly CPSE (Thomson *et al.*, 1992)	32	No sequelae noted
40 CPSE, 25 absence (Scholtes *et al.*, 1996)	65	Good outcome, all but 1

From Drislane FW. Evidence against permanent neurologic damage from nonconvulsive status epilepticus. *Journal of Clinical Neurophysiology* 1999; 16 (4): 323-31

> *Prognosis*: excellent. *Diagnosis*: frequently missed. *Response to AEDs*: excellent. *Recurrence*: frequent. *Outcome*: excellent; no morbidity or mortality.

ii. "de novo" absence status in the elderly

This increasingly recognized entity occurs more frequently in women, and is seen in adults with toxic-metabolic and medication related burdens. Most case series [23, 28-29, 46] show a female predominance with status in 39 of 79 patients due to psychotropic medication, either in excess or on sudden cessation. *"De Novo"* absence rapidly responds to parenteral benzodiazepines and has a low recurrence rate (six out of 41 cases) [21, 47-49]. In the 11 patients with *de novo* ASE reported by Thomas 1992, none had recurrence [29]. Andermann and Robb, however, reported recurrences in some patients [44]. There have been no patients with cognitive decline or deaths.

> *Prognosis*: excellent. *Reponse to AEDs*: good but sometimes delayed. *Recurrence*: occasionally (situation-rated: triggers can be removed). *Outcome*: excellent.

iii. Absence states with degenerative generalized epilepsies; progressive myoclonic epilepsies

Early reports by Livingstone *et al.* [50] described dementia following petit mal status in 6 out 11 patients who were initially of normal intelligence. Brett [51] described deterioration in minor epileptic status and Ohtahara *et al.* [52] described intellectual deterioration in TAS and AASE. Doose and Volzke [53], retrospectively, studied 117 children with primary generalized myoclonic-astatic epilepsy and initially normal intelligence for up to seven years: they described "marked debility or imbecility", but provided no psychological assessments. Doose suggests that unlike animal studies, the duration of sustained abnormal electrical activity in children with NCSE is greater than in the animal models, consequently leading to a more damaging effect [53]. Retarded children remain so, 30% are profoundly retarded and half fail to develop speech [54]. Conversely, 13 children with myoclonic-astatic epilepsy had a "good" outcome [55] with seizure freedom and "normal development in five children". Krumholz [56] avers no clear temporal relationship between AASE and neurologic deterioration in Lennox-Gastaut syndrome, as both seizures and neurologic deterioration may stem from the same progressive underlying encephalopathic process.

> *Prognosis*: guarded to fair. *Response to AEDs*: variable. *Recurrence*: frequent. *Outcome*: variable – some with cognitive decline (difficulty in determining whether this is due to disease or to episodes of AASE).

B) Atypical absence status epilepsy (AASE)

Extracting data on AASE from the literature on NCSE and ASE or dissassociating its effect from associated conditions as in Iiii above, is difficult. Infants and children with nonconvulsive status in the setting of West syndrome or infantile spasms have hypsarrhythmia clinically expressed as a "twilight state". A significant portion of these patients go on to have Lennox-Gastaut syndrome/generalized myoclonic-astatic epilepsies. Patients with AASE described by Ohtahara *et al.* [52]; Doose and Völczke [53]; Stores *et al.* [57]; Fujiwara, *et al.* [58]; Inoue, *et al.* [59], and Thomas [60] highlight the prognostic distinction from ASE, in which AASE arises from a generalized symptomatic or cryptogenic epilepsy, and representing a chronic epileptic encephalopathy. More recently, ring chromosome 20 syndrome with NCSE has been described [60b], almost all with a poor response to AEDs.

Status may last days to weeks, have frequent recurrences and be resistant to parenteral benzodiazepines in these series. Nonconvulsive status epilepticus in children with Lennox-Gastaut syndrome responded poorly to diazepam, with 17 out of 25 improving. Conversely, 51% with AASE reported by Tomson *et al.* [17] promptly improved with benzodiazepines. Tassinari *et al.* [61] found that absence status was far more resistant to therapy in patients with secondary generalized epilepsy than in patients with primary generalized epilepsy, concluding that effectiveness of benzodiazepines in status depends on the type of epilepsy rather than the cause of status. Probably, the cognitive consequences of episodes of AASE alone, in Lennox-Gastaut syndrome are swamped by the effect of other seizure and status types (tonic-clonic seizures), and disease progression. Livingston *et al.* [50] described dementia following absence status in 6 of 11 normal patients. One series by Brett [51] describing minor epileptic status again described evolution to a dementia. In children with myoclonic-astatic epilepsy, Doose [62] found a similar correlation. (Again note the difficulty in isolating the cognitive consequences of AASE from the epilepsy syndrome in which it occurs). As noted in an overview by Shorvon, whether status causes cerebral damage remains undetermined [1]. In their study of 50 children, Stores *et al.* found that 27 of 50 children showed convincing evidence of intellectual or educational deterioration over this period [57].

The studies by Young *et al.* and Litt *et al.* [63, 11] do not meet the traditional criteria for ASE or AASE, and involve ICU patients with multisystem failure.

> *Prognosis*: fair to poor. *Response to AEDs*: relatively refractory (when seen in the setting of epileptic encephalopathy/mental retardation). *Recurrences*: frequent. *Outcome*: frequent cognitive morbidity, but it is difficult to differentiate this from the effects of disease progression and consequences of comorbid seizure types.

IIa) Simple partial non-convulsive status epilepticus (SPSE)

Usually there is a good response to AEDs, but status often recurs. Some cases are refractory to AEDs. Most cases of SE are self-limited.

Overall, prognosis derives from the underlying cause of the particular localization-related status. For the most part, SPSE cases are reported as individual cases [1, 64-68]. (See also earlier chapter on the subject.) "Benign" focal genetic epilepsies involving rolandic, parietal or occipital regions are usually easy to control with good long-term prognosis, and without intellectual or neurologic deterioration. Epilepsy usually remits in the teens. Acquired epilepsia partialis continua is a focal motor status epilepticus and will not be reviewed here.

> *Prognosis*: Usually good to excellent; occasionally poor. *Diagnosis*: frequently missed. *Response to AEDs*: excellent. *Recurrences*: frequent. *Morbidity and mortality*: neglible to absent.

IIb) Complex partial status epilepticus (CPSE)

i. Complex partial status epilepticus of frontal lobe origin (FCPSE)

The first large case series to differentiate CPSE into frontal lobe subtypes was Rohr-Le Floch *et al.* who described 18 patterns, one with recurrence [35]. There are few data on their response to AEDs and sequelae. Thomas *et al.* [17] noted that all five patients had a prompt response to one injection of benzodiazepines. Granner and Lee reported a 60% response rate in FCPSE patients given IV benzodiazepines [25]. Thomas *et al.* [17] noted reponses to IV benzodiazepines in all five patients with CPSE. There are no clear data on recurrence rate or cognitive sequelae.

ii. Complex partial status epilepticus of temporal lobe origin (TCPSE)

Responses to AEDs are variable. Dunne reported gradual improvement to parenteral clonzepam in all cases. Others also report graduated return to baseline over hours to days [21, 25-26, 28].

Most large case series show frequent recurrences in patients with CPSE. The study by

Tomson *et al.* [22] showed that 12 of the 13 CPSE patients when treated, had a recurrence. Ballenger *et al.* [15] reported frequent recurrences in eight patients, and Cockerell *et al.* [10] noted that 17/20 patients had recurrences (See *table IV*).

The studies on outcome in CPSE are more controversial, and most studies were done either prior to delineation of CPSE into frontal or temporal types, or did not differentiate between the two types. The only comparative study of five patients matched with subjects known not to have CSE in the prior-five year period, showed no statistically significant cognitive decline [37]. Apart from this, most of the data are found in abstracts, case reports and books, with several of the patients eventually returning to baseline values [3-8]. Four patients have been reported to have profound and irreversible memory deficits [3, 5, 7]. In a larger series published by Krumholz *et al.* [9], seven of the ten patients described had disorders that could in themselves result in permanent sequelae (e.g. viral encephalitis, strokes, coma or who died without awakening); the three remaining patients with cognitive sequelae persisting at least six months, had CPSE with low antiepileptic drug levels. Other authors have often misquoted this article as representing "cause and effect" as opposed to "co-morbidity" of having CPSE.

Most documented reports of CPSE reveal favorable outcomes with or without successful medical treatment [1, 10, 69]. Of the more than 150 cases of CPSE reviewed by Shorvon, only 3 patients had permanent memory problems as mentioned above [1]. One reported case of CPSE lasting three months, and one lasting four months had benign outcomes, with patients normalizing by six months [69] – All 8 patients reported by Ballenger *et al.* [15], with status lasting < 24 hr returned to baseline. Where information is available, only 1 of eight other patients with CPSE > 24 hr failed to return to baseline [5, 8, 64, 70-74].

Little, if any, morbidity or mortality has been reported in ambulatory patients with CPSE. In a previous abstract by Kaplan of 23 patients seen in the emergency room, the functional outcome at two years showed no deterioration in the index of activities of daily living (ADLs) or in the Glasgow Outcome Scale that could be directly attributable to NCSE [75]. The social or professional "deterioration" occurred only as a result of *co*-morbid factors, or the inability to find employment. The study by Cockerell *et al.* showed that none of 20 patients had cognitive deterioration, five of whom had careful neuropsychological assessment [10].

In summary, when comorbid cognitive insults are excluded (e.g. viral encephalitis, convulsive status epilepticus), less than a dozen documented cases demonstrate lasting cognitive sequelae exist of the hundreds to thousands of CPSE cases that have probably occurred.

> *Prognosis*: CPSE when not associated with comorbid insults: good to excellent. *Response to AEDs*: good to very good, but often delayed. *Recurrences*: frequent. *Outcome*: only very rare cognitive sequelae (< 1% of patients).

III. NCSE presentation by age

i. and ii. See chapters in this book on prognosis for these syndromes

iii. Electrical status epilepticus during slow sleep (ESES) (see also chapters on prognosis in this book)

Tassinari *et al.* [76] found only a temporary improvement in EEG with anti-epileptic drugs Relapses are common [76]. For most patients, status and seizures remit by the mid-teens, but intellectual decline appearing during ESES usually does not completely regress, and many patients have significant persisting cognitive deficits [77-79]. As noted by Shorvon, there are no formal studies of outcome and the long-term effect of continuous electrographic seizure activity on cognition, is unknown [1].

iv. Landau-Kleffner (acquired epileptic aphasia) [see also chapters on prognosis in this book]

Anti-epileptic drugs have an inconsistent effect both on seizures and on electrographic status, however, little effect on language. In patients with persistent EEG seizures or ESES outcome is worse, particularly in the younger patients [80-81]. Several authors suggest that aggressive treatment may improve language, but this has yet to be clearly demonstrated [82-85]. In the short case series by Landau and Kleffner [86], Mantovani and Landau [82] revealed after an interval of 10-28 years that four patients had normalized, one had mild language dysfunction, and four had moderate dysfunction. EEG had normalized. Of the 17 other children reviewed by Shorvon [1] from cases by other authors [81, 87-90], four became normal, nine had moderate language problems, and four had severe aphasias. The bad outcome, however, was connected with a comatose state and anoxia as well as refractory SE, and determined by low-voltage EEG.

v. Minor epileptic status of Brett (see above IB)

vi. Ring chromosome 20 syndrome

Presenting between age 1 day and 14 years, seizures are highly resistant to AEDs, often interspersed with focal and tonic-clonic seizures, and often occur daily. Most patients are mildly to moderately retarded. The effect of NCSE on patients' prognosis is unknown.

vii. Rolandic status (see under IIA)

IV. NCSE presentation with learning delay and mental retardation (see in Sections IB and III)

V. Electrographic seizures and coma

i. Subtle status usually post convulsive status epilepticus (CSE)

In this population, outcome is poor; Treiman *et al.* described 134 patients with subtle SE of whom none regained consciousness during the 12 hour study [91]. Sixty five percent of patients with subtle SE died within 30 days.

ii. With major CNS damage, often with multi-organ failure, (with facial, perioral and/or limb myoclonias), but without apparent preceding CSE

Reports of NCSE in obtunded or comatose patients have varied criteria, some not including focal types; others including non-comatose with comatose patients [11, 33-34, 92]. The response to AEDs in subclinical status is poorer than in most types of NCSE, and particularly, than convulsive SE. Control was achieved only in 40%. Late mortality was 24%. In the 48 patients described by Drislane and Shomer, 88% died; all 29 in coma died [33]. In the study of electrographic status epilepticus in ICUs, Drislane *et al.* further confirmed that generalized electrographic status carried a worse prognosis than focal. Litt *et al.* in a study of 24 critically ill elderly patients without anoxia, found a 52% mortality; all patients with generalized EEG patterns died [11]. Death was ascribed to associated life-threatening medical problems. Intravenous benzodiazepines administration increased the mortality risk and in this report, intensive care (ICU) management did not improve the outcome. Young *et al.* found a 57% mortality (13-23 patients) in the ICU population [63]. The study by Privitera *et al.* [12] showed that outcome in nontonic-clonic status patients (good 41%, worse 36%, died 23%) was similar to the nontonic-clonic SE group (good 49%, worse 14%, died 37%). Privitera *et al.* and Young *et al.* [12, 63] conclude that aggressive treatment with AED or pentobarbital coma does not alter long-term outcomes since most of the brain damage appeared to be due to anoxia. As pointed out by Jordan, concurrent NCSE and acute brain injury synergistically increased morbidity and mortality [13], but again differentiating the morbid effect of multiorgan system failures and severe concurrent brain insult from morbidity from status is problematic. In the study by DeLorenzo *et al.* [27] regarding outcome in a group of NCSE patients that included many with CPSE, morbidity ranged from 6.2% to 62.9%.

> *Prognosis*: poor. *Response to AEDs*: poor. *Recurrences*: few. *Outcome*: particularly difficult to separate co-morbidity from consequent morbidity, but overall high morbidity and mortality.

V. Allied ictal states

i. Confusion with paroxysmal lateralized epileptiform discharges (PLEDs) or PLEDs – plus

ii. Confusion with bilateral independent paroxysmal lateralized epileptiform discharges (Bi-PLEDS)

iii. Confusion with bilateral synchronous epileptiform discharges (BPEDs)

iv. Epileptic encephalopathies: altered mental status with disorganized diffuse or multifocal epileptiform features (e.g. with hypsarrhythmia; "interictal" severe Lennox-Gastaut syndrome; borderline NCSE vs triphasic wave toxic encephalopathies (lithium, baclofen, tiagabine)

These states are not NCSE *per se*.

References

1. Shorvon SD. *Status epilepticus: its clinical features and treatment in children and adults.* Cambridge: Cambridge University Press 1994.
2. Kaplan PW. Assessing the outcomes in patients with nonconvulsive status epilepticus: nonconvulsive status epilepticus is underdiagnosed, potentially overtreated, and confounded by comorbidity. *J Clin Neurophysiol* 1999; 16: 341-52.
3. Treiman DM, Delgado-Escueta AV, Clark MA. Impairment of memory following prolonged complex partial status epilepticus. *Neurology* 1981; 31 (Suppl 4ii): 109.
4. Treiman DM, Delgado-Escueta AV. Complex partial status epilepticus. In: Delgado-Escueta AV, Wasterlain CG, Treiman DM, Porter RJ, eds. Status epilepticus: mechanisms of brain damage and treatment. *Advances in Neurology*, vol. 34. New York: Raven Press, 1983, pp. 69-81.
5. Engel J Jr, Ludwig BI, Fetell M. Prolonged complex partial complex status epilepticus: EEG and behavioral observations. *Neurology* 1978; 28: 863-9.
6. Hilkens PHE, de Weerd AW. Non-convulsive status epilepticus epilepticus as cause for focal neurological deficit. *Acta Neurol Scand* 1993; 92: 193-7.
7. Borchert LD, Labar DR. Permanent hemiparesis due to partial status epilepticus. *Neurology* 1995; 45: 187-8.
8. Escueta AV, Boxley N, Waddell G, Wilson WA. Prolonged twilight state and automatisms: a case report. *Neurology* (Minneapolis) 1974: 24: 331-9.
9. Krumholz A, Sung GY, Fisher RS, Barry E, Bergey GK, Grattan LM. Complex partial status epilepticus accompanied by serious morbidity and mortality. *Neurology* 1995; 45: 1499-504.
10. Cockerell OC, Walker MC, Sander JWAS, Shorvon SD. Complex partial status epilepticus: a recurrent problem. *J Neurol Neurosurg Psychiatry* 1994; 57: 835-7.
11. Litt B, Wityk RJ, Hertz SH, Mullen PD, Weiss H, Ryan DD, Henry TR. Nonconvulsive status epilepticus in the critically ill elderly. *Epilepsia* 1998; 39: 1194-202.
12. Privitera M, Hoffman M, Moore JL, Jester D. EEG detection of nontonic-clonic status epilepticus in patients with altered consciousness. *Epilepsy Research* 1994; 18: 155-66.

13. Jordan KG. Nonconvulsive status epilepticus in acute brain injury. *J Clin Neurophysiol* 1999; 16: 332-40.
14. Niedermeyer E, Ribeiro M. Considerations of nonconvulsive status epilepticus. *Clinical EEG* 2000; 31: 192-5.
15. Ballenger CA, King DW, Gallagher BB. Partial complex status epilepticus. *Neurology* 1983; 33: 1545-52.
16. Guberman A, Cantu-Reyna G, Stuss D, Broughton R. Non-convulsive generalized status epilepticus: clinical features, neuropsychological testing, and long-term follow-up. *Neurology* 1986; 36: 1284-91.
17. Tomson T, Swanborg E, Wedlund JE. Nonconvulsive status epilepticus; high incidence of complex partial status. *Epilepsia* 1986; 27: 276-85.
18. Hauser WA. Status epilepticus, frequency, etiology, and neurological sequelae. In: Delgado-Escueta AV, Wasterlain CG, Treiman DM, *et al.*, eds. Status epilepticus. *Advances in Neurology*, vol. 34. New York: Raven Press, 1983; 3-14.
19. Gastaut H. *Dictionary of epilepsy* Part 1: definitions. Geneva: World Health Organization 1973.
20. Kaplan PW. Behavioral manifestations of NCSE. Epilepsy & Behavior 2002; 3: 122-39.
21. Lee SI. Nonconvulsive status epilepticus-ictal confusion in later life. *Arch Neurol* 1985; 42: 778-81.
22. Tomson T, Lindom U, Nilsson BY. Nonconvulsive status epilepticus in adults: thirty-two consecutive patients from a general hospital population. *Epilepsia* 1992; 33: 829-35.
23. Dunne JW, Summers QA, Stewart-Wynne EG. Non-convulsive status epilepticus: a prospective study in an adult general hospital. *Q J Med* 1987; 62: 117-26.
24. Al-Losi MT, Kaplan PW. The grey zone of non-convulsive status epilepticus. *Epilepsia* 1991; 32 (S3): 93.
25. Granner M, Lee SI. Nonconvulsive status epilepticus: EEG analysis in a large series. *Epilepsia* 1994; 35: 42-7.
26. Kaplan PW. Non-convulsive status epilepticus in the emergency room. *Epilepsia* 1996; 37: 643-50.
27. DeLorenzo RJ, Waterhouse EJ, Towne AR, *et al.* Persistent nonconvulsive status epilepticus after the control of convulsive status epilepticus. *Epilepsia* 1998; 39: 833-40.
28. Fagan JM, Lee SI. Prolonged confusion following convulsions due to generalized nonconvulsive status epilepticus. *Neurology* 1990; 40: 1689-94.
29. Thomas P, Beaumanoir A, Genton P, *et al.* "De novo" absence status of late onset; report of 11 cases. *Neurology* 1992a; 42: 104-10.
30. Kaplan PW. Nonconvulsive status epilepticus. *Sem Neurol* 1996; 16: 33-40.
31. Kaplan PW. Prognosis in nonconvulsive status epilepticus. *Epileptic Disord* 2000; 2: 185-93.
32. Treiman DM, DeGiorgio CMA, Salisbury SM, Wickbobet CL. Subtle generalized convulsive status epilepticus. *Epilepsia* 1984; 25: 653.
33. Drislane FW, Schomer DL. Clinical implications of generalized electrographic status epilepticus. *Epilepsy Research* 1994; 19: 111-21.
34. So EL, Ruggles KH, Ahmann PA, Trudeau SK, Weatherford KJ, Trenerry MR. Clinical significance and outcome of subclinical status epilepticus in adults. *J Epilepsy* 1995; 8: 11-5.
35. Rohr-le-Floch J, Gauthier G, Beaumanoir A. États confusionnels d'origine épileptique: Intérêt de l'EEG fait en urgence. *Rev Neurol* 1988; 144: 425-36.
36. Thomas P, Zifkin B, Migneco O, Lebrun C, Darcourt J, Andermann F. Nonconvulsive status epilepticus of frontal origin. *Neurology* 1999; 52: 1174-83.
37. Dodrill CB and Wilensky AJ. Intellectual impairment as an outcome of status epilepticus. *Neurology* 1990; 40 (Suppl 2): 23-7.
38. Gowers WR. *Epilepsy and other chronic convulsive disorders.* London: Churchill, 1901.
39. Agathonikou A, Panayiotopoulos CP, Giannakodimos S, Koutroumanidis M. Typical absence status in adults: diagnostic and syndromic considerations. *Epilepsia* 1988; 39: 1265-76.
40. Gökyiğit A, Çalişkan A. Diffuse spike-wave status of 9-year duration without behavioral change or intellectual decline. *Epilepsia* 1995; 36: 210-3.
41. DeGiorgio CM, Heck CN, Rabinowicz AL, Gott PS, Smith T, Correale J. Serum neuron-specific emolase in the major subtypes of status epilepticus. *Neurology* 1999; 52: 746-9.
42. Berkovic SF, Andermann F, Guberman A, Hipola D, Bladin PF. Valproate prevents the recurrence of absence status. *Neurology* 1989; 39: 1294-7.
43. Niedermeyer E, Khalifeh R. Petit Mal status ("Spike-wave stupor"). An electro-clinical appraisal. *Epilepsia* 1965; 6: 250-62.

44. Andermann F, Robb JP. Absence status. A reappraisal following review of thirty-eight patients. *Epilepsia* 1972; 13: 177-87.
45. Porter RJ, Penry JK. Petit Mal status. In: Delgado-Escueta AV, Wasterlain CG, Treiman DM, Porter RJ, eds. Status epilepticus. *Advances in Neurology*, vol. 34. New York: Raven Press, 1983: 61-7.
46. Van Sweden B, Mellerio F. Toxic ictal confusion. *J Epilepsy* 1988; 1: 157-63.
47. Schwartz MS, Scott DF. Isolated petit mal status presenting de novo in middle age [letter]. *Lancet* 1971; 2: 1399-401.
48. Goldman JW, Glastein G, Adams AH. Adult onset absence status: a report of six cases. *Clin Electroencephalogr* 1981; 12: 199-204.
49. Vercellete M, Gastaut JL. Les épilepsies débutant après soixante ans. *Rev Electroencephalogr Clin Neurophysiol* 1981; 11: 537-44.
50. Livingston S, Torres I, Pauli LL, Rider RV. Petit mal epilepsy; results of a prolonged follow up study of 117 patients. *JAMA* 1965; 194: 227-32.
51. Brett E. Minor epilepticus status. *Neurol Sciences* 1966; 3: 52-75.
52. Ohtahara S, Ika E, Yamatogi Y, Ohtsuka Y, Ishida T, Ichiba N, Ishida S, Miyake S. Non-convulsive status epilepticus in childhood. *Folia Psychiatr Neurol Jpn* 1979; 33: 345-51.
53. Doose H, Völzke E. Petit mal status in early childhood and dementia. *Neuropädiatrie* 1979; 10: 10-4.
54. Dravet C, Natale O, Magaudda A, Larrieu JL, Bureau M, Roger J, Tassinari CA. Les etats de mal dans le syndrome de Lennox-Gastaut. *Rev Electroencephalogr Clin Neurophysiol* 1985; 15: 361-8.
55. Todt H, Eysold R. Long-term observations. In: Niederdermeyer E, Degen R, eds. The Lennox Gastaut syndrome. *Neurology and Neurobiology*, vol. 45. New York: Alan R. Liss, 1988: 377-86.
56. Krumholz A, Sung GY, Fisher RS, Barry E, Bergey GK, Grattan LM. Complex partial status epilepticus accompanied by serious morbidity and mortality. *Neurology* 1995; 45: 1499-504.
57. Stores G, Zaiwalla Z, Syles E, Hoshika A. Non-convulsive status epilepticus. *Arch Dis Child* 1995; 73: 106-11.
58. Fujiwara T, Watanabe M, Nakamura H, Kudo T, Yagik, Seino M. A comparative study of absence status epilepticus between children and adults. *Jpn J Psychiatry Neurol* 1988; 42: 497-508.
59. Inoue Y, Wara T, Matsuda K, Kubota H, Tanaka M, Yagi K, Yamamori K, Takahashi Y. Ring chromosome 20 and nonconvulsive status epilepticus. A new epileptic syndrome. *Brain* 1997; 120: 939-53.
60. Thomas P. Les états d'absence de l'épilepsie. *Rev Neurol* 1999; 155: 1023-38.
60b. Inoue Y, Fujiwara T, Matsuda K, Kubota H, Tanaka M, Yagi K, Yamamori K, Takahashi Y. Ring chromosome 20 and nonconvulsive status epilepticus.
61. Tassinari CA, Daniele O, Michelucci R, Bureau M, Dravet C. Roger J. Benzodiazepines: efficacy in status epilepticus. In: Delgado-Escueta AV, Wasterlain CG, Treiman DM and Porter RJ, eds. Status epilepticus. *Advances in Neurology*, vol. 34. New York: Raven Press, 1983: 465-75.
62. Doose H. Non convulsive status epilepticus in childhood: clinical aspects and classification. In: Delgado-Escueta AV, Wastertain CG, Treiman DM, Porter RJ, eds. Status epilepticus. *Advances in Neurology*, vol. 34. New York: Raven Press, 1983: 83-92.
63. Young GB, Jordan KG, Doig GS. An assessment of nonconvulsive seizures in the intensive care unit using continuous EEG monitoring: An investigation of variables associated with mortality. *Neurology* 1996; 47: 83-9.
64. De Pasquet EG, Gaudin ES, Bianchi A, De Mendilaharsu SA. Prolonged and monosymptomatic dysphasic status epilepticus. *Neurology* 1976; 26: 244-7.
65. Racy A, Osborn MA, Bern BA, Molinari GF. Epileptic aphasia: first onset of prolonged monosymptomatic status epilepticus in adults. *Arch Neurol* 1980; 37: 419-22.
66. Barry E, Sussaman NM, Bosley TM, Harner RN. Ictal blindness and status epilepticus amauroticus. *Epilepsia* 1985; 26: 577-84.
67. Knight RT, Cooper J. Status epilepticus manifesting as reversible Wernicke's aphasia. *Epilepsia* 1986; 27: 301-4.
68. Primavera A, Bo, GP, Venturi S. Aphasic status epilepticus. *European Neurology* 1988; 28: 255-7.
69. Mikati MA, Lee WL, DeLong GR. Protracted epileptiform encephalopathy: an unusual form of partial complex status epilepticus. *Epilepsia* 1985; 26: 563-71.
70. Hamanaka T. Zum problem des status psychomotorischer anfälle. *Clinical Psychiatry* 1972; 14: 592-603.

71. Markand ON, Wheeler GL, Pollack SL. Complex partial status epilepticus in young children. *Ann Neurol* 1981; 28: 189-96.
72. Hamilton NG, Mathews T. Aphasia: the sole manifestation of focal status epilepticus. *Neurology* 1979; 29: 745-8.
73. Murasaki M. Psychomotor status: case reports and proposal for classification. *Folia Psychiatr Neurol Jpn* 1979; 33: 353-7.
74. Dinner D, Lueders H, Lederman R, Gretter T. Aphasic status epilepticus: a case report. *Neurology* 1981; 31: 388-90.
75. Kaplan PW. Functional outcome following nonconvulsive status epilepticus. *Epilepsia* 1997; 38 (Suppl 8): 224.
76. Tassinari CA, Bureau M, Dravet, C, Dalla Bernardina B, Roger J. Epilepsy with continuous spikes and waves during slow sleep. In: Roger J, Dravet C, Bureau M, Dreifuss FE, Wolf P, eds. *Epileptic syndromes in infancy, childhood and adolescence*. London: John Libbey, 1985, pp. 194-204.
77. Dalla Bernardina B, Fontana E, Michelizza B, Colomaria V, Capovilla G, Tassinari CA. Partial epilepsies of childhood bilateral synchronisation, continuous spike-wave during slow sleep. In: Manelis J, Bental E, Loeber JN, Dreifuss FE, eds. The eighth epilepsy international symposium. New York: Raven Press, 1989, pp. 295-302.
78. Morikawa T, Seino M, Watanabe Y, Watanabe M, Yagi K. Clinical relevance of continuous spike-waves during slow wave sleep. In: Manelis J, Benta E, Loeber JN, Dreifuss FE, eds. The eighth epilepsy international symposium. New York: Raven Press, 1989, pp. 359-363.
79. Jayakar PB, Seisha SS. Electrical status epilepticus during slow-wave sleep: a review. *J Clin Neurophysiol* 1991; 8: 299-311.
80. Bishop DVM. Age at onset and outcome in 'acquired aphasia with convulsive disorder' (Landau-Kleffner syndrome). *J Dev Med Child Neurol* 1985; 27: 705-12.
81. Paquier PF, van Dongen HR, Loonen CB. The Landau-Kleffner syndrome or "acquired aphasia with convulsive disorder": long term follow up of six children and a review of the recent literature. *Arch Neurol* 1992; 49: 354-9.
82. Mantovani JF, Landau WM. Acquired aphasia with convulsive disorder: course and prognosis. *Neurology* 1980; 30: 524-9.
83. Ravnik I. A case of Landau-Kleffner syndrome: effect of intravenous diazepam. In: Roger J, Dravet C, Bureau M, Dreifuss FE, Wolf P, eds. *Epileptic syndromes in infancy, childhood and adolescence*. London: John Libbey, 1985, pp. 192-193.
84. Sawhney IMS, Suresh N, Dhand UK, Chopra JS. Acquired aphasia with epilepsy – Landau-Kleffner syndrome. *Epilepsia* 1988; 29: 283-7.
85. Lerman P, Lerman-Sagie T, Kivity S. Effect of early corticosteroid therapy for Landau-Kleffner syndrome. *Dev Med Child Neurol* 1991; 33: 257-66.
86. Landau WM, Kleffner F. Syndrome of acquired aphasia with convulsive disorder in children. *Neurology* 1957; 7: 523-30.
87. Worster-Drought C. An unusual form of acquired aphasia in children. *Dev Med Child Neurol* 1971; 13: 563-71.
88. Shoumaker RD, Bennett DR, Bray PF, Curless RG. Clinical and EEG manifestations of an unusual aphasic syndrome in children. *Neurology* 1974; 24: 10-6.
89. Deonna T, Beaumanoir A, Gaillard F, Assal G. Acquired aphasia in childhood with seizure disorder: a heterogeneous syndrome. *Neuropädiatrie* 1977; 8: 263-73.
90. Cooper JA, Ferry PC. Acquired auditory verbal agnosia and seizures in childhood. *Speech Hearing Dis* 1978; 43: 176-84.
91. Treiman DM, Meyers PD, Walton NY, Collins JF, Colling C, Rowan AJ, Handforth A, Faught E, Calabrese VP. A comparison of four treatments for generalized convulsive status epilepticus. Veterans affairs status epilepticus cooperative study group. *N Engl J Med* 1998; 339: 792-8.
92. Lowenstein DH, Aminoff MJ. Clinical and EEG features of status epilepticus in comatose patients. *Neurology* 1992; 42: 100-4.

Concluding remarks

Anne Berg, Olivier Dulac, Allen Hauser

Determining the course of epilepsy for a given patient contributes to the therapeutic management, both for the choice of medication and decisions regarding surgery. The early epidemiological studies of the 1960's and 1970's provided a global expectation and some crude indicators of prognosis, both in terms of seizure control and mortality, especially age at onset, seizure type(s), and presence of a presumed etiology. These epidemiological markers, however, only imprecisely identified meaningful subgroups of patients and provided only relatively crude estimates of prognosis based on these factors.

Limitations of this risk factor approach become readily apparent when one considers that the factors that determine the course of epilepsy include not simply the presence of a brain lesion or a genetic predisposition or the stage of brain maturation but the combined effects and the interaction of these factors in a given patient. Furthermore, some lesions still remain difficult to identify, most genetic factors remain to be determined, and the mechanism of the impact of brain maturation on the development of epilepsy, its course and psychomotor consequences remain mostly unknown. Specific seizure types can occur in variety of settings regardless of age at onset and underlying etiology. Finally, the outcome of epilepsy seems to have very little to do with age at onset per se. In short, the early epidemiological studies helped to define the forest, and this was an important, necessary first step. They told us little about what was in that forest, however.

Since the first epidemiological studies, the field of epilepsy has made tremendous strides thanks to advances in clinical and neurosciences. Based upon the results of highly detailed descriptive clinical research largely arising from the French school of pediatric neurology, we now approach epilepsy not as a single disorder but as a multitude of very different disorders or syndromes which, like cancers, have different causes, different implications for treatment, and different outcomes. Increasingly, the concept of syndromes is gaining wider acceptance in clinical practice. This should lead to more accurate initial diagnoses and more appropriate treatment administered earlier in the course of the disorder. This becomes progressively more important as most new antiepileptic drugs are claimed by their promoters to have a wide spectrum of action; however, they demonstrate relatively selective efficacy or even detriment in specific epilepsy syndromes and may possibly affect the course of some forms of epilepsy. The same may be true of methods of rehabilitation. Yet knowledge gained about the existence and definitions of syndromes from small clinical series in tertiary epilepsy centers is of unproven value until it can be validated in larger more representative groups of patients.

Beginning in the 1980s, the new wave of epidemiological studies, largely from continental Europe (particularly France, Holland, and Italy) and some from the United States, have incorporated this more informative and clinically relevant approach into the study of the frequency, causes, and prognosis of epilepsy in the community. The focus in epidemiology has thus shifted from an overly meticulous measure of incidence and prevalence (the extent of the forest) to careful, clinically sound characterization and study of the diversity of the different types of epilepsy in a population (the trees).

A lingering impediment to the use of syndromes both clinically and epidemiologically is two-fold. First, the nosological limits of given syndromes remain too often purely clinical and therefore not reproducible. Second, until now, it has been the epilepsies of infancy, childhood, and adolescence that have been most amenable to identification and characterization with the syndromic approach. The vast majority of adult-onset epilepsies have not yet been sufficiently differentiated for this approach to be of the same value yet in adults although we anticipate this to change with time.

As epidemiologists learn to incorporate clinically relevant information about epilepsy into their studies and as epileptologists begin to incorporate a more scientific approach to their clinical descriptions and definitions of syndromes, the two approaches will increasingly come together to provide a powerful tool for explanatory research into the frequency, causes, prognoses, and consequences of the epilepsies. This book represents the thoughts and discussions of many clinicians and researchers in this field and should provide a basis to help future workers in the field to identify the next round of relevant research questions and how to address them.

Achevé d'imprimer par Corlet, Imprimeur, S.A.
14110 Condé-sur-Noireau
N° d'Imprimeur : 60986 - Dépôt légal : janvier 2003

Imprimé en France